# The Physics, Clinical Measurement and Equipment of Anaesthetic Practice *for the FRCA and FCICM*

# The Physics, Clinical Measurement and Equipment of Anaesthetic Practice *for the FRCA and FCICM*

THIRD EDITION

**Patrick Magee**
Retired Consultant in Anaesthesia
Royal United Hospital, Bath, UK

**Mark Tooley**
Retired Head of department of Medical Physics and Bioengineering
Royal United Hospital, Bath, UK

OXFORD
UNIVERSITY PRESS

OXFORD
UNIVERSITY PRESS

Great Clarendon Street, Oxford, OX2 6DP,
United Kingdom

Oxford University Press is a department of the University of Oxford. It furthers the University's objective of excellence in research, scholarship, and education by publishing worldwide. Oxford is a registered trade mark of Oxford University Press in the UK and in certain other countries.



First Edition published in 2005
Second Edition published in 2011
Third Edition published in 2026



Published in the United States of America by Oxford University Press
546 Fifth Avenue, New York, NY 10036, United States of America.

British Library Cataloguing in Publication Data
Data available

Library of Congress Control Number: 2026940902

ISBN 978–0–19–896037–9

DOI: 10.1093/med/9780198960379.001.0001



The manufacturer's authorized representative in the EU for product safety is Oxford University Press España S.A. of Parque Empresarial San Fernando de Henares, Avenida de Castilla, 2 – 28830 Madrid (www.oup.es/en or product.safety@oup.com). OUP España S.A. also acts as importer into Spain of products made by the manufacturer.

This book is dedicated to our families:
Marie-Suzanne, Lucia, Rosie, William and Patrick Magee
and
Stella, Alissa and Sebastian Tooley

# Foreword to the third edition

In my experience, many healthcare professionals struggle to understand physics and physical principles. Most will have only a rudimentary knowledge of the working principles of the equipment that they use every day, and this applies to physicians, surgeons or nurses, as well as anaesthetists. Patrick Magee and Mark Tooley have very successfully written a textbook that helps the reader to understand the wide range of potentially complex topics relating to the physics, clinical measurement and equipment of anaesthetic practice. The third edition of this book covers the whole of the domain of physics and clinical measurement in the three stages of the Royal College of Anaesthetists (RCoA) 2021 Curriculum for a Certificate of Completion of Training (CCT) in Anaesthetics and in the Faculty of Intensive Care Medicine (FICM) 2021 Curriculum for a CCT in Intensive Care Medicine. This makes it the ideal learning tool for these topics for both the Primary and Final examination for Fellowship of the Royal College of Anaesthetists (FRCA) and for the Final examination for the Fellowship of College of Intensive Care Medicine (FCICM). The section of the book on statistics covers the required statistical knowledge for the Primary FRCA. Although the book has been compiled to ensure full coverage of UK and European anaesthesia and intensive care medicine curricula, the topic is generic and the contents are equally appropriate for healthcare professionals worldwide.

The contents of the book follow a logical sequence that takes the reader from mathematics and statistics through electricity, fluids, and gases to imaging techniques and the function of a variety of items of equipment, including anaesthetic machines and ventilators. The 3rd edition has been updated extensively and now includes sections on videolaryngoscopy, newer ventilators and syringe drivers, and the application of artificial intelligence. The whole book is presented with great clarity: the pages are uncluttered, the tables are easy to read and each chapter is comprehensively illustrated with simple, clear line diagrams that convey succinctly the principles of each topic. The line diagrams of vaporisers and ventilators are particularly informative. Lists of references and further reading at the end of each chapter guide the reader to further information if required.

I have had the pleasure of working with the authors for many years. It is hard to imagine anyone else with more knowledge, experience and enthusiasm for physics and clinical measurement in relation to anaesthesia. Dr Magee obtained a degree in Engineering Science and Biomechanics before going on to train in medicine and specialise in anaesthesia. He was an examiner for the Primary FRCA and is therefore well informed about the level and scope of the knowledge required for that examination. Professor Tooley is a medical physicist (originally, he trained as an electronic engineer), who has spent a significant part of his career working alongside clinical and academic anaesthetists. He is perhaps uniquely placed to understand the application of physics and clinical measurement to anaesthesia.

This book is not just about providing information to pass exams. It will be a valuable resource for those well-established clinicians who wish to refresh their knowledge and understanding of physics, clinical measurement and anaesthetic equipment. This may reflect the need to learn about new monitors or other items of equipment for use in their own clinical practise or it may be driven by the need to enhance knowledge and confidence before attempting to teach trainees. In any event, I expect this book will be in strong demand from trainees, trainers and other experienced clinicians.

Jerry P. Nolan PhD FRCA FRCP FFICM FRCEM (Hon)
Consultant in Anaesthesia and Intensive Care Medicine
Royal United Hospital Bath, UK

# Preface to the third edition

The aim of this book is to help junior anaesthetists who are about to sit the diploma examinations for the Fellowships in Anaesthesia and Intensive Care Medicine of the Royal College of Anaesthetists (FRCA, FFICM), the European Academy of Anaesthesiology and other equivalent international professional anaesthetic qualifications. It is also intended to be a useful revision in the physical sciences for more senior anaesthetic colleagues.

The book will also be of interest to operating department assistants, physician assistants (anaesthesia), hospital-based biomedical engineers and clinical scientists, manufacturers' representatives and those involved in the manufacture, marketing and use of anaesthetic equipment in the UK, the EU, and further afield.

The contents are based on the syllabus of the FRCA and FCICM examinations in mathematics, physics, clinical measurement and monitoring, equipment and safety.

Anaesthetists are a relatively technophilic group of clinicians, but many have either no higher education in mathematics and physics, or at least a decade has elapsed since they have received any such education. In comparison with the other basic sciences of physiology and pharmacology, physical sciences are less popular and less accessible.

The book starts with mathematics, statistics and background physics, not only to enhance the understanding for what follows in the book, but also because these basic sciences are fundamental to many other aspects of medical science. Areas, which in the authors' teaching experience, candidates have found particularly troublesome, such as electricity and electrical safety, have been discussed in some detail in order to clarify. We have endeavoured to make each chapter independent, although frequent reference is made to other chapters where appropriate.

Dr Patrick Magee BSc, MSc, PhD, MB BS, FRCA, was a Consultant Anaesthetist at the Royal United Hospital Bath, who originally graduated in Engineering Science and Biomechanics. He was an honorary Senior Lecturer at the University of Bath in the department of Mechanical Engineering.

Professor Mark Tooley BSc, MSc, PhD, CEng, CSci, FIET, FIPEM, FinstP, FRCP, FREng was a Consultant Clinical Scientist (Medical Physics) at the Royal United Hospital Bath. He was head of the department of Medical Physics and Bioengineering and Director of Research and Development at the Hospital.

He is an Honorary Professor at the University of Bath.

The content of this book is from the relevant parts of the examination syllabus of the Royal College of Anaesthetists and the Faculty of Intensive Care Medicine, but this does not imply any endorsement of this title or its contents by those institutions.

# Contents

1. Mathematics 1
   Graphs 1
   Trigonometry 4
   Calculus 6
   Powers, logarithms, 'e' 11
2. Statistics 17
   Introduction 17
   Categorical data 17
   Numerical data 17
   Quantifying variability 18
   Probability 21
   Hypothesis testing 26
   Power 26
   Parametric methods 27
   Non-parametric methods 28
   Diagnostic tests 29
   Correlation and regression 31
   Comparing groups of categorical data 33
   Meta-analysis 34
   Study design and clinical trials 35
   Evidence-based medicine 36
   Incorrect use of statistics 36
3. Background physics 38
   Introduction 38
   Dimensions and units 38
   Input/output, linearity, drift, hysteresis 40
   Frequency response 41
   Calibration of transducers 42
   Atomic structure 43
   Basic mechanics 44
4. Electricity, magnetism and circuits 48
   Introduction 48
   Electrical properties 48
   Magnetism 49
   Basic electrical circuit rules 50
   Bridge circuits 51
   Alternating and direct voltage/current 53
   Capacitors and inductors 54
   Transformers 55
   Other electrical analogies 56

5. Electronics and biological signal processing 58
Introduction 58
Filters 58
Amplifiers 60
Signal processing 64
Digital signal processing 64
Electrodes and transducers 65

6. Electrical safety 69
The electricity supply 69
Electrical safety features 69
Earth faults 72
Microshock 74
Circuit breakers 74
Earth-free supplies 76
Other safety issues of electricity 76

7. Behaviour of fluids (liquids and gases, flow and pressure) 78
Fluid flow behaviour 78
Theory of flow measurement devices 80
Pressure 83
Partial pressure 85
Diffusion 86
Osmosis 87

8. Thermodynamics: heat, temperature and humidification 89
Introduction 89
The gas laws 89
Specific heat capacity 92
Latent heats of vaporisation and of crystallisation 93
Temperature 93
Thermometry 94
Heat transfer 94
Keeping patients warm 95

9. Solubility, vaporisation and vaporisers 98
Introduction 98
Solubility of molecules in liquids 98
Solubility of gases in gases 99
Vaporisation 100
The basis of vapour production by a vaporiser 102
Vaporisers 104

10. Ultrasound and Doppler 110
Introduction 110
Properties of ultrasound 110
Visualisation of needle positioning 113
Doppler 113

Measurement of absolute blood flow 117
High-power ultrasound 117
Conclusions and future directions 117

11. Principles and standards of anaesthetic monitoring 119
Introduction 119
Recommendations for standards of monitoring 121

12. Blood pressure measurement 127
Introduction 127
Non-invasive blood pressure measurement 127
Direct measurement of blood pressure 131
Components of the monitoring system 132
Resonance and damping 134
Other blood pressure measurements 140

13. Cardiac output measurement 143
The pulmonary artery catheter 143
Echocardiography 145
Pulse contour analysis 146
Transthoracic electrical impedance 147

14. Gas pressure, volume and flow measurement 149
Introduction 149
Gas pressure measurement 149
Gas volume and flow measurement 150

15. Pulse oximetry 160
Pulse oximetry 160

16. Respiratory gas analysers 165
Introduction 165
Refractometry 166
Infrared spectroscopy 168
Mass spectrometry 169
Raman spectroscopy 171
Piezoelectric gas analysis 171
Paramagnetic oxygen analyser 172
Polarography and fuel cells 174
Nitric oxide (NO) measurement 175
Preoperative exercise testing 175

17. Blood gas analysis 177
Introduction 177
The $pO_2$ electrode 177
The pH electrode 177
The $pCO_2$ electrode 178
Derived variables from a blood gas machine 178
Errors in blood gas measurement 179
Temperature and blood gas analysis 179

Transcutaneous blood gas analysers 179
Intravascular blood gas analysers 179

18. Electrophysiology and stimulation 181
Introduction 181
The electrocardiogram 181
The electroencephalogram 184
Evoked responses 187
Monitoring neuromuscular blockade and the electromyogram 190

19. Monitoring depth of anaesthesia 194
Introduction 194
Depth of anaesthesia monitors using the EEG 194
Depth of anaesthesia monitors using the AER 198
Depth of anaesthesia monitors using the ECG 199
Artificial intelligence and depth of anaesthesia monitoring 199

20. Pacemakers and defibrillators 202
Introduction 202
Pacemakers 202
Defibrillators 204

21. Surgical diathermy 210
Introduction 210
Current density 210
Surgical effects and associated waveforms 210
Electrodes 212
Safety of diathermy 213
Interference with other equipment 214

22. Gas supply and the anaesthetic machine checklist 215
Supply of anaesthetic gases 215
Pressure regulators, gas flow control and anaesthetic machine safety features 219
The anaesthetic machine and equipment checklist 220

23. Airway management devices 225
Introduction 225
The artificial airway 225
The facemask 226
The laryngeal mask airway 227
The I-gel 228
The cuffed oropharyngeal airway 229
The endotracheal tube 229

24. Aids to intubation 236
The laryngoscope 236
Fibre optics 236
Videolaryngoscopy 238

25. Breathing systems 241
Introduction 241
The Mapleson classification of semi-closed rebreathing systems 241
Humphrey ADE system 247
Venturi systems 247
The circle system 247

26. Artificial ventilators 253
Respiratory mechanics during ventilation 253
Ventilator mechanics 253
Testing 258
Some ventilator types 259
Intermittent blowers 260
Intensive care ventilators 262
Manual resuscitators 265
Portable ventilators 265
Other methods of gas exchange 265

27. Intravenous pumps and syringe drivers 270

28. Environmental safety 274
Fire and explosion 274
Atmospheric pollution and anaesthetic gases 274
Scavenging systems 275

29. Imaging and radiation 278
Introduction 278
Radioactive decay 278
Production of X-rays 279
Imaging 280
Magnetic resonance imaging 283
Lasers 287

30. Cleaning and sterilisation of equipment 290
Two different processes 290

31. Medical training using simulators 292
Introduction 292
Simulation centre environments 292
Model-driven patient simulators 293
Mathematical modelling 294
Patient types 295
Scenario scripts 295
Scenarios 296
Surgical skills laboratory 296
Simulated or standarised patients 296
Hybrid training 297
Virtual and augmented reality training 297

*Index* 299

# Chapter 1 **Mathematics**

The chapter links with: Chapters 2, 3, 5 and 7.

## Graphs

### *The straight line*

Graphs are used to represent pictorially or clarify a relationship between two variables, say $x$ and $y$, or $t$ and *function* ($t$). If $x$ and $y$ are related by the *linear* equation $y = mx + c$, then the graphical relationship is a straight line as in Figure 1.1, where $m$ is the slope, a constant value for a straight line and $c$ is the value of $y$ when $x = 0$. Figure 1.2 shows the relationship when $m$ and $c$ take negative values. Note that if $c = 0$, the line passes through the origin, 0, of the $x$–$y$ axes.

Examples of other linear relationships that can be represented in this way include the following (the bracketed symbols are the variables equivalent to $x$ and $y$ given here):

$v = u + a\,t$; (variables are $t$ and $v$), where $u$ is the starting velocity of an object that is subjected to acceleration $a$ for time $t$, after which its velocity is $v$.

$F = m\dfrac{d^2x}{dt^2}$ (variables are $\dfrac{d^2x}{dt^2}$ and $F$), where a force $F$ acts on a mass $m$, causing an acceleration $\dfrac{d^2x}{dt^2}$.

$Q = k\Delta P$; (variables are $\Delta P$ and $Q$), where, in laminar fluid flow, flowrate $Q$ is proportional to pressure drop $\Delta P$.

$V_o = V_i - i\,R$; (variables $i$ and $V_o$), where the output voltage of an electrical circuit $V_o$ results from an input voltage $V_i$ and a current $i$ flowing through a resistance $R$.

$\omega t = \theta$; (variables $t$ and $\theta$), where an object travelling at angular velocity $\omega$, travels through an arc of angle $\theta$ after time $t$.

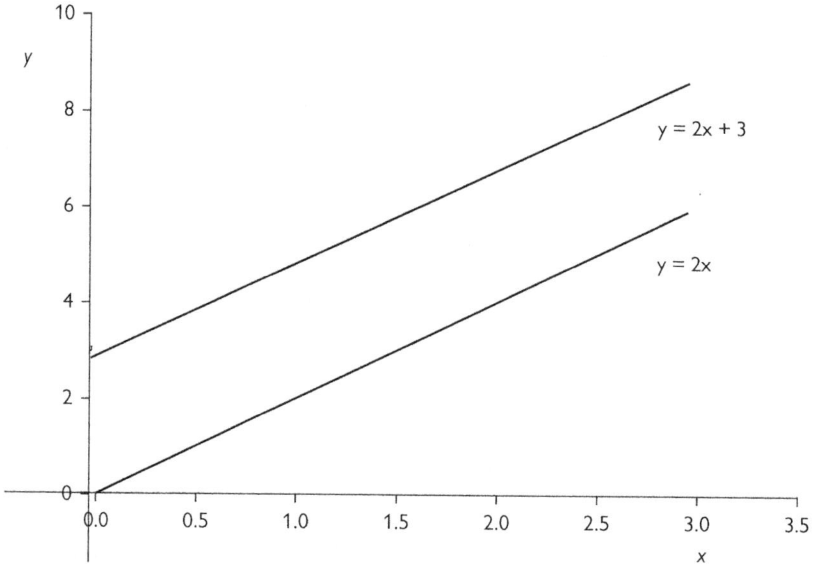


**Fig. 1.1** The straight line of the type $y = mx + c$.

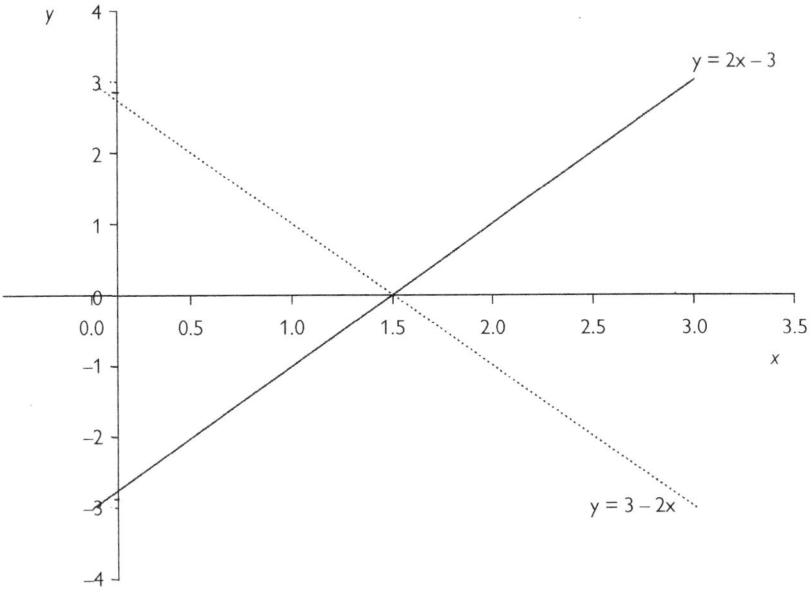


**Fig. 1.2** More straight lines of the type $y = mx - c$ and $y = c - mx$.

## *The parabola*

The relationship between two variables need not be linear as those drawn previously, but the one may be related to the square of the other, such as $y = mx^2$, producing a parabolically shaped curve, passing through the origin 0.

If the curve is displaced upwards by an amount equal to $c$ on the $y$-axis, the equation becomes $y = mx^2 + c$, and if displaced sideways along the positive $x$-axis by an amount equal to $a$ the equation becomes $y = m(x - a)^2$. These are shown graphically in Figure 1.3.

Examples of such relationships might include the following:

$\Delta P = kQ^2$ where $\Delta P$ and $Q$ are the pressure drop and flow respectively in a region of turbulent flow.
$V = k'X^2$ where $V$ is the velocity at a distance $X$ radially from the long axis of a pipe in which there is laminar flow.

## *Other graphical relationships*

The relationship between two variables may be even more complex, but nevertheless expressible in mathematical form. For example, if $y$ is expressed as a polynomial

$$y = m_1x^3 + m_2x^3 + m_3x + c,$$

then it will look as in Figure 1.4.

Computers will now fit such curves to experimental data points and produce the appropriate equation describing the relationship. The purpose of such graphical information is to predict the way the variables will behave under different circumstances. If the point at which this information is required lies on the curve within the data point set, it is called 'interpolation', and if it lies on the curve outside the

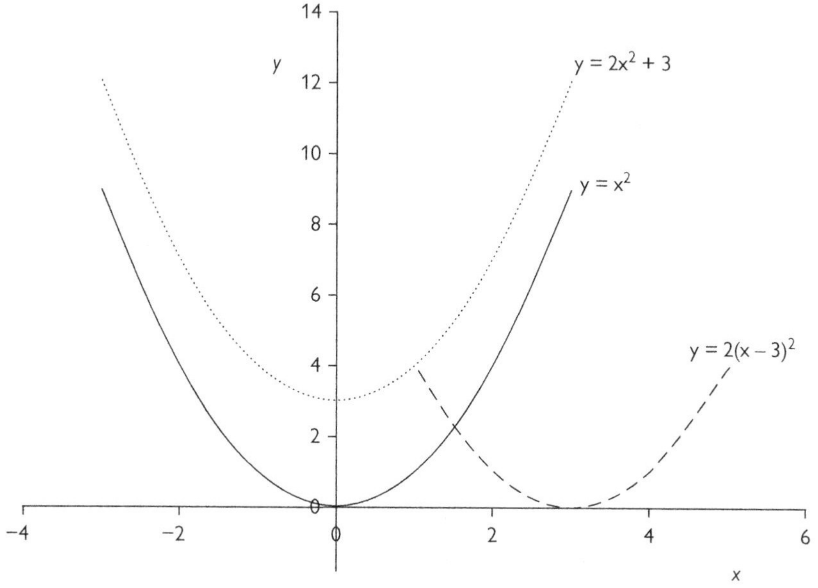


**Fig. 1.3** Parabolas of the type $y = mx^2$, $y = mx^2 + c$, and $y = m(x - a)^2$.

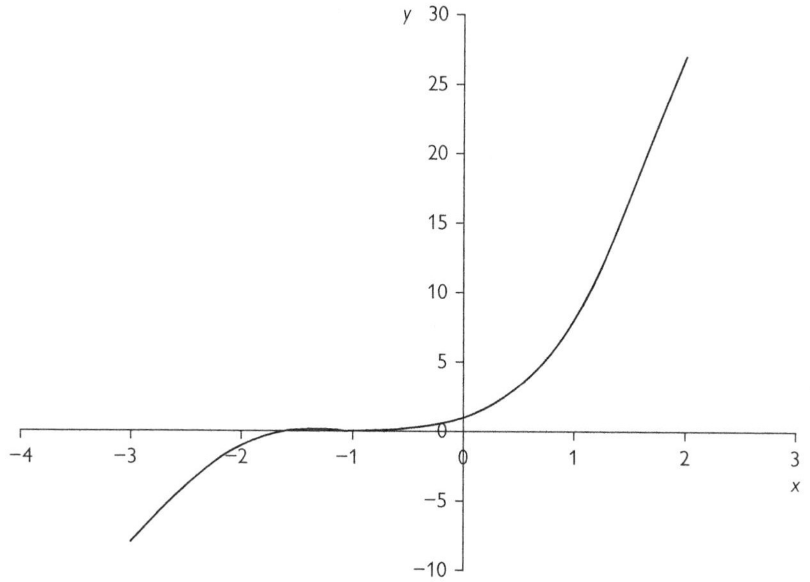


**Fig. 1.4** The polynomial $\boldsymbol{y = m_1x^3 + m_2x^2 + m_3x + c}$.

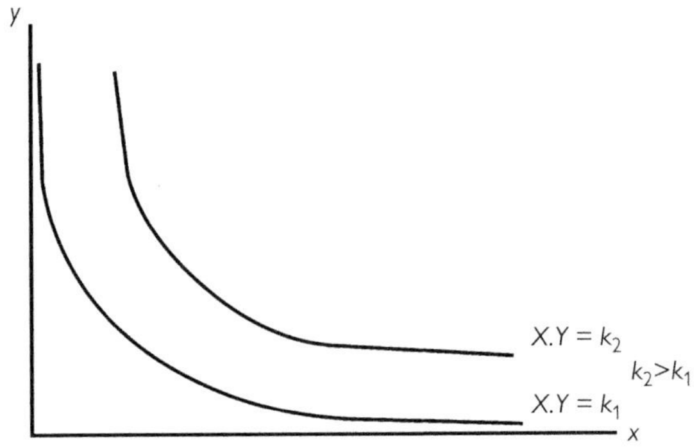


**Fig. 1.5** Rectangular hyperbolae of the form $xy = k$, where $k_2 > k_1$.

data points it is called 'extrapolation'; extrapolation is necessarily potentially less accurate than interpolation, unless the data are known to fit the curve exactly.

### *The rectangular hyperbola*

A circle is a special case of an ellipse, and a hyperbola differs from an ellipse only in a single sign in its algebraic equation. A special case of a hyperbola is a *rectangular hyperbola*, whose equation is of the form $xy = k$, and it is worth dwelling on briefly, since there are numerous examples in anaesthesia. These include the following:

> $PV = nRT$, the universal gas law, where $P$ is pressure, $V$ is volume, $T$ is the absolute temperature of the gas, and the other symbols are constants.
>
> $VF = K(P_{E,CO_2})^{-1}$ where $V$ is the patient's minute ventilation, $F$ is fresh gas flow in a breathing system, and $K(P_{E,CO_2})$ is a constant whose value depends on the value of $(P_{E,CO_2})$.

Another example is the shape of the strength/duration curve of excitation of a muscle or nerve. The rectangular hyperbola resembles the curve in Figure 1.5.

## Trigonometry

Figure 1.6 shows a triangle with one right angle (90°) between two sides of length $x$ and $y$, with the third side of length $r$, from which some simple and widely applicable relationships can be stated.

If the angle between, say $x$ and $r$, is designated $\theta$, then the ratios of different side lengths to each other, namely $y/r$, $x/r$, and $y/x$ are defined as follows:

$$\sin\theta = \frac{y}{r},\ \cos\theta = \frac{x}{r},\ \tan\theta = \frac{y}{x}.$$

Some useful numerical examples include sin 30° = cos 60° = ½, sin 90° = cos 0° = 1, tan 45° = 1. Inverse ratios of *sin, cos* and *tan* are, respectively, *cosec, sec* and *cotan.*

In the triangle OAP, if OP is also the radius of length $r$ of a circle, an arc of which is shown, and on which a point P lies, then the coordinates of point P can be described as both $(x, y)$ and $(r, \theta)$, where $\theta$ is the angle formed with the $x$-axis by the circle radius. Looking at Figure 1.6, where point P lies on a curve at a constant distance $r$ from the origin 0, the following relationship for any right-angled triangle is deduced:

$$x^2 + y^2 = r^2.$$

From Figure 1.6, this is identical to $r^2 \cos^2\theta + r^2 \sin^2\theta = r^2$ or $\cos^2\theta + \sin^2\theta = 1$, another important trigonometric relationship.

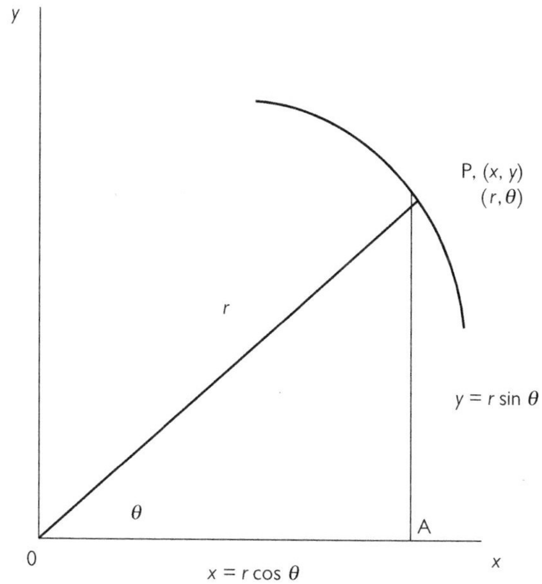


**Fig. 1.6** A point P expressed as both $(x, y)$ and $(r, \theta)$.

As shown in Figure 1.7, if a point P describes a circle by rotating round its circumference at constant angular velocity $\omega$, and it sweeps out an angle $\theta$ in time $t$, then $\theta = \omega t$; furthermore the path of the vertical amplitude $y$ can be traced on a screen with a time base and its motion is given by $y = A \sin \omega t$, where $A$ is the maximum amplitude, occurring when $\theta = \omega t = \pi/2$ radians or 90°.

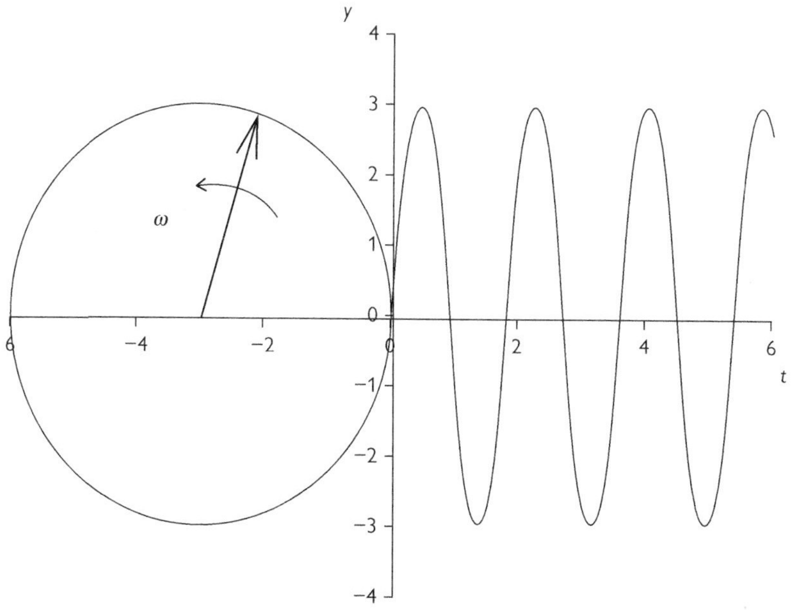


**Fig. 1.7** Simple harmonic motion. A point rotating around a circle on a moving horizontal time axis traces out a sine wave.

The path traced is a *sine wave*, described by the same equation.

Physical examples of such sine waves include electromagnetic radiation, alternating current, clock pendulum movement, a vibrating mass and spring system, and the path swept out by a lung function generator. The motion generated in this way is called *simple harmonic motion*.

Different wave forms, with different amplitudes and frequencies, can be superimposed. These are harmonics that make up a more complex, non-sinusoidal waveform, such as the arterial pressure or ECG waveform. Conversely, these complex waveforms can be analysed by being broken down into their constituent sinusoidal components of different frequencies and amplitudes, some of which may be out of phase with each other. This is known as *Fourier analysis*, the significance of which is that in order to reproduce a waveform faithfully, a piece of monitoring equipment has to be able to reproduce all components, from lowest to highest amplitudes, and from lowest to highest frequencies, with minimum distortion and phase shift. This will be further discussed in Chapter 3.

# Calculus

## *Differentiation*

This term refers to the rate of change of a function with respect to a variable. The slope of a straight line, or the rate of change of $y$ with respect to $x$, has already been described as $m$, a constant. But, if the line is a curve where $y$ is a function of $x$, i.e. $y = f(x)$, with a varying slope, then the slope at a given point is the instantaneous rate of change of $y$ with respect to $x$, or algebraically:

$$slope\ f(x) = \delta y \,/\, \delta x,$$

where $\delta y$ and $\delta x$ are very small changes in $y$ and $x$ respectively.

This is shown in Figure 1.8. As the intervals of change $\delta x$ become vanishingly small the term $\delta y/\delta x$ becomes a calculable term called the *first differential* of $f(x)$, or dy/dx. Looking at specific functions, if

$$y = mx + c \quad \text{then} \quad dy \,/\, dx = m$$
$$y = kx^2 + c \quad \text{then} \quad dy \,/\, dx = 2kx$$

In general, if $y = a(x + b)^n + c$ then $dy/dx = na(x + b)^{[n-1]}$.

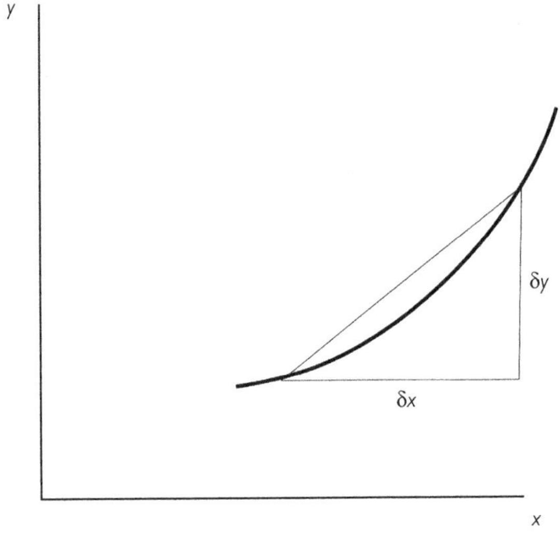


**Fig. 1.8** Instantaneous slope $\delta y/\delta x$ of a curve $y = f(x)$.

The derivation of these expressions can be found in any calculus text.

A physical example where this is relevant is in an expression to estimate distance travelled with respect to time; its rate of change or differential is velocity. The function can be differentiated a second time to give acceleration. For example, if the distance travelled in time $t$ is $y$, where $y = m\,t + c$, then the velocity, $dy/dt = m$, a constant, and the acceleration $d^2y/dt^2 = 0$, since differentiating the constant $m$ gives zero. Also, information can be gleaned about maxima and minima on curves where the slope $dy/dx$ is zero, and where the rate of change of the slope $d^2y/dx^2$ is negative or positive respectively. This is shown graphically in Figure 1.9.

Consider a practical example of this. The velocity $v$ of fluid flowing in a tube of diameter $2a$, where the flow is laminar, shown in Figure 1.10, is described by

$$v = V_{max}\frac{(a^2 - x^2)}{a^2},$$

where $V_{max}$ is the maximum value of $v$, occurring at $x = 0$ in the midline of the tube, and where $v = 0$ at the tube walls, where $x = \pm a$.

$$dv\,/\,dx = \frac{V_{max}}{a^2}(-2x) = 0$$

when $x = 0$, i.e. the tube midline, and

$$d^2v\,/\,dx^2 = \frac{V_{max}}{a^2}(-2) < 0,$$

i.e., a maximum value (rather than a minimum).

## *Integration*

This is the opposite process to differentiation. If we integrate $d^2y/dx^2$ with respect to $x$, we get $dy/dx$, and if we integrate again we get $y$. If we integrate yet again, we are calculating the area under the $x$–$y$ curve.

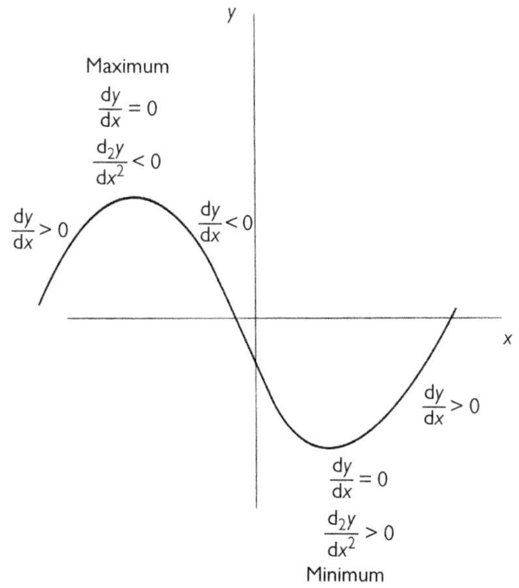


**Fig. 1.9** Maxima and minima on curves.

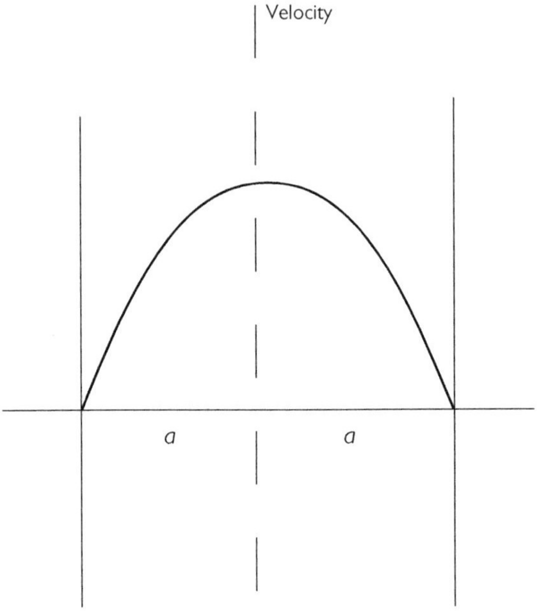


**Fig. 1.10** Velocity profile across a tube in which fluid is flowing.

Figure 1.11 shows a short section of a curve, with two points identified $(x, y)$, and $\{(x + \delta x), (y + \delta y)\}$.The area of the elemental rectangle shown is thus $(y + ½\delta y).\delta x \cong y.\delta x$, ignoring the smallest terms.

The sum of all such elemental rectangles, ignoring small terms, is written as $\Sigma\, y\delta x$.

As $\delta x \Rightarrow 0$, this becomes the integral of $y$ with respect to $x$, written mathematically as $\int y\,dx$, the area under the curve between certain limits of $x$, for example, if

$$y = xn, \text{ then } \int y dx = \frac{x^{(n+1)}}{(n+1)} + constant$$

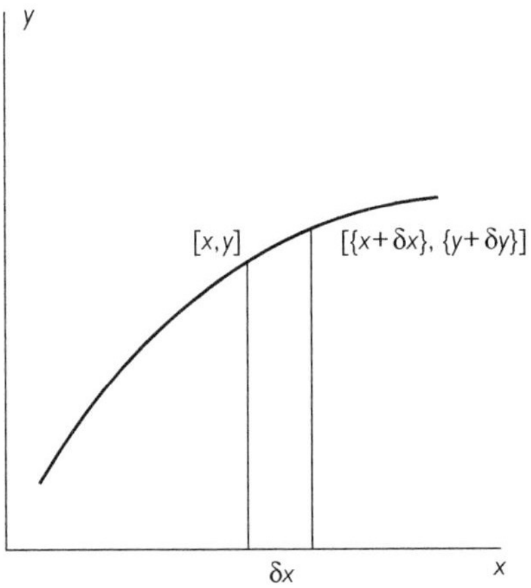


**Fig. 1.11** Area under a small element of curve.

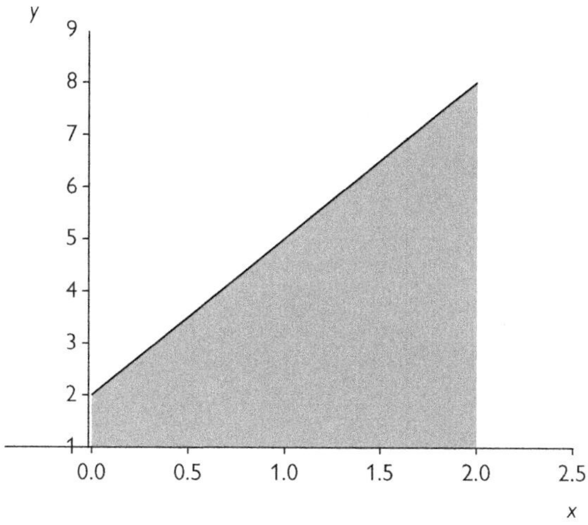


**Fig. 1.12** Area under the straight line $y = 3x + 2$, no limits specified.

The constant is necessary, since differentiating a constant gives zero, so back integration needs the constant to be re-established. Its value is determined by integrating between defined limits of $x$.

For example, suppose $y = 3x + 2$, shown in Figure 1.12, then

$$\int y.dx = \int (3x + 2)\,dx = 3\frac{x^2}{2} + 2x + constant$$

As the figure shows, some additional information is needed to calculate the constant, since it is otherwise unknown how many elemental rectangles are being summed together in order to calculate the area under the curve. This is usually dealt with by stipulating boundaries, say between $x = 1$ and $x = 4$. Then the area under the curve is:

$$\int_{x=1}^{x=4} (3x + 2)dx = \left[\frac{3x^2}{2} + 2x\right]_{x=4} - \left[\frac{3x^2}{2} + 2x\right]_{x=1} = 28.5.$$

Figure 1.13 shows this.

A clinical example of the use of integration is in the use of the thermodilution catheter to measure cardiac output. The computer associated with the device plots the curve of temperature change (shown in Figure 1.14) as measured at the thermistor tip of the catheter against time, and the expression for cardiac output is of the form

$$cardiac\ output = \frac{constant_1 \times thermal\ capcity\ of\ the\ injectate}{constant_2 \times \int(temperature\ change).d(time)}$$

Notice therefore that the larger the integral (area under the curve), the smaller the cardiac output because area under the curve is the denominator. Figure 1.14 shows the plotted curve.

## *Differential equations*

The idea of describing rates of change of processes using differential notation has already been introduced. A simple differential equation is shown below; it says 'the rate of decrease of a substance $y$ with respect to a variable $t$ is proportional to the amount of $y$ which is left':

$$\frac{dy}{dt} = -ky \text{ or } \frac{dy}{dt} + ky = 0,$$

whose solution is $y = A_1\ e^{-k.t}$.

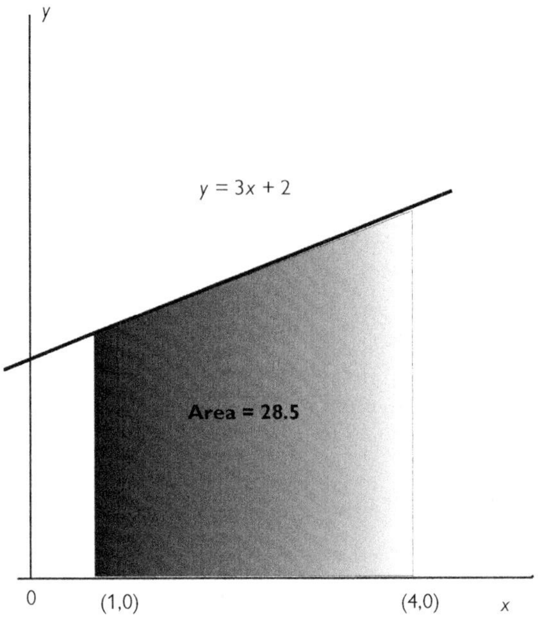


**Fig. 1.13** Area under the straight line $y = 3x + 2$, limits specified.

This is a mathematical way of describing an exponential process, of which there are many examples in medicine such as plasma drug concentration as redistribution occurs; the negative exponent in the first equation indicates a decreasing process rather than an increasing one.

The concept of simple harmonic motion, which has also been introduced, can be expressed in words as 'acceleration is proportional to displacement and opposes it' and it can be expressed in terms of a differential equation as:

$$\frac{d^2y}{dt^2} = -ky \text{ whose solution is whose solution is } y = A \sin \omega t.$$

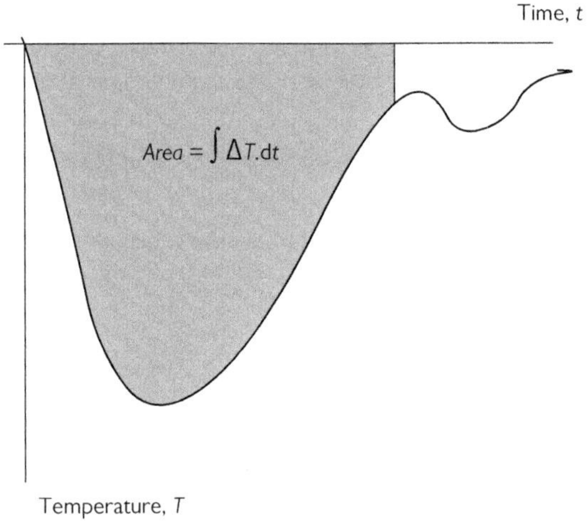


**Fig. 1.14** Area under a thermodilution curve, used to calculate cardiac output.

This describes, for example, the motion of a mass on a spring. More generally, the behaviour of engineering and physiological systems can be described by similar differential equations such as:

$$A\frac{d^2y}{dt^2}+B\frac{dy}{dt}+Cy=D,$$

where the first, second and third terms on the left-hand side are frequently acceleration, velocity and displacement terms respectively, and the term on the right-hand side is often a forcing function, which might be zero.

This can describe, for example, the motion set up in a vibrating catheter system to reproduce an arterial waveform with damping. These sorts of differential equations often have solutions that contain multiple exponential expressions.

## Powers, logarithms, 'e'

Very large or very small numbers can be conveniently expressed as powers. Since humans use 10 as the computing base, numbers are expressed as powers of 10, i.e.

$$10^0=1, 10^1=10, 10^2=10\times 10=100,$$

$$\ldots 10^6=10\times 10\times 10\times 10\times 10\times 10=1000000.$$

The verbal prefix 'kilo-' means $10^3$, and 'mega-' means $10^6$.

Likewise,

$$\frac{1}{10}=10^{-1}, \frac{1}{1000}=10^{-3}(\text{prefix 'milli-'}),$$

$$\frac{1}{1000\,000}=10^{-6}(\text{prefix 'micro-'}), 10^{-9}(\text{prefix 'nano-'}).$$

These apparently very small quantities appear in electronics and biochemistry, often because of the way these units are derived. For example the unit of electrical capacitance is the farad; it is a very large unit, defined as the charge in coulombs stored in a conductor per unit voltage across it ($C = Q/V$); therefore picofarads ($10^{-12}$) are often preferred. Likewise the unit of resistance is the ohm ($\Omega$), and it is a small unit; we therefore often refer to megaohms ($10^6$).

If $y = 1\,000\,000 = 10^6$, then 6 is the power to which 10 is raised to get 1 000 000. In this case therefore, 6 is the *logarithm to base 10* of $10^6$. If we replace 6 with the algebraic term $b$, then in general terms: if

$$y=10^b,$$

then

$$\log_{10} y=b.\log_{10} 10=b.1=b.$$

In words this would read 'log to base 10 of $y$ equals $b$ (times log to base 10 of 10)'. Log to a base of itself is 1. Logarithms therefore allow easier number representation and manipulation, particularly of very large or very small numbers.

For example, if

$$y=100\,000\,000=10^8=10^2\times 10^6,$$

$$\begin{aligned}\log_{10}(10^2\times 10^6)&=\log_{10} 10^2+\log_{10} 10^6\\&=2\log_{10} 10+6\log_{10} 10\\&=2\times 1+6\times 1\\&=8\\&=\log_{10} 10^8.\end{aligned}$$

Hence powers of 10 multiplied together result in a number whose powers are added, i.e.

$$10^a \,.\, 10^b = 10^{(a+b)}, \text{ and} \log_{10} = 10^{(a+b)} = (a+b).$$

Likewise

$$\log_{10}(a\,.\,b) = \log_{10} a + \log_{10} b.$$

and

$$\log_{10}(a\,/\,b) = \log_{10} a - \log_{10} b.$$

For example,

$$\begin{aligned}\log_{10}(10^6/10^2) &= \log_{10} 10^6 - \log_{10} 10^2\\ &= 6-2\\ &= 4\\ &= \log_{10} 10^4.\end{aligned}$$

An example of the use of logarithms in a clinical measurement setting is the *decibel*, a logarithmic ratio of power or amplitude (voltage or current) in relation to the electronic gain (amplification) of biomedical electronic equipment (see Chapter 4).

By definition

$$\textit{power gain in decibels (dB)} = 10\log_{10}.\frac{\textit{output power}}{\textit{input power}}$$

and

$$\textit{voltage (or current) gain} = 20\log_{10}.\frac{\textit{output voltage (or current)}}{\textit{input voltage (or current)}}$$

Graphical use of logarithms can be made by representing log *x* plotted graphically against log *y* (a log–log plot) or *x* against log *y* (semi-log). Pharmacological variables are often presented in this way.

Negative logarithms also have a meaning:

$$-\log_{10} a = \log_{10}(1/a) = \log_{10}(a^{-1}).$$

In acid base balance, the concept of pH uses negative logarithms: by definition

$$\text{pH} = -\log_{10}[\text{H}^+].$$

Normal hydrogen ion concentration,

$$\begin{aligned}[H^+] &= 40 \text{ nanomol l}^{-1}\\ &= 40\times 10^{-9}\text{mol l}^{-1}.\end{aligned}$$

Therefore,

$$\begin{aligned}-\log^{10}[\text{H}^+] &= -\{\log_{10} 40 + \log_{10} 10^{-9}\}\\ &= -\{\log_{10} 10 + \log_{10} 4 + \log_{10} 10^{-9}\}\\ &= -\{1.0 + 0.6020 + (-9)\} \approx 7.40.\end{aligned}$$

Instead of base 10, it is possible to choose other number bases, which can be used to express both large numbers and logarithms. For example if a base of 2 is chosen (binary),

$$2\times 2\times 2 = 2^3 = 8$$

and

$$\log_2 8 = 3.$$

If a general base *a* ($a > 1$) is chosen, such that $y = a^x$, which is a general exponential function, then it can be shown that the gradient, d*y*/d*x* of the curve is of the form:

$$\frac{dy}{dx} = m.\,y = m.\,a^x,$$

where $m$ is a constant with different values depending on the base, $a$.

If $a \leq 2$, then $m < 1$; and if $a \geq 3$, then $m > 1$. Imagine a base then, which has the property $m = 1$. This would mean that the rate of change of this function at every point is equal to the value of the function at that point.

This base is the natural exponential, e, where e = 2.7183. This seems a bizarre choice at first, but mathematically e also has the property of being represented by the very tidy power series:

$$e^x = 1 + x + \frac{x^2}{2\times 1} + \frac{x^3}{3\times 2\times 1} + \ldots \frac{x^n}{n(n-1)\ldots 2\times 1}.$$

Furthermore, the graphical representation of $e^x$ very adequately describes many changes in physiological and engineering systems. The property that $m = 1$ for e means the rate of change of this function is equal to the amount left and can be expressed mathematically as

$$\frac{d}{dx}(e^x) = e^x.$$

Such a curve is shown in Figure 1.15.

Logarithms to base 'e' can be used, when they are called natural logarithms, $\log_e x$ or $\ln x$, i.e.

if $x = e^y$, then $y = \log_e x$ or $\ln x$.

The fact that the rate of change of a substance is proportional to the amount of substance present is sufficient to define an exponential function, and describes the behaviour of a range of natural

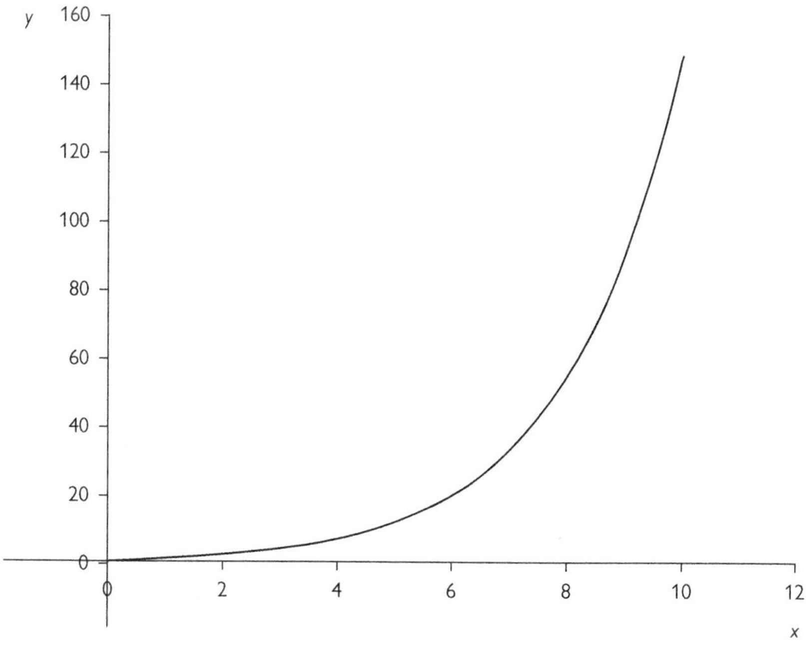


**Fig. 1.15** Curve $y = e^{0.5x}$.

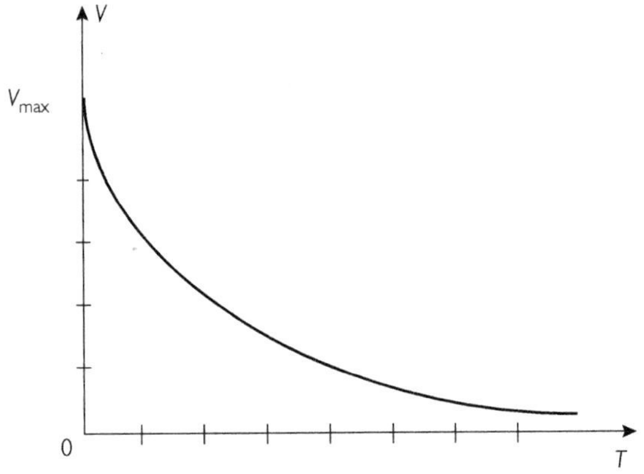


**Fig. 1.16** Decaying exponential curve with the equation $V = V_{max}.e^{-0.5t}$ .

phenomena. For example, a rectangular bath full of water starts to empty as the plug is removed; the (volumetric) rate of emptying of the bath is proportional to the height of water '*h*' left in the bath at time '*t*', and this is proportional to the pressure, $\rho\, g\, h$, which is driving the emptying process, where $\rho$ and $g$ are constants (see later).

Expressed mathematically,

$$-\frac{d}{dx}(volume\ left) = constant_1 \times p.g.h,$$

the minus sign indicating volume decrease with height; i.e.

$$k_1 \frac{dh}{dt} = -k_2.h.$$

The curve describing this behaviour is shown in Figure 1.16, and can be described by an equation like $V = V_{max}.\, e^{-kt}$ where $V$ is volume, $V_{max}$ is maximum volume, $k$ is a constant and $t$ is time. It could equally well apply to lung emptying.

Lung filling also occurs in an exponential fashion, and Figure 1.17 shows the form of the curve whose equation is $V = V_{max}\ (1 - e^{-kt})$.

The reduction in plasma concentration of a drug or dye, or the fall in blood temperature after a thermodilution bolus, also follows an exponential pattern prior to any recirculation. The half-life, $t_{½}$, is the time taken for the concentration of the drug to fall from $C_{max}$ to ½.$C_{max}$. The time constant $\tau$ (tau), is the time elapsing for the function to fall to zero if the rate of decay had remained at its initial value, which corresponds to falling to a value of $C_{max}/e$ on the exponential curve. Figure 1.18 shows this.

To calculate $t_{½}$:

$$\text{If } C = C_{max}.\, e^{-k.1}, \text{ then when } C = ½.C_{max},$$

$$\frac{1}{2} = e^{-kt1/2},$$

therefore

$$\begin{aligned} t_{1/2} &= -\frac{1}{k}.\log_e.\frac{1}{2}, \\ &= 0.693 / k. \end{aligned}$$

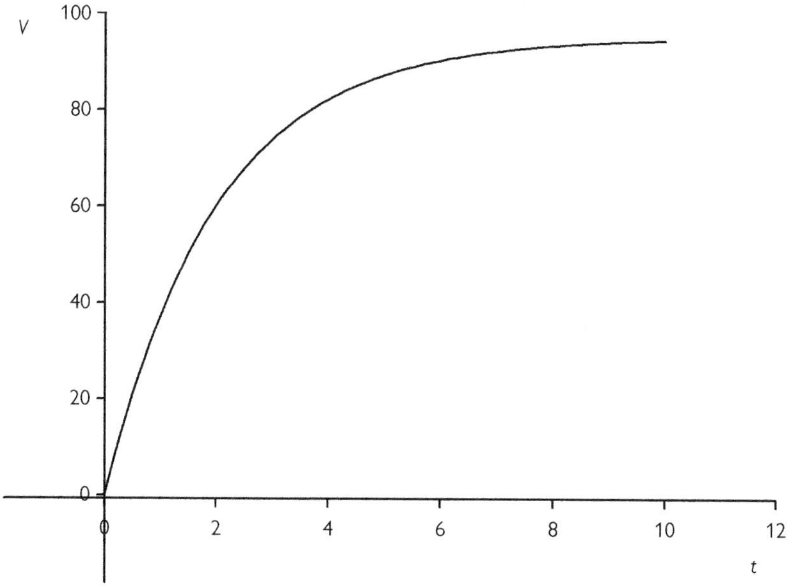


**Fig. 1.17** Exponential curve describing lung filling with the equation $V = V_{max}(1 - e^{-0.5t})$.

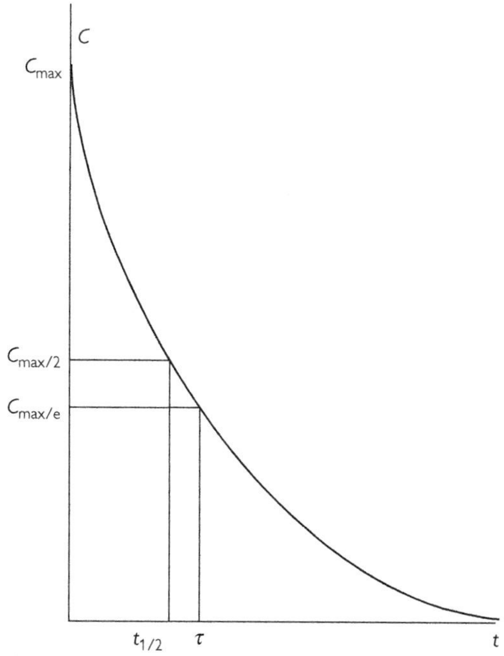


**Fig. 1.18** Exponential decay in drug plasma concentration $C$, and its relationship to time constant and $\tau$ (tau) and half-life $t_{½}$.

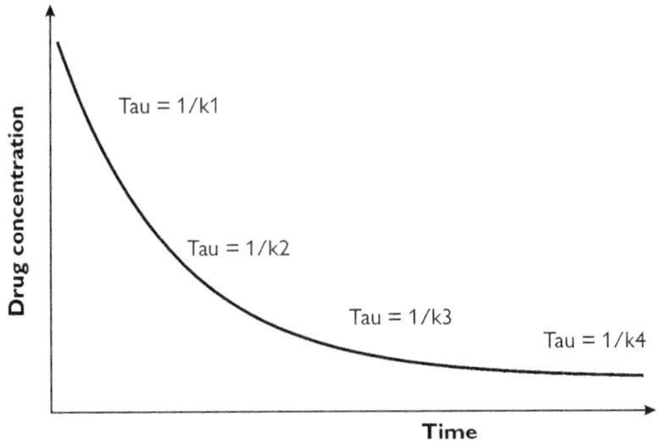


**Fig. 1.19** Exponential decay of drug concentration in a multi-compartment pharmacokinetic model, with equation $C = C_1 e_1^{-k_1 t} + C_2 e_2^{-k_2 t} + C_3 e_3^{-k_3 t} + C_4 e_4^{-k_4 t}$.

The slope of the exponential decay curve is $dC/dt = -kC_{max}e^{-kt} = -kC_{max}$ when $t = 0$. The tangent to this curve has the equation $C = C_{max}(1 - kt)$. $\tau$, the time constant, is defined by the point on this line at which $C = 0$, so $\tau = 1/k$, at which time $C = C_{max}/e$ on the curve.

As a rule of thumb, after one time constant there is a fall to 0.37 $C_{max}$ of the initial value; after $2\tau$, $C$ has become 0.135 $C_{max}$; after $3\tau$, $C$ is 0.05 $C_{max}$. The degradation process is normally considered complete after four time constants.

Note that if the equation $C = C_{max}.e^{-kt}$ is written in logarithmic form:

$$\log_e C = -kt.\ \log_e C_{max},$$

then the resulting semi-log plot of $\log_e C$ plotted against $t$ is a straight line with a (negative) slope $-k$, which makes its interpretation easier.

Many pharmacokinetic and other processes are complex, involving multiple exponential curves, whose equations might be something like:

$$y = A_1 e^{-k_1 t} + A_2 e^{-k_2 t} + \cdots,$$

shown graphically in Figure 1.19, which might represent a drug concentration in a multi-compartment model with different time constants.

## *Further reading*

**Arcole, A. and Roe, P.** (2011) Mathematical relationships in anaesthesia and intensive care medicine, *CEACCP*, **11**(2), pp. 50–5.

**Cruickshank, S.** (1998) *Mathematics and Statistics in Anaesthesia*, Oxford Medical Publications, Oxford.

# Chapter 2 **Statistics**

This chapter contains: categorical and numerical data, quantifying variability, probability, the Normal distribution, hypothesis testing (parametric and non-parametric), diagnostic tests, meta-analysis, correlation and regression, comparing categorical data, evidence-based medicine, power calculations, study design and clinical trials, and inappropriate use of statistics.

The chapter links with: Chapters 1, 3, 5 and 19.

## Introduction

This chapter will provide background to enable the reader to understand basic statistics and be able then to follow more complex statistical ideas. Although statistics is more than the mere analysis of data, it is a subject largely about data, so this will be discussed first. Data can be categorical or numerical, and in these two classifications there are various different types of data.

## Categorical data

### *Data that can be put into two categories*

This is the allocation of the individual to one of two categories. Often these relate to the presence or absence of some attribute. These data also have many other names such as binary, dichotomous and attribute data. Examples of such categorisations for patients include:

- Male/Female
- Smoker/Non-smoker
- Anaesthetist/Surgeon
- Married/Single.

Each of these can only be one or the other – they could be coded '1' or '0' to be *binary* (or on, off). For example, male = 0, female = 1, or vice versa.

### *Data that have more than two categories*

Many classifications require more than two categories, such as blood group, type of doctor, country of birth. Also the two categories, such as described previously, might be expanded into several categories. For example, the married/single could be expanded to married/single/divorced/separated/widowed. This sort of data is called *nominal* data, where there are several categories, but with no logical order.

When there is a natural order (such as in seniority), the data are then called *ordinal* data. For example, anaesthetists could be divided into: 'Foundation year 1', 'Foundation year 2', 'speciality doctor', consultants', 'senior consultants' and 'professors'. Ordinal data can be reduced to two categories, with possibly a considerable loss of information (e.g. 'consultants', 'resident doctors').

## Numerical data

Discrete numerical data are where the observation takes exact numerical values. Counts or events are discrete values. For example: number of children, number of ectopic beats in a time period and so on. Continuous (or analogue) data are usually obtained by some form of measurement. Examples are body temperature, blood pressure, height and weight. These values have an infinite number of possibilities, depending on the measurement interval, and variation. Although there are infinite possibilities, measurement systems usually round the continuous data up, or down, to discrete values. Blood pressure is often rounded up to the nearest 5 mmHg, for example.

### *Linear and non-linear scales*

Continuous data, such as heart rate can be displayed as a point on a linear scale. A linear scale increases at a constant rate and each interval between adjacent numbers is the same (as shown in Figure 2.1(a)). In some measurements, where a wide range of values is encountered, it can be useful to display numbers in a non-linear way. For example, in flowmeters capable of large flows, it would be impossible to measure low flows with any degree of confidence. The normal form of non-linear scale is the logarithmic scale in which each increment on the scale corresponds to a proportional increase in the amount measured (as shown in Figure 2.1(b)). This can allow accuracy at small values but also large values can be displayed. Logarithms are discussed in more detail in Chapter 1.

### *Graphical displays of data*

It is normally only possible to automatically display data graphically if the variable concerned has an electrical signal associated with it. This signal is normally digitised and displayed on a computer screen as a straightforward signal against time, or in the frequency domain or, where relevant, in other display forms such as histograms or pie diagrams. The digitisation and computers are described in Chapter 5. Data can also be presented as a scatter diagram. This is one of several ways and is a simple graph where the values of one variable are plotted against those of another. An example of this is shown in Figure 2.2. It should be noted that in this example drug concentration is a continuous variable, whereas infusion rate is a discrete one.

Simple graphical ways of summarising a complete set of observations are by means of a histogram and a pie chart. In the histogram, the number (or frequency) of observations is plotted for different values or groups of values. Figure 2.3 shows a histogram of the number of children being given immunoglobulin M plotted against the plasma IgM concentrations.

A pie chart is very useful for displaying the proportions that go to make up a whole, in the form of a circle split up into sectors. For example using some of the data for the histogram, the proportion of children having five different serum concentrations can be shown as a pie chart, as in Figure 2.4.

## Quantifying variability

In anaesthesia, when measurements are taken from patients regarding their height, weight, blood pressure, there is a wide range of values recorded and a wide spread of values between patients. Parameters are needed to describe these data sets. The simplest method used for describing a set of observations of a numerical variable (e.g. height) is to calculate the average.

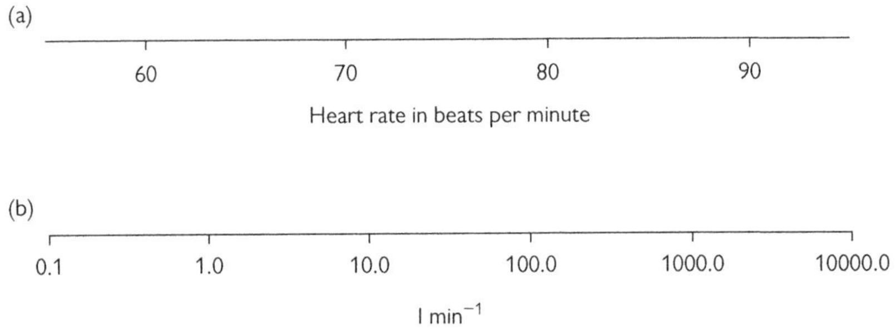


**Fig. 2.1** Examples of linear (a) and non-linear (b) scales.

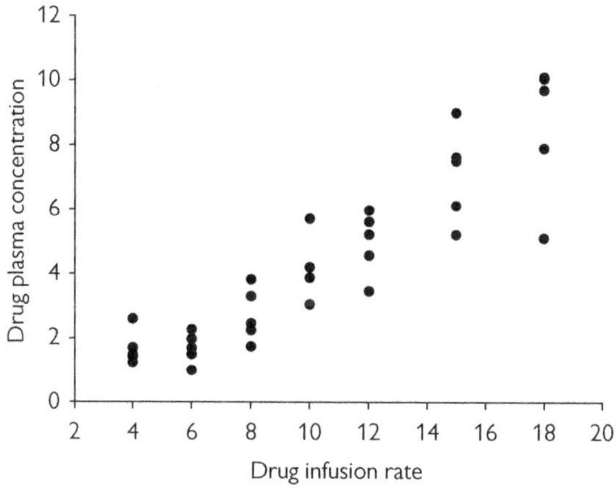


**Fig. 2.2** Example of a scatter diagram. The *y*-axis is plasma concentration and the *x*-axis is infusion rate.

## *Averages*

The most used average to do this is the *arithmetic mean*, normally referred to as simply the *mean*. This is the sum of all the observations divided by the number of observations. For example, if the data set of heights from 11 patients was 1.55, 1.62, 1.65, 1.72, 1.75, 1.76, 1.80, 1.80, 1.80, 1.85, 1.86 m, then the mean will be the sum of these heights divided by 11 (the number of patients), which is 1.74 m. This mean does not give any indication of the spread or *variance* of the values or whether the values are spread equally along the number axis or clustered together. This will be explored later.

Other measures to describe averages are the *mode* and the *median*. The mode is the most frequently occurring observation in a data set. In the height data set used above, the sample mode is 1.80 m, as this height has three observations and the other height values have only one observation each. The median is the middle value of the set of measurements when they are placed in order according to their numerical value, or *ranked* in order. In the above example of heights, the numbers are ranked in ascending height values, and so the middle value, or median, will be the 6th value, which is 1.76 m. If there were an even number of observations, then the median would be the average of the middle two values.

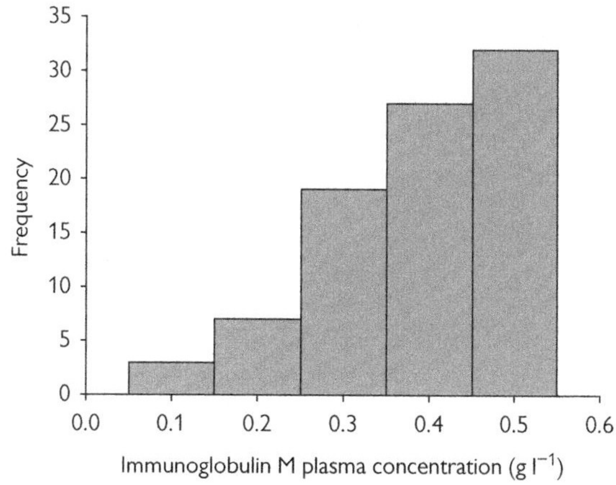


**Fig. 2.3** Example of a frequency histogram of IgM plasma concentrations (Isaacs *et al.*, 1983).

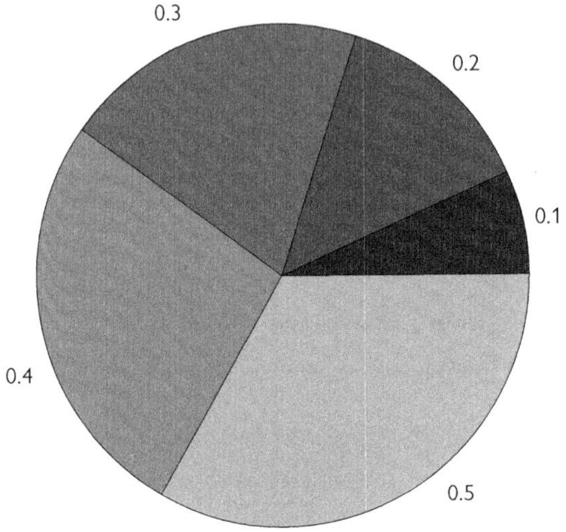


**Fig. 2.4** Pie chart showing five plasma concentrations from Figure 2.3 and the proportion of children having those levels. The numbers in each sector are the plasma concentrations in g $l^{-1}$.

## *Variability*

Graphical methods are important for examining the variability of data, but it is also necessary to be able to quantify the amount of variability in the data. This numerical value, in conjunction with the mean, would provide an informative, but brief, summary of a set of data. There are three main approaches to giving the variability a numerical value: the *range*, the *centiles*, and a numerical measure of the dispersion around the mean.

The range, which is the simplest variability measure, is quoted as the lowest and highest values of a series of numbers. Obviously outliers, or unusual values, will confuse the issue and make the spread of values appear greater than it really is. The situation can be improved by giving two numbers that encompass most, rather than all, of the data values. For example, the range between which 90% of the observations lie can be calculated - this would then omit the outliers. This is called the *central range.* The data set can be further split into *centiles*, or *percentiles*. If the data set is ranked from lowest value to highest value, then halfway along is the 50% centile (or median). For example, if there are 100 data points, set out and ranked in ascending order, then the 5% centile will be the 5th data value. The 95% will be the 95th and so on. For other data sets, interpolation may be needed. The central range discussed above is the range between 5% and 95% of the data values. As an example, using the data shown in the histogram of Figure 2.3, then this data could be ranked as follows:

$$\{0.1,\ 0.1,\ 0.1,\ 0.2,\ 0.2,\ 0.2,\ 0.2,\ 0.2,\ 0.2,\ 0.2,\ \ldots\}.$$

As shown in Figure 2.3, to finish the data set, nineteen 0.3 values would be added, then twenty-seven 0.4 values, and then finally thirty-two 0.5 values. The 5% value (of the data set) would be worked out by:

$$0.05 \text{ (the 5\%)} \times 89 \text{ (the total number of concentrations plus 1)}$$
$$= (3+7+19+27+32+\mathbf{1}) \times 0.05 = 4.45.$$

So the 5% value is the 4.45th value, but there is no 4.45 value, so the 5% value will be halfway between the 4th and the 5th values. In this set, both of these values are the same and so the 5% value is 0.2. In a similar calculation, the 95% value is 0.5. Therefore, in this data set the 5% and 95% centiles are 0.2 and

0.5 g $l^{-1}$. All other centiles can be calculated in the same manner. The difference between the 25% and the 75% values is called the *inter-quartile range*, which again can be used to describe variability in a more useful way than just the total range.

### *Variance and standard deviation*

A mean ($\overline{x}$) has been calculated for the data set, and all the data points ($x_i$) may have values similar to the mean value, i.e. their differences may be small. In this situation, there is a low spread or *variance*. All the data points may have large differences between the mean and the points and then there will be high variance. A numerical value can be worked out for this variance by first working out the difference from each of the data points to the mean. If all these values were added together, to get some 'feel' for the variance, then this would not be useful as the sum might be zero, as some differences would be negative and some equally positive. If the differences are squared (to remove the negatives) and then summed, then this provides an indication of the spread. The average of these 'squared differences' gives a measure of individual deviation from the means. The calculated sample variance can be written as:

$$\frac{\sum_{i=1}^{n}(x_i - \overline{x})^2}{n-1}$$

If the data set is a sample from a larger population (for example, the measured heights of ten adult female anaesthetists, the variation in the sample will, on average, be less than the population as a whole. If the population varies (in this case, adult female anaesthetists), the estimate of the population variance is made by multiplying the sample variance by n/n–1, where n is the number of observations in the sample. As the sample size increases, the estimate of the population variance is closer to the sample variance. The estimated population variance can be written as:

$$\frac{\sum_{i=1}^{n}\left(x_i - \overline{x}\right)^2}{n-1}$$

To put the *variance* in the same units as the mean, the equation needs to have its square root taken, and this result is then called the *standard deviation*. An easier form (which is mathematically the same, only rearranged) for calculation purposes is:

$$s = \sqrt{\frac{\sum x_i^2 - \frac{1}{n}(\sum x_i)^2}{n-1}}.$$

For most circumstances, the large majority (95%) of a set of observations will be within ± two standard deviations of the mean. This statement depends on the *shape* of the distribution. If a histogram is drawn of some data (see Figure 2.5), then it is symmetrical if each side of the mode (the most commonly occurring value, in this example 0.7) has a similar shape. If it is not symmetrical, it is called a skewed distribution and an example is shown in Figure 2.6. This figure shows positive skewness where there is a long right-hand tail, and this is most common skewed distribution, often occurring where there is a 'hard stop' value which cannot be measured (for example, patient weight in kg must be greater than zero). Negative skewness is where there is a long left-hand tail. The data may be able to be transformed mathematically by using, for example, logarithms of each data point, and this may give a more symmetrical picture. The shape and properties of distributions will be introduced further in the next section on probability.

## Probability

The probability of some outcome can be interpreted as the proportion of times that a certain outcome would occur if the experiment were repeated a large number of times. The probability that a baby will be a girl can be estimated by observing what proportion of a large population of babies are girls.

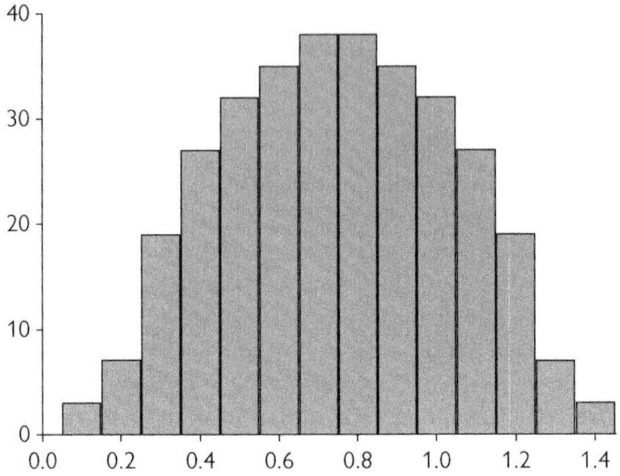


**Fig. 2.5** Symmetrical frequency distribution.

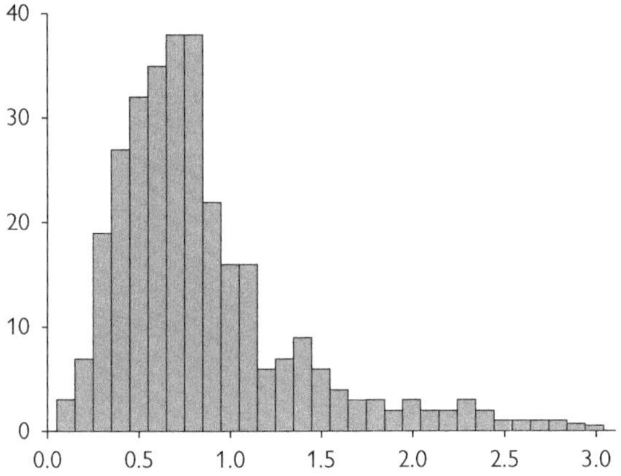


**Fig. 2.6** Unsymmetrical frequency distribution with positive skew.

Probability lies between 0 and 1. Something that cannot happen has the probability of 0 and something that is certain has the value of 1. There are rules about probabilities: for a given event, for any two outcomes that might happen, the probability of either occurring is the *sum* of the individual probabilities, as long as they cannot occur at the same time (they are exclusive). For example, if the probability of an individual being an anaesthetist is 0.01 and that of being a physicist is 0.02, then the probability of being either an anaesthetist or a physicist is 0.03. It follows that the sum of *all* possible occupations must add up to 1, since all the occupations must occur. If two or more different events happen that are independent of each other (the outcome of one tells us nothing about the other event), then to obtain the probability of a combination of specific outcomes, the individual probabilities are multiplied. For example, if there are three people in a library, the probability that they are all anaesthetists is 0.01 × 0.01 × 0.01, i.e. 0.000 001. If the events are not independent (for example, the anaesthetists might be colleagues who have arrived together), then the multiplication rule does not apply, and the calculations are more complex.

## Probability distributions

Many statistical methods are based on the assumption that the observed data are a sample from a distribution that has a known shape. If this assumption is reasonable, then statistical methods of analysis are called parametric analyses and are simpler to use than those from a sample without such a distribution. They are also more powerful—that is, they are more likely to detect differences. Those methods that make no assumptions about distribution shape are called non-parametric methods. The most commonly used distribution for continuous variables is called the Normal distribution (or Gaussian).

## The Normal distribution

Histograms (an example was shown in Figure 2.3) have already been discussed as a graphical method of showing the frequency with which different values of a variable occur in the data set. If the midpoint of each band in Figure 2.5 is joined up then the resultant curve will be a frequency polygon, as shown in Figure 2.7. The shape of the curve is bell shaped, symmetrical and has one peak. Its shape is loosely similar to the Normal distribution, which is a probability distribution that has one peak and is symmetrical. This distribution (unlike the one in Figure 2.7) has no upper and no lower limit - it is defined for all values to infinity. The height of the frequency curve is the probability density. As with the histogram of observed data, the Normal distribution is used by considering areas. The total area under the curve is always 1.0. A restricted area gives the probability between the values within the restricted area. For example, the probability of the whole range or area occurring is certain or 1, and the area to the left of the median is 0.5. Therefore the probability of being below the median is 0.5 or 50%.

The Normal distribution is completely described by two parameters - the mean ($\mu$) and the standard deviation ($\sigma$). For example the distribution in Figure 2.8 has a mean of 10 and a standard deviation of 2.

If we assume that in the population, some variable (for example blood pressure) has a Normal distribution, then the probability of a certain value (or pressure) occurring can be estimated from the area under the curve. For example, the probability of the pressure being between one standard deviation

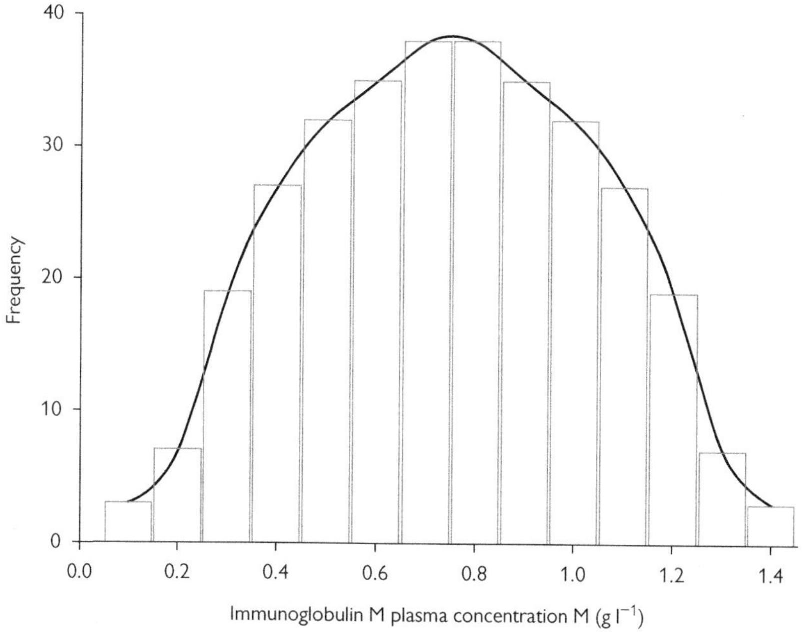


**Fig. 2.7** Frequency distribution, showing bell-shaped curve.

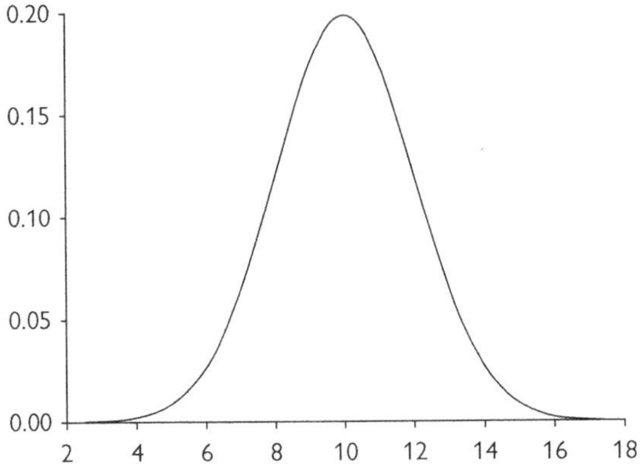


**Fig. 2.8** Normal distribution with a mean of 10 and a standard deviation of 2.

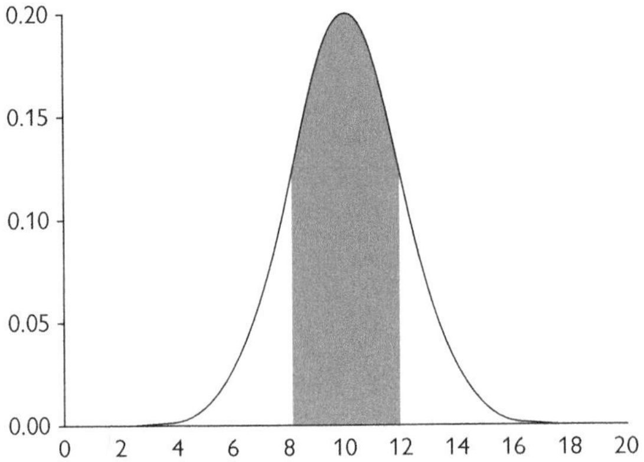


**Fig. 2.9** Normal distribution (mean of 10, standard deviation of 2) showing area between mean plus one standard deviation (12) and mean minus one standard deviation (8).

on one side of the mean (12 in the figure) to one standard deviation the other side (8 in the figure) is 68% of the area under the curve, or 0.68. This is illustrated in Figure 2.9. Conversely being outside it (i.e. greater or less than one standard deviation) is the difference between the total area (1) and this value, i.e. 1 - 0.68, or 0.32.

## *Sample and population means*

When a mean of a sample of data points is used to estimate the mean of a certain variable, it is not known how good this estimate of the mean is and how near in value it is to the true mean of the complete population from which the sample has been drawn. If, for example, the complete population of the UK has its resting blood pressure taken, then this extremely large data set will have a true mean $\mu$ and a true standard deviation $\sigma$. A subset of the population (for example 10 patients) can have their blood pressure taken and this sample will have its own mean ($\bar{X}_i$) and standard deviation ($s_i$), which may well be very different from the population values. Figure 2.10 shows this in schematic form, with the top box representing the complete population and the smaller boxes below representing small samples, taken at random from the population. Each of these samples will have their own mean and standard deviation.

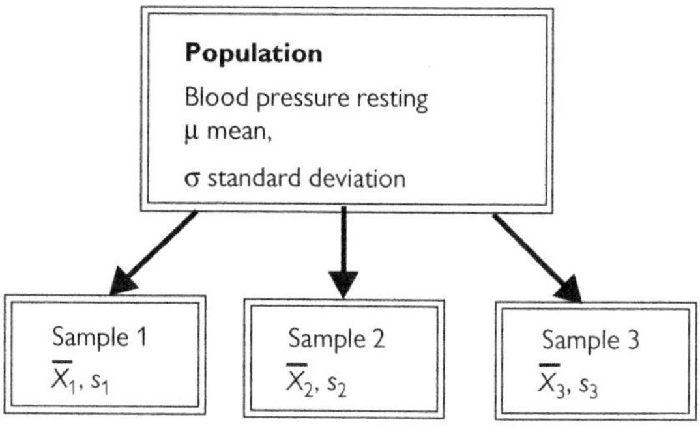


**Fig. 2.10** Diagram showing the mean and standard deviation of the whole population with random sample sets drawn from this, each having a mean ($\overline{X}$) and standard deviation ($s$).

The mean of Sample 1 (a small number of patients) will be a certain value and is probably different from the mean of Sample 2 and so on. If the number of patients in each sample is very large, then the sample mean will become closer to the population mean. If the number of patients in each sample is small, then it is likely that this sample could be less representative of the population mean. If all the means of Sample 1, Sample 2, Sample 3 and so on are calculated and the *grand* mean of these sample means is calculated, it will be found that this grand mean is in fact the population mean, $\mu$, with a standard deviation of:

$$\sigma(\textit{the population standard deviation}) / \sqrt{(\textit{the number of patients in each sample})}.$$

The standard deviation of the means of the samples (of size $n$) is termed the *standard error of the mean* (SEM), and the best estimate of it is obtained using the patients drawn from one of the single sample sets of data:

$$s(\textit{the sample standard deviation}) / \sqrt{(\textit{the number of patients in the sample})}.$$

The standard deviation quantifies variability in the population and the SEM quantifies uncertainty in the estimate of the mean. In 95% of samples, the mean obtained from the sample is within two (actually 1.96) standard errors (SE) of the true population mean. The interval from the population mean −2 SE to the population mean +2 SE is known as the 95% confidence interval. The 99% confidence interval would be obtained by using ±3 SE (actually 2.58). However, these multiples of the SE are only true if the data are normally distributed and the number of patients in each sample is large (large is normally taken to be greater than 30). If the sample size is small, then the standard deviation of the sample (which is used to estimate the standard deviation of the population) may become very different from the true population value. For the small sample size, a multiplier of more than two is needed to calculate the 95% confidence intervals for the mean, because there is a greater imprecision involved. The 95% confidence interval of the total population can be obtained from a Normal distribution table found in statistical textbooks and this table quotes 1.96 SE. Because of this imprecision, the confidence intervals will be wider for samples containing small numbers of data points, and a different distribution is needed to calculate the intervals. This distribution is called the *Student's t-distribution*. For example, for a sample containing five patients, the 95% confidence interval will be, using the t-distribution, ±2.57 SE. The Student's t-test makes use of comparing the confidence intervals of two sets of data using the t-distribution, and this will be discussed in the next section. The confidence intervals of two sets of data can be compared to see if they overlap or a hypothesis test can be used. An important parameter of the t-test is the number of *degrees of freedom*. This is a strange concept, but is defined as the *size of the sample – the number of estimation parameters* (*here, standard deviation*). So for a sample of 10 patients, the degrees of freedom will be $n - 1 = 9$.

## Hypothesis testing

Hypothesis testing is a way of determining whether some observed effect is likely to be real, or simple due to chance. The null hypothesis is that any differences are due to chance variation in samples -there is no difference in the population from which the samples are drawn. The *P* value is the probability of getting a difference between the two samples as large or larger as is observed, if the null hypothesis is true (i.e. the two samples are the same). The cut-off values for *P* can be chosen to be any value, but are normally taken to be 0.05 or 0.01. If the *P* value is higher than the cut-off value, then there is no evidence to reject the null hypothesis (i.e. there is insufficient evidence that the difference is not due to chance variation); if it is below, then the null hypothesis is unlikely to be true and is rejected. A value of $P = 0.01$ means there is a 1% probability of obtaining the data that is actually observed if the null hypothesis is true, i.e. it is much more likely that the two samples are from different populations. If the null hypothesis is rejected (at a particular cut-off value for P), then a statistically significant difference is detected.

Before the statistical test is carried out, a cut-off value for *P* must be set. When the *P* value is generated, then it is either below the cut-off or above it. If it is below this value, then this is called the critical region and the null hypothesis is rejected. This of course can be the correct interpretation and the sample sets are from different populations. Or this rejection might be incorrect when the null hypothesis is in fact true. This is a Type I error, an $\alpha$ error, or false positive (i.e. reject the null hypothesis when it is in fact true). If the P value is greater or above the cut-off value, then this is the acceptable region and the null hypothesis is not rejected. This may be because the sample sets are from the same population. However, it may also be that the samples are from different populations (i.e. the null hypothesis is false) but that the test has not detected the difference. In this case, there is a Type II error, a $\beta$ error, or false negative (i.e. don't reject the null hypothesis when it is in fact false). A summary of hypothesis testing, giving all the possible outcomes from a test, is shown in Figure 2.11.

## Power

The power of a test is the probability that a study of a given size would detect as statistically significant a real difference of a given magnitude. The actual required sample size can be calculated using appropriate statistical software (for example, SPSS or Python) or by using tables, such as Altman (1980). The

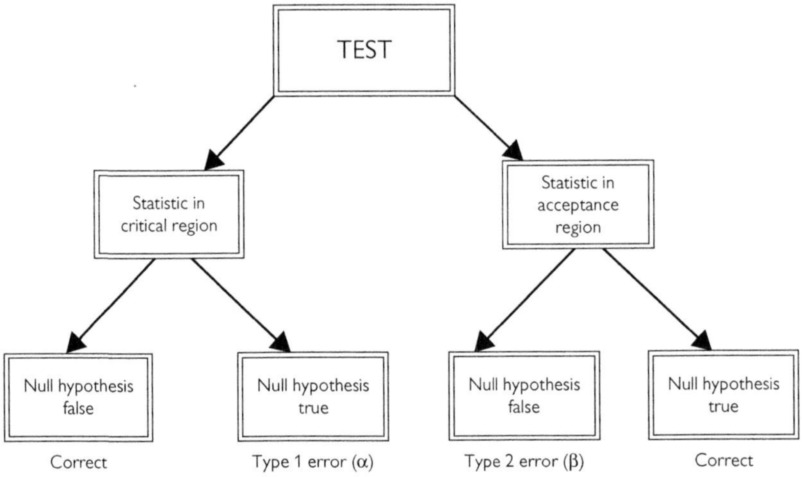


**Fig. 2.11** Test flow diagram.

power is 1–β or 100(1–β)%, where β is the probability of making a Type II error. With the appropriate sample size used, there is a high chance of detecting as statistically significant a worthwhile effect, if it exists, and to be reasonably sure that no benefit exists if it is not found in the experiments. The greater the power (and the sample size), the surer it is that both of these are the case. It is common practice to require a power of between 80 and 90%.

There are four items that need to be specified or estimated to carry out sample size calculations, either to insert into the appropriate software or to use with the table mentioned earlier. These are the minimum difference, or effect, that represents clinical importance, the population standard deviation, the desired Type I error (normally set at <0.05) and the desired power (based on the Type II error). Normally, the minimum difference and the standard deviation are combined to give the standard difference (min difference/standard deviation), which is used in the nomogram mentioned earlier; a line drawn from the left y axis of the standardised difference to the right y axis of the power required will pass through a straight line giving the sample number required. When planning research and the sample size, the standard deviation of the population of interest might not be known. Estimates for this may be obtained by using published data, or, more commonly, by carrying out a small pilot study to provide a useful estimate for standard deviation and the standard difference. Columb and Atkinson (2016) explain this well.

# Parametric methods

## *Student's t-tests*

A test can be carried out of the null hypothesis, that the mean from a sample is from a population with a known mean. If the data sets are large (>100, for example), then the Normal distribution is used, otherwise a distribution called the Student's t-distribution is used (as discussed previously). The test, called a *one-sample t-test* uses the test statistic:

$$t = (\textit{sample mean} - \textit{known mean}) / (\textit{SE of sample mean}).$$

This test uses the t-distribution, which becomes close to the Normal distribution when the numbers in the data set are large. The t value will be 0 when the means are the same: it is likely that the sample is from the given population. As the difference between the sample mean and the known mean increases, the t value increases and it becomes more likely that the null hypothesis is not true, and the sample is from a different population. Normally it does not matter whether the difference between the means is positive or negative, and then a *two-sided* t-test is used. The t statistic can be translated into a *P* (probability) value, using appropriate software (e.g. SPSS mentioned earlier). For example, a population has a mean systolic blood pressure of 120 mmHg, and in our sample of nine patients having a certain anaesthetic, the mean blood pressure is 110 mmHg with a standard deviation of 10.6. This gives a test statistic of:

$$t = (110 - 120)/10.6/3), \text{ which gives } t = 2.8$$

In this example, the *P* value is *calculated* (from statistical tables) to be 0.05. If the null hypothesis cut-off is 0.05 (i.e. $P < 0.05$), then the calculated *P* value is not less than the cut-off, so the null hypothesis is not rejected, but only just! If the cut-off was set at 0.01, then the null hypothesis would not be rejected.

The *paired t-test* is an extension of the one-sample test, and is a special case of the *two-sample* t-test. Paired data can result when the same individuals have been studied more than once and also when each member of the sample has been individually matched to another in the other sample. An example could be women who take their blood pressure before and after their menstrual periods. One sample would consist of all the women before and the other sample would consist of all the women after. Each woman would be paired with herself, before and after. With paired data, the interest is in the average difference between observations and the variability of these differences. The *within-subject* differences are important. The test statistic value is now calculated as (with $n - 1$ degrees of freedom):

$$t = (\textit{mean of differences between each before and after subject}) / (\textit{SE difference}).$$

The other two sample t-test is where the two samples are truly independent, i.e. there is no pairing and the number of samples in each group can be different. The mean difference between the two groups and the variability between subjects is important. The test statistic is calculated (with $n_1 + n_2 - 2$ degrees of freedom), where Sample 1 contains $n_1$ patients, and Sample 2 contains $n_2$:

$$t = (\textit{mean of first group} - \textit{mean of second group}) / (\textit{SE}(\textit{mean } 1 - \textit{mean } 2)).$$

# Non-parametric methods

## *Wilcoxon signed rank sum test*

Non-parametric tests are used in cases where it cannot be assumed that the data are drawn from a particular family of distribution. The one-sample t-test requires the data to be well-approximated by a normal distribution. Where this assumption does not hold, a non-parametric test can be used, called the Wilcoxon signed rank test (though this does require the data to be from a symmetric distribution, i.e. that the mean and median of the underlying distribution are equal).

As with the one-sample t-test, the null hypothesis is that the data are drawn from a distribution with a particular known mean. If this null hypothesis is true, then on average, there would be an equal number of observations greater than and less than the set value. The signed rank test calculates how likely it would be to observe the data values if the null hypothesis is true. The test method calculates the difference from each data point to the set value. In the example in Table 2.1 the set value is 100 mmHg. Once each difference is calculated, then the differences are ranked in order (i.e. the least magnitude is position 1, the next position 2, etc.) but the signs are ignored for the ranking. Any differences that are the same will have their ranks averaged, e.g. 1.5 and 5.5 in the example. Once the ranks have been worked out, the 'negative' rank numbers are added together. These are differences –7 and –10 in the example, which give ranks 3 and 5.5. These add up to 8.5, and this value gives a $P$ value of 0.05. The probability of getting our data if the null hypothesis is true is 0.05, which is likely to be rejected.

**Table 2.1** Blood pressure values of ten patients with rank order of differences (ignoring their signs) from a set value of 100 (mmHg)

| Patient | Blood pressure (mmHg) | Difference from 100 (mmHg) | Ranks |
|---|---|---|---|
| 1 | 80 | 20 | 10 |
| 2 | 85 | 15 | 9 |
| 3 | 87 | 13 | 8 |
| 4 | 89 | 11 | 7 |
| 5 | 90 | 10 | 5.5 |
| 6 | 92 | 8 | 4 |
| 7 | 95 | 5 | 1.5 |
| 8 | 95 | 5 | 1.5 |
| 9 | 107 | –7 | 3 |
| 10 | 110 | –10 | 5.5 |

### *Mann–Whitney U test*

This is another non-parametric test, an alternative to the t-test for comparing data from two independent groups (the test is also called the Mann–Whitney–Wilcoxon), where the null hypothesis is that the two samples are drawn from populations with the same median. The test is also used when the variances of the two populations of data are significantly different (the F test will determine this, which is the ratio of the variances), but alternatively, a modified t-test called the Welch test could be used in this situation. The Mann–Whitney ranks both groups together as illustrated in Table 2.2, and then the sum of the ranks of each group is compared (comparing columns 1 and 3, which give totals of 19.5 and 35.5). If the null hypothesis is true, then the sum of each rank of the separate groups will be similar. The more different they become, the more likely the null hypothesis is false. Again, distribution tables are used to find the *P* values.

## Diagnostic tests

In a diagnostic test, patients can be classified into two groups, according to the results of an investigation or test. For example, two groups could be if a patient is awake or asleep. A measurement that can be used to detect whether the patient is awake or asleep during anaesthesia is an index obtained from the *electroencephagram* (EEG), obtained from a depth of anaesthesia monitor. A *threshold* value is set so that if the EEG index is above this, then the patient is assumed to be awake, and below this the patient is assumed to be asleep. Ideally this value of the threshold would discriminate completely between the two groups but usually perfect discrimination is not possible. Different values of the threshold would give better or worse discrimination. *Sensitivity* is the proportion of true positives (i.e. patients who are in fact awake) that are correctly identified by the test. This is also known as the true positive rate. *Specificity* is the proportion of true negatives (i.e. patients who are in fact asleep) that are correctly identified as negative (i.e. asleep) by the test. This is also known as the true negative rate. Table 2.3 shows a useful summary of this and is known as a *confusion matrix*

**Table 2.2** Blood pressure values from two groups of patients

| Group 1 rank | Group 1 values (mmHg) | Group 2 rank | Group 2 values (mmHg) |
|---|---|---|---|
| 1 | 80 | | |
| 2 | 85 | | |
| 3 | 87 | | |
| | | 4 | 89 |
| | | 5 | 90 |
| 6 | 92 | | |
| 7.5 | 95 | | |
| | | 7.5 | 95 |
| | | 9 | 107 |
| | | 10 | 110 |
| Sum = 19.5 | | Sum = 35.5 | |

**Table 2.3** Representation of a diagnostic test

| Test result | Actual condition | | |
|---|---|---|---|
| | Positive (patient is awake). | Negative (patient is asleep) | |
| Positive (EEG = awake) | True positive (correct) = a | False positive = b | total positive tests a + b |
| Negative (EEG = asleep | False negative = c. | True negative (correct) = d | total negative tests c + d |
| | total actual positives | total actual negatives | |
| | a + c | b + d | |

Sensitivity is defined as: true positives/total actual positives, a/(a + c). Specificity is defined as: true negatives/total actual negatives, d/(b+d).

## *Receiver operating characteristics curves*

Receiver operating characteristics (ROC, first used in testing radar receiver installations) curves are a graphical representation of how robust a diagnostic test (for example, the EEG test described above) is and is a plot of the true positive rate (sensitivity) against the false positive rate (1-specificity). The ROC curve is a plot of the sensitivities and specificities at different thresholds (for example, different values of the EEG index for determining awake and asleep). An ROC curve shows the trade-off between sensitivity and specificity (any increase in sensitivity will be accompanied by a decrease in specificity). The closer the curve follows the left-hand border and then the top border of the ROC space, the more accurate the test. The closer the curve comes to the 45-degree diagonal of the ROC space, the less accurate the test. The area under the curve is a measure of test accuracy or the *goodness* of the test. Three ROC curves are shown in Figure 2.12, and show worthless, good and excellent tests. Different diagnostic tests (for

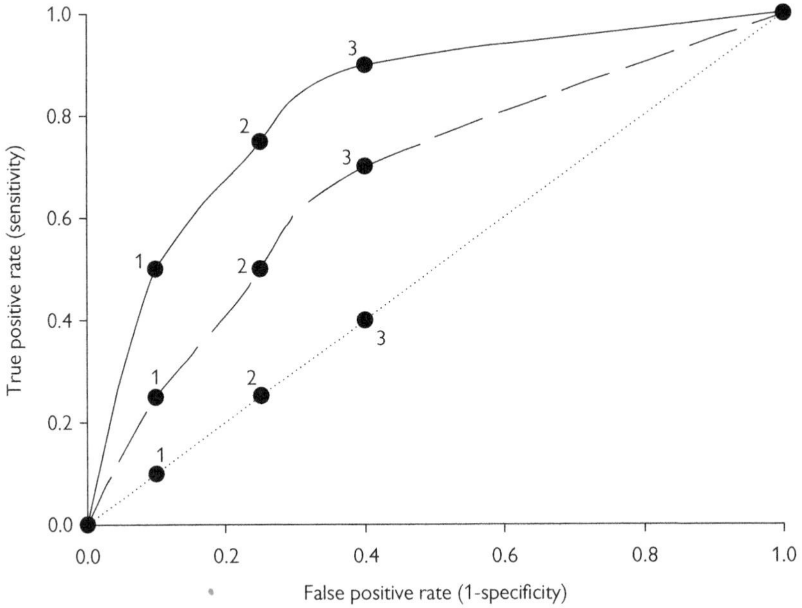


**Fig. 2.12** Three receiver operating characteristics curves. The dotted is a worthless test, the dashed a good test, and the solid line an excellent test. The 1, 2 and 3 represent different threshold values.

example, different EEG indices) will have different curves. The area under the curves will be different and allow some comparison between methods.

### Analysis of variance

It is not a good idea to compare multiple groups of data using multiple t-tests; this is because the performance of multiple tests increases the chance of a Type I error, resulting in an increased chance of falsely concluding that there is a real difference when there is not. It is essential instead to use *analysis of variance* (ANOVA). This is an extension of using the ideas discussed using two samples or groups of data into three groups or more. The simplest form is *one-way analysis of variance* where there is a single way of classifying individuals (e.g. types of ventilation). When there are two classifiers (or factors) (e.g. where each patient also receives more than one treatment), then *two-way* analysis of variance is used, and so on. This discussion will deal only with one-way analysis of variance. The principle behind ANOVA is to put the total variability of a set of data into components according to different sources of variation. The variation between the samples within each group is compared with the variation between the groups. If the groups of data are from the same parent population, then the ratios of these two variances should be near 1.0, and the larger this number (or 'F' ratio) is, then the more unlikely that the null hypothesis is true. The assumption for this test is that the data are normally distributed.

As an example, if three groups of patients are on different types of ventilation, then a measure could be their oxygen saturation after 5 minutes. If the groups contain 8, 9 and 7 patients, then the total number of patients would be 24. Initially the total *sum of squares* is calculated by summing the 24 deviations from the overall mean (of the 24 patients). This result would be broken down into two parts: the *within-groups* and the *between-groups*. For the within-groups calculation, the sum of squares would be made by summing the 24 observations from the mean in its own group (group 1 patients have their deviation from the mean of group 1, group 2 from the mean of group 2 and so on). The between-groups would be calculated by the sum of the squares of the mean difference of each group from the overall mean. If the complete data were from the same population, then these two variances would be similar, and the null hypothesis would be accepted. The greater the difference between the two variances, the more likely that one or more of the groups are from different populations.

## Correlation and regression

### Correlation

Correlation is a measure of association between two variables. Figure 2.13 shows a scatter diagram of two variables, $x$ and $y$, and 10 observations. The degree of association between the points is measured by the correlation coefficient ($r$), which is how much the data points deviate (their perpendicular distance) from a line of best fit. This is illustrated in Figure 2.13, and the equation is:

$$r = \frac{\Sigma\,(x-\bar{x})(y-\bar{y})}{\sqrt{\left[\Sigma((x-\bar{x})^2\,\Sigma(y-\bar{y})^2\right]}};$$

$r$ can have values between −1 and 1, and is zero if the variables are not associated at all. Perfect positive correlation, $r = 1$, is shown in Fig. 2.14(a) and this is where the increase in one variable gives an exact linear increase in the other variable. Negative association ($r$ is negative) is when higher values of one variable are associated with lower values of the other. $r = -1$ is a perfect negative association and is shown in Fig 2.14(b). A positive correlation of 0.8 is shown in Figure 2.14(c), and −0.8 is shown in Figure 2.14(d). The coefficient is based on a linear trend and the fit is normally by the least squares method.

A significance test can be used to determine whether the observed correlation could be simple due to chance (based on the t-test).

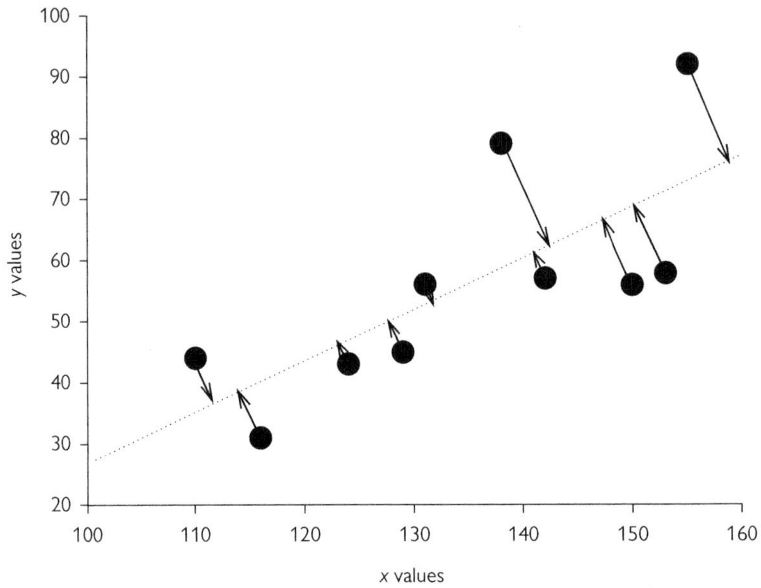


**Fig. 2.13** Graph showing ten observations with line of best fit drawn and also illustrating the perpendicular distance from each data point to the line.

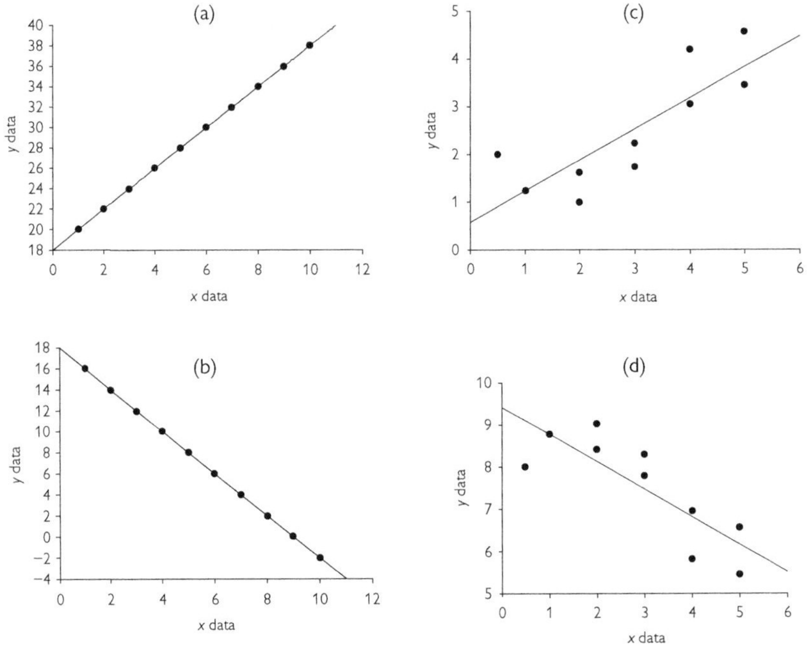


**Fig. 2.14** Scatter graphs showing different correlations. (a) $r = 1$; (b) $r = -1$; (c) $r = 0.8$; (d) $r = -0.8$.

### *Linear regression*

This both describes the relationship between the two variables and gives the equation of the straight line that predicts how the *y* variable (the dependent or response variable) alters with a change in the *x* variable (the independent or predictor variable). The equation of the regression line is:

$$y = mx + c,$$

where *c* is the intercept, and *m* is the slope of the line (see Chapter 1). The fit is using the least squares fit, which is to minimise the sum of the squared vertical distances of the points from the line. A test statistic can be used to determine whether the gradient is statistically different from zero. The distance of each sample from the line is called the *residue* and the residual variation is the amount of variation of the points from the line and is a measure of the *goodness of fit* of the line. A measure used in regression is $R^2$ (square of the correlation coefficient), which is the sum of squares explained by regression as a percentage of the total sum of squares. A high value of $R^2$ indicates that the majority of the variability in one variable is explained by the other.

There are non-linear relationships as well, such as polynomials. The simplest one being a quadratic, and an example of this is shown in Figure 2.15, which shows drug effect against drug concentration. Instead of being modelled with the equation for a straight line, the regression equation is:

$$drug\ effect = a(concentration)^2 + b(concentration) + c.$$

## Comparing groups of categorical data

### *The analysis of frequency tables*

A general way of showing frequency of events is to use a table (contingency table) where each cell of the table corresponds to a particular combination of characteristics relating to two or more classifications. A two-way contingency table, which relates to two categorical variables, will be discussed. An example

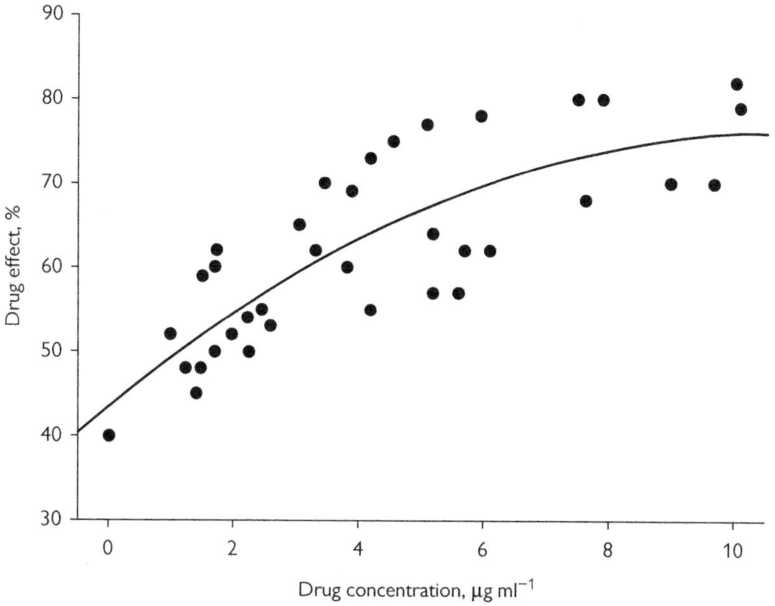


**Fig. 2.15** Graph showing example of non-linear regression, $R^2$ = 0.65.

**Table 2.4** Two-way frequency table showing coffee consumed by type of anaesthetist or trainee

| | Cups of coffee per day | | | | | | |
|---|---|---|---|---|---|---|---|
| Type of anaesthetist or trainee | 0 | 1 | 2 | 3 | 4 | 5 | Total |
| Medical student | 0 | 0 | 1 | 3 | 1 | 0 | 5 |
| Foundation year 1 | 0 | 0 | 0 | 1 | 4 | 10 | 15 |
| Speciality doctor | 0 | 2 | 3 | 5 | 20 | 10 | 40 |
| Consultant | 5 | 10 | 10 | 20 | 5 | 0 | 50 |
| Total | 5 | 12 | 14 | 29 | 30 | 20 | 110 |

of a two-way frequency table is shown in Table 2.4, which shows coffee consumed by grade of anaesthetist. The analysis of the frequency tables is (largely) based on hypothesis testing: the null hypothesis is that the there is no association between the two classifications (coffee and medical grade) in the relevant population (anaesthetists). The observed frequencies are compared with what is expected if the null hypothesis is true. The calculations are based on the expected frequencies on the distribution of the variables of the whole sample, as indicated by the row and column totals. The combination of row and column categories are called cells. The test statistic is calculated:

$$\sum (observed - expected)^2 \, / \left(expected\right).$$

Obviously the larger this value, the more likely that the null hypothesis is not true.

### *Expected frequencies*

If the null hypothesis is true and the two variables are unrelated (independent), then the probability of an individual being in the particular row (i.e. specialty doctor) is independent of which column they are in (i.e. coffee consumption). The probability of being in a particular cell of the table is the product of (being in the row) and (the column) containing that cell. These probabilities are estimated using the observed proportions. For example, there were five medical students in the department where there was a total of 110 anaesthetists/medical students, so the proportion of medical students is 5/110 = 0.045. Similarly, the proportion of staff consuming no coffee was the same, 5/110 or 0.045. If the grade of staff and coffee consumption are independent, then the expected proportion of the whole sample that are medical students and drink no coffee is the product of these proportions: 5/110 × 5/110 = 0.002. To get the expected frequency in that cell of the table, this is multiplied by the total number of staff in the department to get: 0.002 × 110 = 0.23. This procedure is done for each cell, and the expected table of grade and coffee is shown in Table 2.5.

When the null hypothesis is true, the statistic $X^2$ has a Chi-squared distribution (the $X$ would have Normal distribution). The data will have a cut-off where the null hypothesis is rejected – that is, where there is evidence that the amount of coffee is related to career grade.

## Meta-analysis

Meta-analysis is a statistical procedure that integrates the results of several independent studies that are considered possible to combine. Well-conducted meta-analysis can provide a more precise estimate of treatment effect, but badly conducted analysis may be biased owing to the exclusion of relevant studies or inclusion of inadequate studies. Misleading analysis can generally be avoided if a few basic principles are observed. The analysis can be considered as an observational study of all the evidence from all previous studies. The steps involved in the process are really similar to general research

**Table 2.5** Expected table of coffee consumed by grade of anaesthetist

| | Cups of coffee per day | | | | | | |
|---|---|---|---|---|---|---|---|
| Type of anaesthetist or trainee | 0 | 1 | 2 | 3 | 4 | 5 | Total |
| Medical student | 0.22 | 0.54 | 0.63 | 1.3 | 1.35 | 0.9 | 5 |
| Foundation year 1 | 0.68 | 1.6 | 1.9 | 3.9 | 4 | 2.7 | 15 |
| Speciality doctor | 1.8 | 4.4 | 5 | 11 | 11 | 7 | 40 |
| Consultant | 2.3 | 5.5 | 6.4 | 13 | 13.6 | 9 | 50 |
| Total | 5 | 12 | 14 | 29 | 30 | 20 | 110 |

The hypothesis test is based on how alike these tables are. The test statistic $X^2$, is calculated as:

$\sum \frac{(O - E)^2}{E}$, where $O$ is observed and $E$ is expected

studies, where the problem to be addressed is set out, the data is collected and analysed, and the results are reported.

For any meta-analysis, a detailed research protocol should be carried out in advance, that states the objectives, the hypothesis to be tested, and the criteria for selecting (or rejecting) relevant studies. The criteria for studies to be included are very important, and relate to the quality and design of the trials. Ideally only proper controlled, blinded trials with proper randomisation should be included. It can sometimes be difficult to assess the quality of a study to be included, as occasionally the published information on the quality of the study can be sparse. It has also to be decided whether to include only published studies in the analysis. Either way (to include or not to include) can produce difficulties, as using only published studies can result in distorted results due to publication bias, but also unpublished results may distort the results due to the lack of peer-review. Unpublished results can be included, however, if care is taken in assessing the quality of the study.

Before studies are combined analytically, it can be useful to combine the various studies graphically using a common scale to assess the degree of similarity between the studies.

There can be difficulties in meta-analysis in combining the data from all the different studies. A simple arithmetic average of the results from all the trials would give misleading results, as the results from smaller trials are more subject to chance variations and these studies should be given less weight. Methods used to combine trials use a weighted average of the results, in which the larger trials have more influence than the smaller ones. The variability between the various studies is also considered in the combining process, and this can be a complicated process.

## Study design and clinical trials

All medical research is carried out in relation to one or more objectives, which should be defined in the design of the research. This is often neglected but it is the foundation of quality research. It is better to consult a statistician at this early stage, rather than the later analysis phase.

Research can be observational, either prospective (in the future) or retrospective (in the past). In these studies, no intervention is carried out, the population of interest is just observed and studied. They include surveys, case–control studies and cohort studies. The other type of study is experimental, and this is always prospective. This is where some intervention is carried out on the population of interest and normally compared against a control, placebo, or another known effective drug or device. Sample sizes should be calculated so as to achieve the desired power, as discussed earlier. Groups being compared should be as similar as possible, in terms of demographics and other parameters, to minimise bias.

### *Clinical trials*

Clinical trials can consist of comparing drugs or medical devices and are usually carried out in four phases. In drug trials, phase 1 involves looking at the clinical pharmacology and toxicity of the drug under investigation. Phase 2 is about the initial clinical investigation. Phase 3 is the full-scale evaluation or treatment, and phase 4 is the post-marketing surveillance. For medical device studies, there is the pre-clinical phase, where the device is tested in the laboratory or in animal studies. Phase 1 involves the use of a small number of human subjects in a pilot study. Phase 2 is a larger, powered study, and phase 3 examines patient safety and effectiveness. The important thing is that two (or more) groups are studied using similar populations, but with different treatments or medical devices.

In clinical trials, random allocation is ideal, but sometimes this is not achieved or possible. If randomisation cannot be achieved, then research can be systematic, by using, for example, patients' dates of birth, to select them. The outcome being sought should be decided in advance, such as the effect or treatment on a physiological variable.

Ideally, 'blinding' should be used in a trial. In a single-blind trial, one group, typically the patients, is unaware of the treatment or device they are being given. In a double-blind trial, both the researchers and the patients (the participants) do not know the device or the treatment being used. The gold standard is a double-blind, placebo-controlled, randomised trial.

Any clinical trial must have appropriate ethics approval, which can be from the health research authority or, in early device trials, from an appropriate university ethics service. The research protocol should be written before any studies are carried out, and the sample size determined, either for the correct power, or for a small pilot to calculate the sample size, as discussed earlier.

## Evidence-based medicine

Evidence-based medicine is where individual clinical expertise is integrated with the best external evidence. It is about the conscientious, explicit and judicious use of current best evidence in making decisions about the care of individual patients. The best evidence can come from both clinically relevant basic sciences and patient-centred research. External clinical evidence can make previously accepted diagnostic tests or anaesthetic procedures invalid and replace them with new ones that are more accurate, safer and more effective. However, evidence-based medicine is not restricted to randomised trials and the meta-analysis discussed earlier. It involves tracking down the best external evidence to answer the various clinical questions and combining this with the best clinical care.

## Incorrect use of statistics

Statistical methods can be misused or misinterpreted to give a favourable result when it doesn't exist, or to give an incorrect negative impression. There can be bias in the data collection, for example, just studying white males, and not the full diversity of interest in a clinical variable. There can be selective sampling, where inconvenient data are not collected, or cherry picking only data that fit an inappropriate hypothesis, or just not using all the data. Sometimes the focus might only be on the average of the population, without considering the variance or distribution. Issues can be confusing in an exploration study of pilot data using a controlled powered experiment. There can be the misuse of correlation where many variables have been recorded, and only a select few have been used, to get a significant result, which appears to show an association between two variables, which is misinterpreted as a correlation. Patients may drop out of a study, or the study is not randomised, or the treatment effect is overestimated. There can be confusion using statistical significance with importance, which are very different. Significance indicates the likelihood that an observed result is not due to chance, whereas importance refers to the practical relevance of the result, regardless of its significance.

As mentioned earlier, there can be problems with carrying out too many t-tests and getting an incorrect and significant result, which proves to be incorrect. A study that has too few samples, i.e. incorrectly powered, can give a misleading result, especially any text implies that it is powered correctly. These errors in the use of statistics may not be deliberate, and highlight why it is important to consider what sources of bias might exist in a proposed study, and to assess whether these can be corrected for.

## *References*

**Altman, D.** (1980) Statistics and ethics in medical research: III How large a sample, *Br. Med. J.*, 281, pp. 1336–8.

**Columb, M.O. and Atkinson M.S.** (2016) Statistical analysis: sample size and power estimations, *BJA Educ*, **16**(5), pp. 159–61.

**Isaacs, D., Altman, D. G., Tidmarsh, C. E., Valman, H. B.**, and **Webster, A. D.** (1983) Serum immunoglobulin concentrations in preschool children measured by laser nephelometry: reference ranges for IgG, IgA, IgM, *J. Clin. Pathol.*, **36**(10), pp. 1193–6.

## *Further reading*

**Altman, D. G.** (1991) *Practical Statistics for Medical Research*, Chapman and Hall, London.

**Bland, M.** (2000) *An Introduction to Medical Statistics*, 3rd edn, Oxford University Press, Oxford.

**Cruickshank, S.** (1998) *Mathematics and Statistics in Anaesthesia*, Oxford University Press, Oxford.

**Egger, M., Davey Smith, G.**, and **Phillips, A. N.** (1997) Meta-analysis: principles and procedures, *BMJ*, **315**, pp. 1533–7.

# Chapter 3 **Background physics**

This chapter contains: dimensions and units; input, output, linearity, drift and hysteresis; frequency response; calibration of transducers; atomic structure; basic mechanics.

The chapter links with: Chapters 1, 4, 5, 7 and 29.

## Introduction

This chapter covers the background physics that is not otherwise covered in the relevant chapters associated with the equipment discussed. It is a useful introduction to some loosely related, but widely applicable concepts.

## Dimensions and units

Any measurement made by the anaesthetist can be simplified and made easier to understand if it is represented by its basic dimensions. Dimensions are the basic components of equations and are independent of the units used. For example a common term in physics and medicine is velocity, which has the dimensions of length per unit time, written dimensionally as $[L][T]^{-1}$. This means that, independent of the measurement system used, the measurement of velocity requires that the numerical value of a length be divided by the numerical value of a time. Equations or graphical axes can be predicted and their validity can be checked by dimensional analysis. Each side of an equation can be represented in basic dimensions and both sides should balance. The dimensions needed to describe most events are mass [M], length [L], time [T], and temperature [θ]. An example of dimensional analysis is described later in this chapter but first units must be discussed. All measurements need to have their correct unit and symbol attached to them. Equations have a unique language and the syntax must be correct for communication within the international community. In the past many different systems of units were used; one was Imperial, another c.g.s. The Système International (SI) of units was established in 1960 and is now the recognised system of measurement communication. For completeness the base quantities are shown and some useful derived physical quantities are shown in Table 3.1.

In the SI system the combination of basic units involves multiplication and division but multiplication is shown as a space and division is shown as a negative superscript. For example, velocity, in metres per second, is m $s^{-1}$. Prefixes to the name of each unit are usually in multiples of $10^3$ and $10^{-3}$. There are a few non-SI units that are still used in medicine, (not just anaesthesia) and these seem resilient to change. One is the millimetre of mercury (mmHg) for intravascular pressures (100 mmHg = 13.3 kPa), and total and partial gas pressures. The standard atmosphere (1 atm = 101 kPa) and the wavelength unit, the ångstrom (Å = $10^{-10}$ m) are also still used.

As an example of dimensional analysis, Poiseuille's equation will be examined, which is applicable to blood flow analysis. This states that flow, the rate of change of volume with respect to time, $\Delta V/\Delta t$, is dependent on the fourth power of the radius of the vessel. Resistive forces act against the flow of the liquid and this term is called dynamic viscosity η and its units are kg $m^{-1}$ $s^{-1}$. Its dimensions are:

$$[\eta]=[M]\,[L]^{-1}\,[T]^{-1}$$

A thought experiment suggests that the rate of flow of volume depends in some way on the pressure gradient along the tube $\Delta p/l$, on $r$, the radius of the tube and on $\eta$. This can be written as:

**Table 3.1** SI base units and derivations

| Physical quantity | Name | Symbol | SI derived unit |
|---|---|---|---|
| length | metre | m | base |
| mass | kilogramme | kg | base |
| time | second | s | base |
| electric current | ampere | A | base |
| temperature | kelvin | K | base |
| amount of substance | mole | mol | base |
| luminous intensity | candela | cd | base |
| frequency | hertz | Hz | $s^{-1}$ |
| force | newton | N | m kg $s^{-2}$ |
| pressure, stress | pascal | Pa | N $m^{-2}$ |
| energy, work | joule | J | Nm |
| power | watt | W | J $s^{-1}$ |
| electric charge | coulomb | C | s A |
| electric potential | volt | V | W $A^{-1}$ |
| absorbed dose | gray | Gy | J $kg^{-1}$ |
| dose equivalent | sievert | Sv | J $kg^{-1}$ |
| temperature | degree Celsius | oC | K |

$$\frac{\Delta V}{\Delta t} = k\left(\frac{\Delta p}{1}\right)^{x} \eta^{y}\, r^{z}.$$

The dimensions of the left side of the equation are written ($dV = [L]^3$, $1/dt = [T]^{-1}$):

$$\frac{\Delta V}{\Delta t} = [L]^{3}\,[T]^{-1}.$$

For part of the right side of the equation, pressure is force ($F$), per unit area ($A$) and force is mass ($m$) multiplied by acceleration ($a$):

$$\frac{\Delta p}{1} = \frac{F}{(A\,1)} = \frac{ma}{(A\,1)}.$$

This can be written with dimensions:

$$[M][L][T]^{-2}[L]^{-2}[L]^{-1}$$
$$= [M][L]^{-2}[T]^{-2}.$$

Since the dimension of $r$ is [L], the right side becomes:

$$= \left([M]\,[L]^{-2}\,[T]^{-2}\right)^{x}\,\left([M][L]^{-1}[T]^{-1}\right)^{y}\,(L)^{z}.$$

Equating both sides using powers of [L] the equation becomes:

$$3 = -2x - y + z.$$

Equating powers of [M], the equation becomes:

$$0 = x + y.$$

Equating powers of [T], the equation is:

$$-1 = 2x - y.$$

therefore $x = 1$; $y = -1$ and $z = 4$.

These were three equations to solve for the three unknowns. This gives the original equation as:

$$\frac{\Delta V}{\Delta t} = k\left(\frac{\Delta p}{l}\right)\eta^{-1}r^4,$$

which is a form of the Hagen–Poiseuille equation.

# Input/output, linearity, drift, hysteresis

Many measurements in anaesthesia can be simplified to a black box in which an input is applied to a system, a transfer function acts on the input, and a modified output is produced which is the product of the transfer function and the input. This is illustrated in Figure 3.1.

For clinicians, it is less important to know how the transfer function is carried out, than to know its function. One aspect of a system that is important, especially in such a system as converting a transducer output to a useful value, is its linearity (and non-linearity). A linear system is one where the same function (e.g. amplification of a certain gain) is applied to the whole range of the input values, whereas in a non-linear system the function applied to the input changes throughout the range. If the relationship between the input and output obeys the following three rules the system is said to be linear.

- If the input increases *N* times, the output must also increase *N* times.
- A sinusoidal input gives a sinusoidal output of the same frequency.
- The output does not depend on the previous history of inputs; this can be expressed as no memory or no *hysteresis*.

*Hysteresis* causes distortion (non-linearity) and can occur in measurement in medicine, especially using certain transducers. If hysteresis is present, the signal output from a transducer, produced by a physiological condition such as temperature, can differ depending on whether the temperature is increasing or decreasing. Also hysteresis can occur naturally, for example in the lung. Figure 3.2 shows the curve of pressure against volume for the lung, the difference between the curves of expansion and deflation shows hysteresis, and this area represents the energy spent overcoming airway and tissue resistance.

*Drift* is where there is slow change in the output signal where there is no actual change in the variable being measured. This effect can appear to be at random but there is normally some underlying cause. This can be, for example, in a strain gauge pressure transducer (see Chapters 5 and 12). When this is first switched on, there will be some slight heating of the resistors in the transducer, due to current passing through them. This will alter the balance and affect the output. Normally, this drift will stabilise as the tiny heating effects equilibrate.

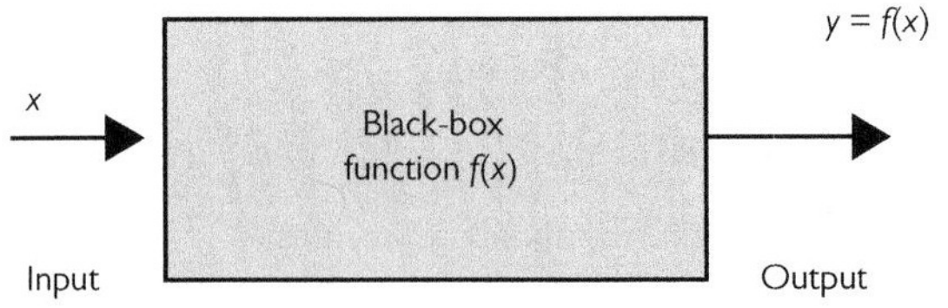


**Fig. 3.1** Diagram showing black-box concept.

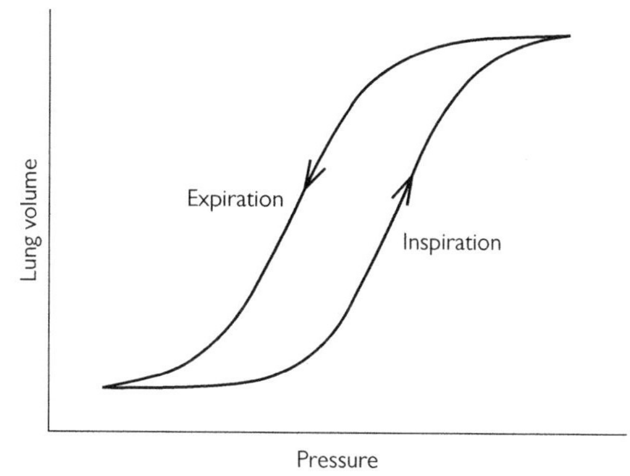


**Fig. 3.2** Inspiration-expiration loop showing hysteresis.

## Frequency response

Another important aspect in a system is the frequency response. Signals described with respect to time (the time domain) are typically those where a physiological signal such as blood pressure or the electroencephalogram (EEG) are represented as a voltage signal, either continuous or sampled, against time. Time domain signals can also be transformed or represented in the frequency domain. The frequency domain is where the amplitudes of the frequency components are plotted against frequency. This can have advantages with the analysis of the signals, by presenting the information in a different manner and this can unmask hidden details. An example of a simple spectrum of a square wave is shown in Figure 3.3.

Any complex waveform may be represented as the algebraic sum of a number of sine or cosine waves. This is usually a fundamental frequency and a number of *harmonics* that are multiples of this frequency. For example, a square wave, as shown in the centre of Figure 3.3 has a fundamental frequency, which has the same frequency as the fundamental sine wave, and an infinite number of odd harmonics. In reality a reasonable version of a square wave can be made up of several harmonics, as shown in the left-hand diagram of Figure 3.3. The diagram shows the harmonic make-up of the square wave with three odd harmonics included and the *spectrum* (the plot of the amplitude of the frequency

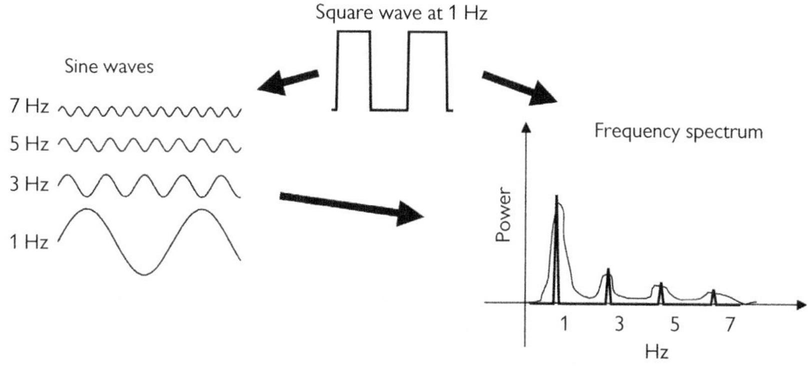


**Fig. 3.3** Figure showing a square wave and its frequency components. See text for details.

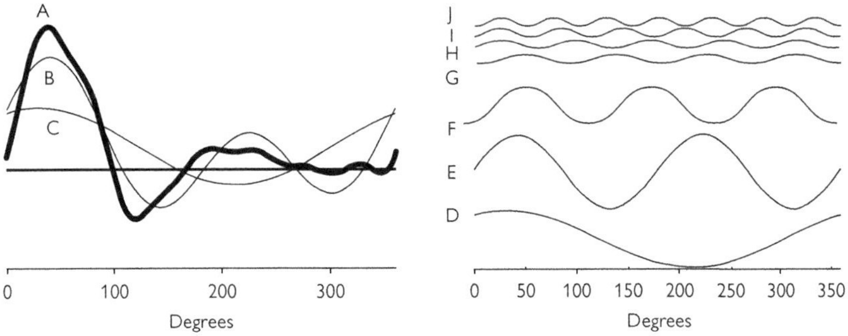


**Fig. 3.4** Physiological velocity waveform from the common femoral artery. Wave A is the waveform produced with eight harmonics (sine waves), B is the wave with the fundamental and 2nd harmonic. C is the fundamental frequency. On the right of the figure, D–J are the fundamental and 2–7th harmonics, respectively. Data are from Evans *et al.* (1989).

components against the frequency in Hz) of the square wave shown in the right-hand diagram. The amplitude of each frequency component in the spectrum is related to the amplitude of each sine wave component in the left-hand diagram.

A physiological example of the harmonic make-up of a signal is shown in Figure 3.4. This figure shows a blood flow waveform plotted in the time domain, obtained from a common femoral artery. Eight harmonics can be used to represent a good approximation of the femoral arterial flow waveform.
In the square wave example, each odd harmonic wave starts at the same point, or *phase*, in time (zero degrees) and these are added to produce the square wave. In the femoral artery example, the harmonics are consecutive and each one has a different starting point, or phase, in the sine wave cycle (0–360 degrees). These are again added together to produce the desired waveform. The figure illustrates each harmonic with its correct phase shift, apart from the 8th harmonic, which is too small to visualise. It should be noticed that if the number of harmonics is reduced to two (waveform B), then there is considerable distortion in the resultant waveform. Any amplifier processing this signal must have sufficient bandwidth to include at least the eight harmonics. This will be discussed in more detail later.

A waveform such as the EEG is very complicated but still each time period can be broken down into different frequencies, with each frequency having a different amplitude and phase. This process is carried out by a mathematical method using *Fourier* series. This is also used in the *digital domain* by using Fourier transforms, which is just a digital version of the Fourier series. These topics will be discussed again, in context, in the section on signal processing in Chapter 5.

## Calibration of transducers

It is highly desirable for the electrical output of a transducer to be linearly proportional to the amplitude of a physiological event. The act of applying a physiological event (real or simulated) of known amplitude and measuring the transducer output is known as calibration. The transducer output may be voltage, current, or a digital value. A correct calibration procedure consists of both static and dynamic calibrations. As an example of the procedure, the calibration of an arterial blood pressure measuring system will be considered. Using a column of mercury to correlate mmHg to voltage carries out static calibration. The blood pressure transducer is assumed to be linear throughout its working range and so a single point calibration could be used along with *zeroing*. It is prudent to check the linearity by carrying out several point calibrations, at least one at each end of the working range. Dynamic calibration tests the frequency response of the system. What is wanted is a perfect electrical equivalent of the arterial pressure at the output of the amplifier. As discussed above, any arterial waveform is a complex

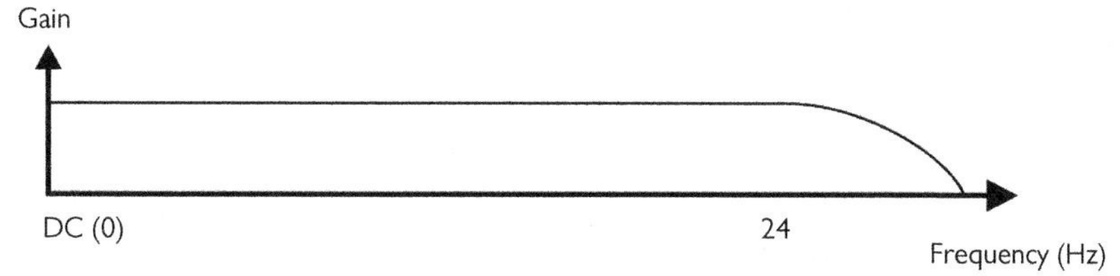


**Fig. 3.5** Graph of the required amplitude frequency response for measurement in the arterial system.

wave consisting of many frequency components. The system under calibration must be capable of accurately passing all frequency components from the arterial site to the output of the amplifier, with no amplitude or phase (time) distortion. To give an example of the frequency response required, the highest heart rate that is sometimes encountered is 180 beats per minute, which is equivalent to a frequency of 3 Hz. Fourier analysis shows that the arterial waveform is sufficiently constructed using eight harmonics and so the system must have a flat response (i.e. all harmonics have the same amplitude and phase shift) from DC to 24 Hz (i.e. 3 × 8 harmonics). This is illustrated in Figure 3.5, showing the constant gain of the system from DC to 24 Hz.

A mechanical sine-wave generator applied to the transducer can carry out this dynamic calibration from the transducer to the amplifier. This is shown in Figure 3.6. The sine-wave generator will sweep (either manually or automatically) from DC until the highest frequency of interest, typically a few hundred Hz. The output from the reference amplifier should show a flat response throughout the sweep range (as demonstrated in the output from the reference amplifier), and the calibration side should ideally show a flat response in the working frequency range (typically 0–24 Hz), and any resonant peak (see Chapter 12) should appear beyond this, as demonstrated in the diagram. At higher frequencies, the response will fade.

A transducer can be calibrated perfectly and the amplification following it can be perfect. There can be problems with how the transducer is connected to the physiological event, and this must be given some thought. If the transducer, or connecting amplifiers, are non-linear, then multiple calibration points throughout the working range must be made to construct a calibration curve.

## Atomic structure

All matter can be broken into a limited number of substances, the atomic elements. There are just over a hundred elements and the basic building block in all of these is the atom.

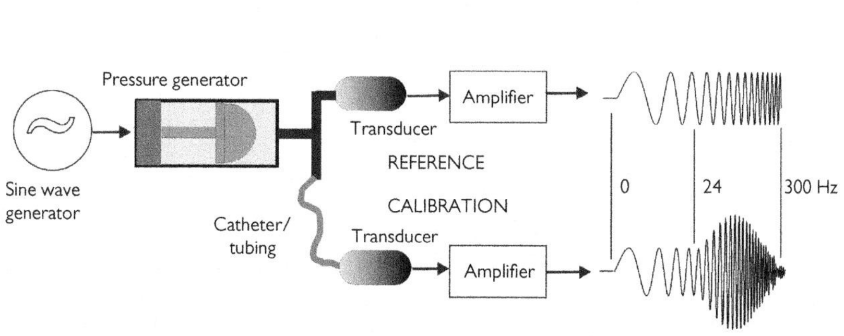


**Fig. 3.6** The dynamic calibration of a transducer and catheter system. The reference transducer records directly from the pressure generator and the calibration side is connected to the catheter measuring site. The waveforms show examples of the outputs from the amplifiers, showing flat waveforms from 0 to 24 Hz, and resonance between 24 and 300 Hz on the calibration waveform.

A simplified model of an atom consists of a nucleus of protons and neutrons, with electrons in orbit around the nucleus. The characterising difference between elements is the number of protons, called atomic number, Z, that the atoms contain. The nucleus will be positively charged due to the protons, creating an attractive electrostatic force between the nucleus and the electrons. The electrons occupy discrete orbits or *shells* around the nucleus, which occur at different discrete energy levels. By convention, the binding energy of electrons in an atom is negative. Electrons in the shell nearest the nucleus have the lowest energy (the ground state) and successive shells have electrons of progressively increasing energy as the distance from the nucleus increases. The nucleus has a diameter of approximately $10^{-14}$ m, and the whole atom a diameter of $10^{-10}$ m. There are a limited number of energy shells and the total number of electrons in a shell is restricted. The shells are known by the letters K, L, M, etc. as shown in Figure 3.7, and the maximum number of electrons in these shells are 2, 8 and 18 respectively. The atom is electrically neutral, since the electrons will balance the protons. The atomic number determines the electron structure of the atom and therefore its chemical properties. The combined number of protons and neutrons is the atomic mass number, *A*. The normal terminology is that *A* is written as superscript and the proton number *Z* is written as a subscript. So, for example, helium is $^{4}_{2}$He, meaning 2 protons and 2 neutrons, and therefore 2 electrons.

All the nuclei of the atoms of one particular element have the same number of protons, but the number of neutrons can vary. Isotopes are atoms of the same element that have different numbers of neutrons and many are artificially produced. For example, $^{12}_{6}$C refers to a stable carbon atom with $A = 12$ and $Z = 6$. Carbon 15 still has $Z = 6$, but has three more neutrons, which make it unstable and radioactive. It is called a radionuclide.

In each atom the outermost or valence shell is concerned with the chemical, h2thermal, optical and electrical properties of the element. If an atom gains or loses an electron, the electric charge no longer balances. An atom that loses or gains an electron becomes an ion and the process is known as ionisation.

# Basic mechanics

## *Mass, weight and force*

The mass of a substance is the amount of it, and the SI unit is the kilogram (kg), which is often how mass is described. Units such as pounds (lb) or stone are archaic in the UK and EU, and should not be used. Another way of thinking of the amount of the substance is its volume, the SI unit of which is $m^3$, or litre where 1000 L = 1 $m^3$. The relationship between mass and volume is density, where density is mass per

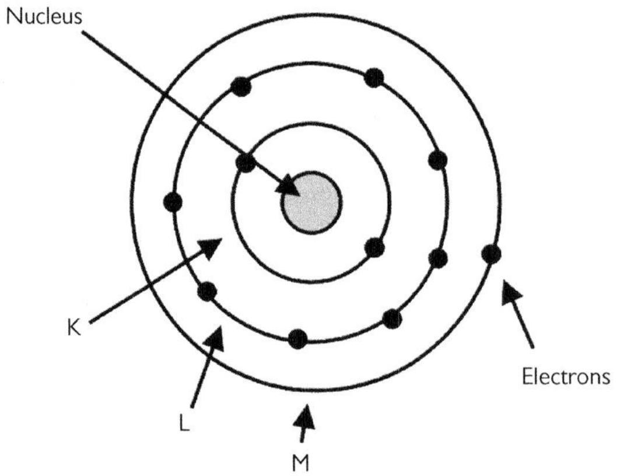


**Fig. 3.7** Electron shells in an atom.

unit volume in kg $m^{-3}$. A very dense substance such as mercury weighs 13 600 kg $m^{-3}$, while air weighs 10 000 times less at 1.3 kg $m^{-3}$.

So what is the difference between mass and weight? On the surface of the Earth, the force of attraction between an object of mass *m* kg, and the centre of the Earth is $m \cdot g$ newtons, where *g* is the acceleration due to gravity at the Earth's surface. Colloquially, this force of attraction is often referred to as *weight*, whose value is *m* kg wt or *m.g* newtons. In a 'weightless' or microgravitational environment, where the effect of *g* has been eliminated by the laws of orbital mechanics, the same object would have the same mass *m*, but its weight would be zero. Astronauts walking on the Moon had the same mass as their Earth mass, but their weight was one sixth of their Earth weight due to the smaller gravitational acceleration on the moon.

As mentioned above, weight is a special sort of force. Force *F* is a term whose units are newtons and, where it causes a given mass *m* to move with acceleration *a*, in the absence of other forces, such as friction, then:

$$F = m.a$$

This is Newton's second law of $a = g$ , force *F* becomes identical to the weight. Another way of expressing Newton's second law of motion is that

$$force = rate\ of\ change\ of\ momentum, or\ F = d(m.v)/dt.$$

Newton's first law of motion states that every body stays at rest or in uniform motion (constant velocity) unless acted on by such a force. The third law is that every action (or force) must have an equal and opposite reaction. Thus, your weight on the ground is balanced by the reactive force from the ground. A force of action from a missile propulsion system has the equal and opposite reaction of acceleration of the missile.

Pressure is force per unit area with units of [kg].[m $s^{-2}$]/[$m^2$], or N $m^{-2}$, or Pa. Pressure will be discussed in detail in Chapter 7 on Behaviour of Fluids. The pressure generated by a ventilator can be a force or weight acting on a bellows over a cross-sectional area. The same concept applies to car brakes, where a force from the driver's foot on the pedal acts over a small piston surface area, causing a high pressure on the brake. A classical anaesthetic example is the fixed force from a thumb on a syringe plunger will create a higher pressure at the outlet of a 2 ml syringe than a 20 ml syringe.

## *Energy and work*

When a force *F* moves an object a distance *d* in the same direction as *F*, then an amount of work *F.d* N m (joule) is done. This is shown schematically in Figure 3.8 as the area under the *F–d* curve. *F* might be the result of a ventilator bellows pressure *P* acting over the bellows cross-sectional area *A*. Hence $F = P.A$ and work = *P.A.d* joules.

Work is transferred directly into energy. This may be potential energy, when an object is given the potential to do further work, or to kinetic energy, when movement takes place. In a process involving interchange between work and energy, some work is converted into thermal energy, and is usually lost to the surroundings.

Energy can also be lost by being absorbed by interacting surfaces. However, if the distance *d* that the object of mass *m* is moved is a vertical height *h*, the potential energy of the object is *m.g .h* joule. If the object were then allowed to fall freely under gravity, and most of the potential energy was recovered as kinetic energy $\frac{1}{2}m v^2$, with some energy loss from air resistance, where *v* is the final velocity, then

$$\tfrac{1}{2}.m v^2 \le m\, g\, h.$$

Figure 3.9 attempts to show the relationship between this form of work and energy.

The ventilator bellows that produced work *PAd*, converts this to energy in inflating the lung to a volume *V*, through a pressure change $\Delta P$. At the end of inspiration the potential energy of the lung would be $V\Delta P$, although some losses will have occurred in overcoming airway resistance and elastic forces in the lung. This expression would also represent the respiratory work done by the patient if he

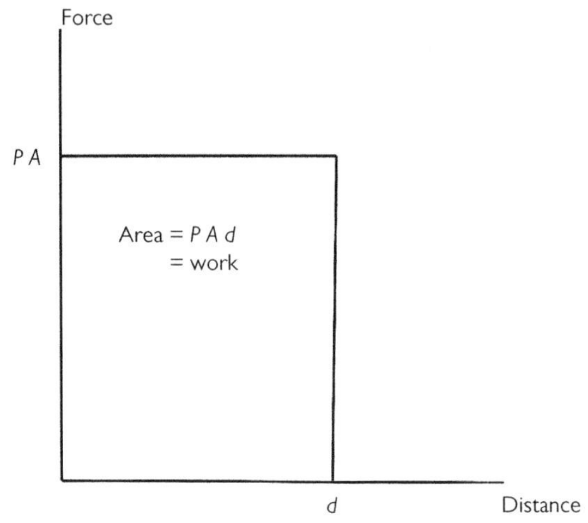


**Fig. 3.8** The work done in moving a ventilator bellows of cross-sectional area *A* through a distance *d*, by applying a pressure *P* (see text).

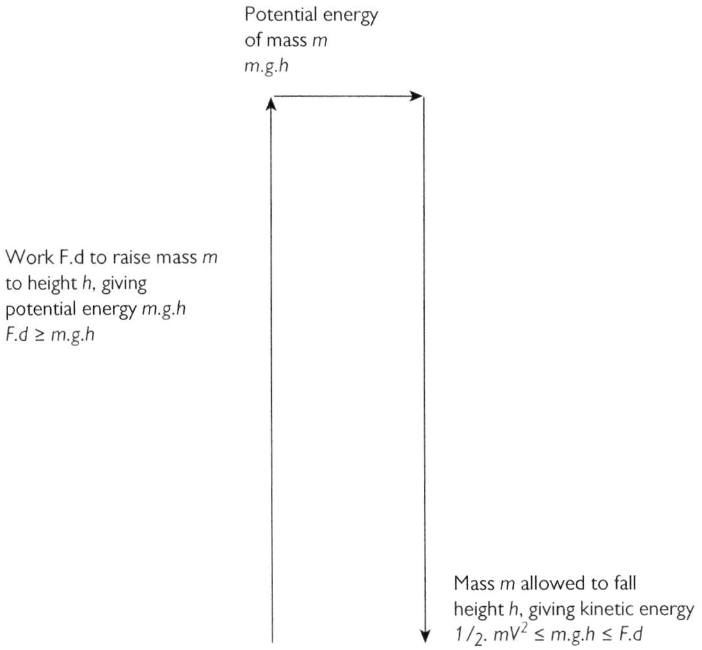


**Fig. 3.9** Exchange of work and energy.

or she had inflated her own lung. A short exercise will reveal that the units of pressure × volume are the same as those of work or energy. Notice from Figure 3.2 that the expiratory pathway on this loop is not the same as the inspiratory pathway. The difference is called *hysteresis* and represents heat dissipation.

## *Power*

Power is work or energy per unit time, and therefore a 'powerful' device is one that is capable of giving high energy or work per unit time. The units are N m $s^{-1}$, or J $s^{-1}$ or W. Electrical power is measured as voltage × current, and is converted into light, heat, power transmission or other electro-mechanically useful activity. For example, an electric motor converts electrical power or energy into mechanical power or work, and a generator does the converse.

## *Reference*

**Evans, D. H.**, **McDicken, W. N.**, **Skidmore, R.** and **Woodcock, J. P.** (eds) (1989) *Doppler Ultrasound*, JohnWiley & Sons Ltd, Chichester.

## *Further reading*

**Dorrington, K. L.** (1989) *Anaesthetic and Extracorporeal Gas Transfer*, Oxford Medical Engineering Series, Oxford Science Publications, Oxford, pp. 4–7.

**Hill, D. W.** (1976) *Physics Applied to Anaesthesia*, Butterworths, 3rd edn, pp. 226–8.

**West, J. B.** (1979) *Respiratory Physiology, the Essentials*, 2nd edn, Williams and Wilkins, p. 67.

# Chapter 4 **Electricity, magnetism and circuits**

This chapter contains: electric charge, current, voltage, power, analogies, magnetism, circuit rules, bridge circuits, alternating and direct current and voltage, capacitors, inductors, transformers.

This chapter links with: Chapters 3, 5, 6, 10, 12, 18, 20 and 21.

## Introduction

Electricity is a broad term that includes a variety of phenomena resulting from the flow (or presence) of electric charge. It is a complex subject, but this chapter will provide the necessary background for simple electric circuits here, and the following chapters on electronics, biological signal processing, and electrical safety.

## Electrical properties

### *Electric charge*

Electric charge is a property of certain subatomic particles. Charge originates in the atom (see Figure 3.7 in Chapter 3), in which its most familiar carriers are the proton and electron. By convention, electrons carry a negative charge while protons carry a positive charge. The protons are located in the centre of the atom and the electrons are in motion outside of the nucleus in orbits. In simplistic terms, the protons are trapped inside the nucleus making it difficult for them to 'escape'. Under certain conditions, however, electrons can escape, and the movement of them is 'electricity'. Charge may be transferred between bodies, either by direct contact, or by using a conducting material such as copper or wire. *Static* electricity refers to the imbalance of charge on a body, usually caused by friction when two dissimilar materials are rubbed together, transferring charge from one to the other. Charge is measured in coulombs (C) and one coulomb contains $6.24 \times 10^{18}$ electrons.

### *Electric current*

The movement of this electric charge is known as an electric current, and the magnitude of this is measured in amperes. One ampere flowing for one second passes a coulomb of charge. So the current ($I$) = C s$^{-1}$. By historical convention, conventional current flows from the most positive part of a circuit to the negative and this concept is continued in this text and most others (but in fact the actual flow of the electrons is in the opposite direction). Current flowing through a wire causes many observable effects, for example heating and *magnetism*. Magnetism will be discussed later.

### *Voltage or volts*

Voltage was historically called *tension* or *pressure*, which captured the concept well, and a water analogy (discussed later) can further help with this understanding. Voltage is the electric potential energy per unit charge, measured in joules per coulomb (V, volts = J C$^{-1}$). It can also be referred to as the electric potential, noting that it is a per unit charge quantity. It is the difference in voltage that is meaningful. The difference in voltage measured when moving from point A to point B is equal to the work that would have to be done, per unit charge, to move the charge from A to B.

When a voltage is generated by a battery, or by a *magnetic force* (see later in this chapter), this generated voltage is called an *electromotive force* (EMF). The EMF represents energy per unit charge (voltage) that has been made available by the generating mechanism but it is not a force as such. The term is useful to distinguish voltages that are generated from the voltage changes that occur in a circuit as a result of energy dissipation, e.g. in a light bulb (or resistor).

### *Power*

The power *P* (work done per second, in watts, J $s^{-1}$) consumed by a circuit is:

$$V\,(\mathrm{J\,C^{-1}}) \times I(\mathrm{C\,s^{-1}})$$

### *Water analogy*

A simple analogy to help understand voltage is that of water flowing in a closed circuit of pipework, driven by a mechanical pump. The voltage difference between two points corresponds to the water pressure difference between the two points. If there is a water pressure difference between two points, then the water flow (due to the pump) from the first point to the second will be able to do work, such as driving a *turbine*. In a similar way, work can be done by the electric current driven by the voltage difference due to the *battery*: for example, the current generated by the battery can light a bulb in a circuit. If the pump isn't working, it produces no pressure difference, and the turbine will not rotate. Equally, if the battery is flat, then it will not light the bulb.

This water flow analogy is a useful way of understanding many electrical concepts and is also further discussed later. In such a system, the work done to move water is equal to the pressure multiplied by the volume of water moved. Similarly, in an electrical circuit, the work done to move electrons or other charge-carriers is equal to the electrical pressure multiplied by the quantity of electrical charge moved. Voltage is a convenient way of measuring the ability to do work. In relation to flow, the larger the pressure difference between two points (voltage difference or water pressure difference) the greater the flow between them (either current or water flow).

As discussed earlier voltage usually means voltage difference. Obviously, when using the term voltage in the shorthand sense, it must be clear about the two points between which the voltage is specified or measured. When using a *voltmeter* (a special device that gives a voltage reading on its numerical display) to measure voltage difference, one lead of the voltmeter must be connected to the first point and the other to the second point.

A common use of the term voltage is in specifying how many volts are dropped across a device such as a light bulb. In this case, the voltage or, more accurately, the voltage drop across the device, can usefully be understood as the difference between two measurements.

## Magnetism

Magnetism is the effect that is observed when the north and south ends (poles) of a bar magnet attract or repel neighbouring ferromagnetic items. Two bar magnets brought into close proximity to each other show that opposite poles attract each other and like poles repel.

A wire carrying an electric current also behaves like a magnet by inducing a *magnetic field* around it. Therefore magnetic fields can be created using electrical power, and can be used to provide mechanical force, as in an electric motor. Conversely, if a wire is moved through a magnetic field, an electric current is induced in the wire proportional to the wire's speed of movement. Therefore mechanical force, or movement, can create electric current in this way, as in a dynamo, or in a power station.

If the current-carrying wire is coiled, a more intense magnetic field is created, because each wire in the coil that carries current induces a magnetic field around it. The close proximity of the coils to each other magnifies the flux density as many times as there are coils. If the single current-carrying wire, which induces flux $\phi$ (in Webers), is coiled into $N$ coil turns, then the flux thus induced is $N\,.\phi$ (Weber). An elongated coil ensures uniformity of the magnetic field along its length. The coil can have an air core or an iron core. The high magnetic permeability of iron compared with that of air means that the flux

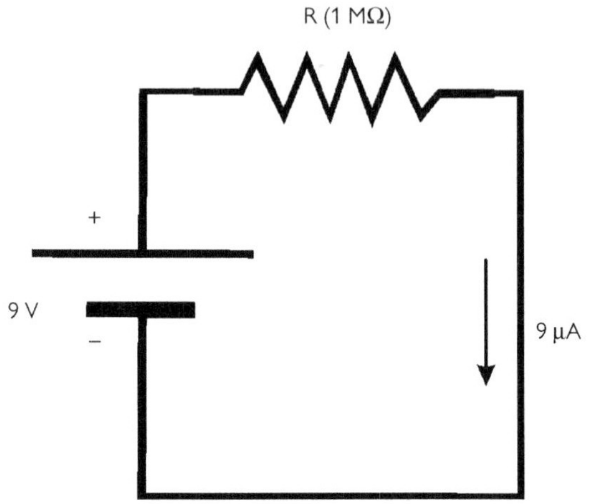


**Fig. 4.1** Simple circuit with battery of 9 V and resistor of 1 MΩ.

density $B$ of such a coil will be greatly enhanced for a given magnetic field strength $H$, since $B = \mu H$. If the wire is coiled around an iron core in a toroidal form, the flux density is further enhanced because of the high permeability of iron.

A changing magnetic field induces a voltage in the coil proportional to the rate of change of the magnetic field, and the induced voltage opposes the change of magnetic flux that produced it. The transformer uses this property and transfers electrical energy from one circuit to another by means of a magnetic field linking both circuits, and this is discussed later in this chapter.

## Basic electrical circuit rules

Ohm's law states that the current ($I$) in *amperes* flowing through a conductor of *resistance* ($R$) measured in *ohms* ($\Omega$), is proportional to the electromotive force (*voltage*, $V$) in volts. For a constant voltage, $V = IR$. This law gives the basis for solving most basic electrical circuits. Current flows through a component when a voltage is supplied across it. A simple circuit showing a battery (voltage) across a resistor is shown in Figure 4.1. If the battery voltage is 9 V, and the resistance is 1 M ($10^6$)Ω, then the current through the circuit will be $9/(1 \times 10^6)$ A, which is 9μA.

There are some basic rules about voltage and current in simple circuits:

1. The sum of currents into a point equals the sum of currents out of it.
2. Components connected in series have the same current going through each of them.
3. Components connected in parallel have the same voltage across each of them. Each parallel limb can consist of a number of components in series.
4. When two resistors $R_1$ and $R_2$ are connected in series the total resistance ($R_t$) is the sum of $R_1$ and $R_2$. This can be shown by the following: The voltage across both will be $V$, and the current will be the same through both resistors. Therefore $V_1$ will be $IR_1$ and $V_2$ will be $IR_2$. The two voltage drops across the resistors will be equal to the total $V$, so:

$$V = IR_1 + IR_2 = I(R_1 + R_2)IR_t.$$

Therefore $R_t = R_1 + R_2$.

5. When the two resistors are connected in parallel the total resistance ($R_t$) is the reciprocal of ($1/R_1$ + $1/R_2$). This can be shown by the following. The voltage across both resistors will be $V$, and the total

current flowing before the branch is $I$. The current through $R_1$ will be $V/R_1$ and the current through $R_2$ will be $V/R_2$. The sum of the current flowing through the two resistors will be equal to the total current $I$, so

$$V/R_1 + V/R_2 = V(1/R_1 + 1/R_2) = I.$$

$I$ is also equal to $V/R_t$. Therefore $1/R_1 + 1/R_2 = 1/R_t$. The effect of putting resistors in parallel is to decrease the total resistance to below the value of the lowest resistor.

### *Voltage dividers*

Resistors can be usefully used as voltage dividers. This is illustrated in Figure 4.2.

In this diagram $V_{out} = V_{in}R_2/(R_1 + R_2)$. This is solved as follows: $V_{out} = IR_2$ and $V_{in} = I(R_1 + R_2)$, therefore $V_{out} = V_{in}R_2/(R_1 + R_2)$.

## Bridge circuits

Circuits based on voltage dividers can be expanded to form bridge circuits, typically the Wheatstone bridge. An example is shown in Figure 4.3.

These circuits can be found in many medical devices. The circuit shown can be thought as two voltage dividers in parallel (A and B in the diagram). If $R_1 = R_4$ and $R_3 = R_2$, then both points x and y will be at the same potential. Both voltage dividers A and B will divide the battery voltage by the same amount. Therefore the voltage between x and y will be zero, i.e. the bridge is in balance. If $R_3$ is replaced with an unknown resistance such as a thermistor or a strain gauge as shown in Figure 4.4, then $R_2$ can be substituted with a variable resistance, similar in value to the $R_3$. Again the bridge can be balanced by adjusting $R_2$ so that the voltage between x and y is zero. If a sensitive voltmeter is connected between x and y, then a very small change in resistance $R_3$ can be measured. In this way the tiny change in, for example, pressure transducers that employ strain gauges can be detected. The bridge in effect balances out the resting potential (which can be a large voltage), so that tiny pressure signals can be further amplified by other components, as discussed later.

The bridge can be made doubly sensitive by having a second strain gauge added on the opposite side of the bridge, as shown in Figure 4.5. In the pressure transducer example, both strain gauges are under strain under resting conditions. As pressure is put on the transducer one strain gauge will compress whilst the other will expand, making one increase its resistance and the other decrease.

If the supply potential to the bridge changes, or there is noise on the supply, then this does not affect the balance of the bridge (both voltages on either limb go up or down the same amount). In a similar manner, temperature changes will have little effect on the bridge, as the temperature change will affect each arm of the bridge equally. This property is the reason why the bridge circuit is used in medicine, to maintain accuracy in a measured signal in the face of potentially unwanted changes elsewhere. The

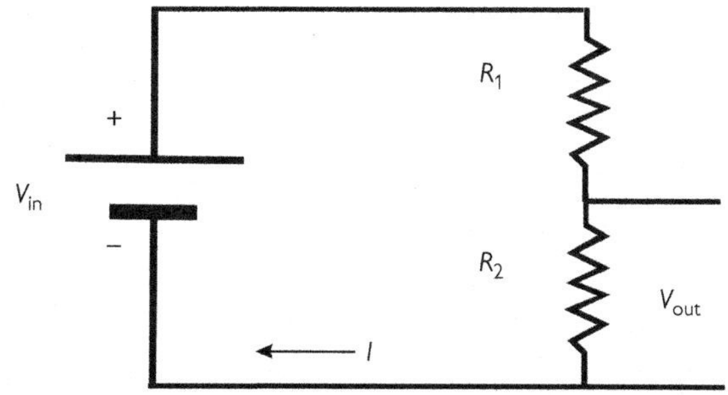


**Fig. 4.2** A voltage divider.

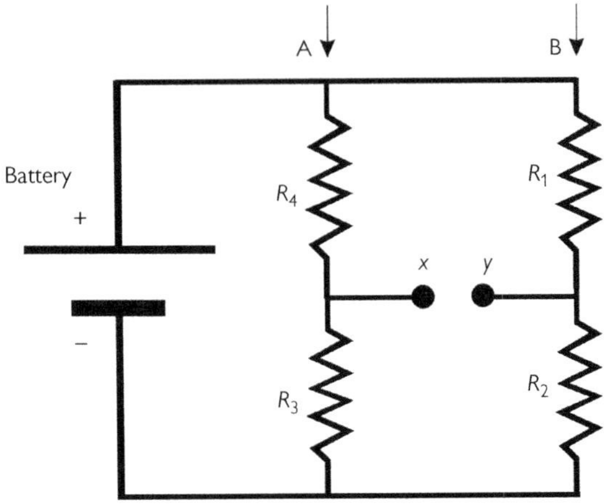


**Fig. 4.3** A bridge circuit.

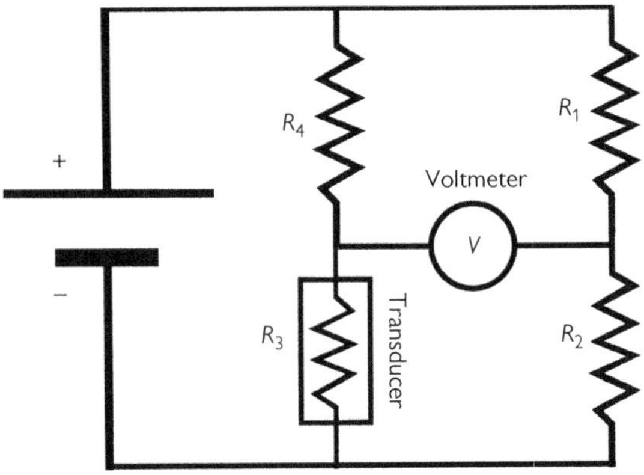


**Fig. 4.4** Bridge circuit with strain gauge replacing $R_3$.

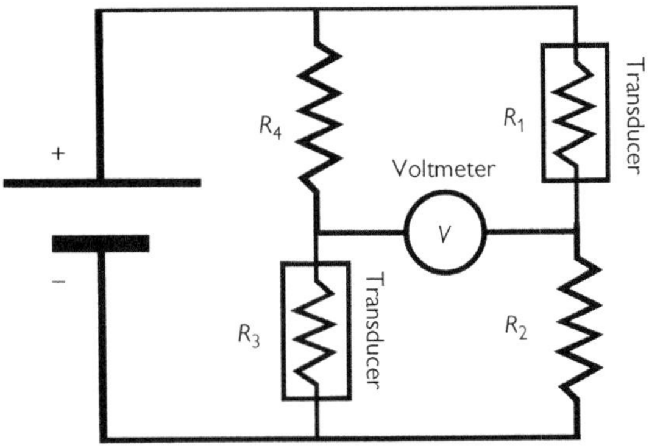


**Fig. 4.5** Bridge circuit with two strain gauges replacing $R_3$ and $R_1$.

bridge can also remove the level of the resting baseline pressure, and therefore make it incredibly sensitive to tiny changes from this baseline pressure.

## Alternating and direct voltage/current

Two types of current flow exist in electric circuits: when the voltage source (or current) is at a constant level, and the flow of current is in a constant direction. This current flow is defined as *direct current* (DC). The other is *alternating current* (AC), where the signal (the voltage or the current) oscillates around zero in a rhythmical manner, as in a sine wave. Part of Figure 4.6 shows a 50 Hz domestic UK mains sine wave (the solid waveform). The AC wave needs to be quantified, and there are several possible ways of doing this. The mean of the wave is not useful as this is zero. The peak values could be used (+325 V, –325 V) but these are seldom used. The normal way that the 50 Hz wave is quantified is by using the *root mean square* (RMS) of the waveform. This is the value that would give the same heating effect (a resistor or electric fire) if the same value of DC voltage were supplied. For example, if 325 V AC peak (230 RMS) were applied to an electric fire, then the same amount of heat would be obtained if 230 V DC were to be applied to the same electric fire. The RMS value is really the average of the heat-producing parts of the waveform and since the negative and positive parts of the wave both produce the same heating effects, they can be taken as going in the same direction, as described by the dashed waveform. The AC voltage is converted to RMS by first squaring the waveform. This has the effect of *converting* the negative parts of the waveform to positive values (the dashed waveform). The mean is taken (the average of the waveform, the 'heating' effect) and it is then square rooted to take account of the squaring at the first stage of the procedure.

The domestic electricity supply alternates at 50 Hz in the UK and 60 Hz in the US. (The voltage in the US is 110 V RMS.) These frequencies are used as they are the most efficient for power transmission, but by unhappy coincidence these frequencies fall into the range that is the most dangerous for the human body. This is discussed further in Chapter 6. Other forms of alternating current oscillate above

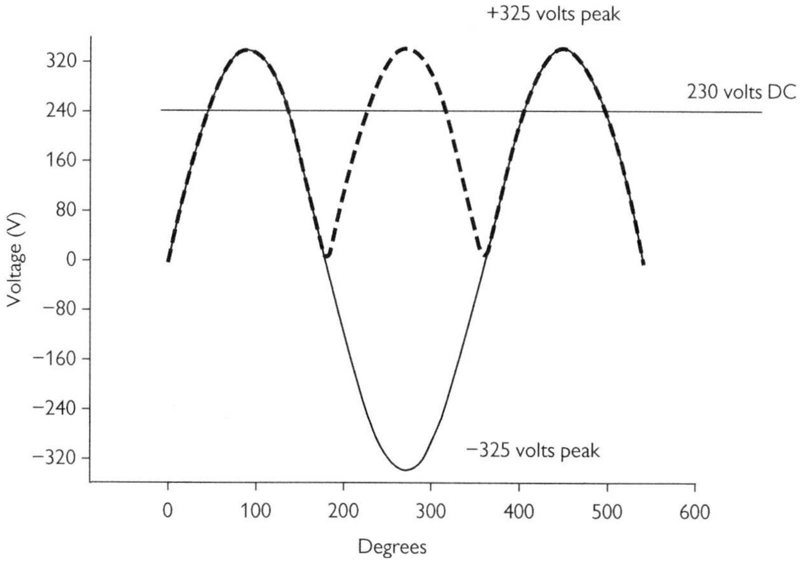


**Fig. 4.6** Domestic UK mains supply wave (solid curve) plus rectified mains supply (dashed wave). The 230 V DC level is shown.

a DC level, e.g. a blood pressure signal obtained from a pressure transducer, which was discussed in the last section.

## Capacitors and inductors

Two important components in electrical and all electronic circuits are the capacitor and the inductor. The capacitor consists of two conductor plates separated by an insulator (which could be air or a solid material). An inductor consists of a number of turns of a wire conductor wound around a core of normally magnetic material. The capacitor and inductor behave very differently depending on whether AC or DC is applied across them. If a constant (DC) voltage is applied (by closing the switch) across a capacitor, via a source resistance as shown in Figure 4.7, the capacitor will charge up exponentially from zero volts to the DC value across it and the current will decrease exponentially with a time constant of $RC$ seconds (in Figure 4.7, $RC$ = 1 s).

The steady state current (i.e. DC) through an inductor, as connected as shown in Figure 4.8, will be limited only by the resistance of its coil but a change of current produces a change in the magnetic field around the coil, which in turn generates a voltage in the coil with the opposite polarity to the driving voltage, which opposes the change in current. It therefore *slows down* any change of current. Figure 4.8 shows that when DC voltage is applied to the inductor (by closing the switch), the effect is the opposite to that which occurs with a capacitor. The time constant in this case is $L/R$ seconds.

In an AC circuit (a similar circuit to Figure 4.7, but the battery is replaced by the AC source) the voltage across the capacitor is constantly changing direction and the current and voltage never reach steady state conditions as in the DC case. The current through a capacitor is proportional to the rate of change of voltage and so when a sinusoidal voltage waveform is applied (starting at zero), the current is at a maximum at the start of the cycle. As the capacitor charges up, the current decreases and the voltage increases. The minimum of the voltage cycle is the peak of the current waveform where the rate of change approaches zero. The current waveform peaks before that of the voltage, and therefore the voltage *lags* the current by a quarter of the whole cycle (360 degrees), or 90 degrees. This is illustrated in Figure 4.9.

The magnitude of the current increases as the frequency increases. The resistance to current flowing is inversely proportional to frequency and is called *reactance*. It is calculated as $X_c = 1/(2\pi fC)\Omega$, where $f$ is the frequency of the supply waveform in Hz.

The current and voltage relationships with an inductor are different and in this case the voltage peak occurs before the current peak and so the voltage *leads* the current by 90 degrees as illustrated in Figure 4.9. The inductive resistance or reactance is $X_L = 2\pi fL\Omega$, where $L$ is the inductance in H (Henry).

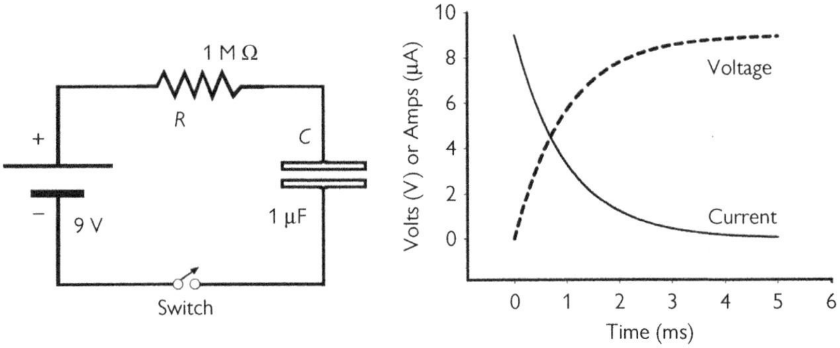


**Fig. 4.7** Capacitor charging circuit showing components and the corresponding current and voltage waveforms across the capacitor C.

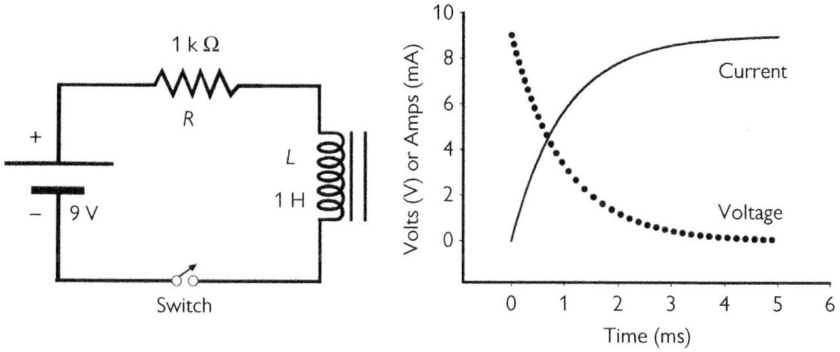


**Fig. 4.8** Inductor circuit showing components and the corresponding voltage and current waveforms.

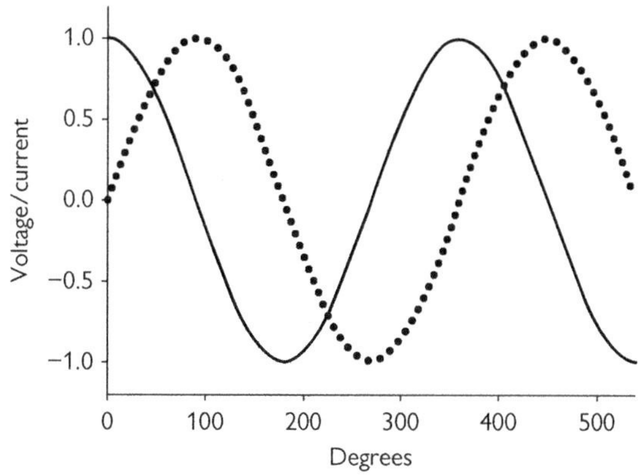


**Fig. 4.9** Voltage waveforms across circuit components and the corresponding current waveforms, showing the relative phase relationships. Across a capacitor, the voltage waveform is the dotted wave and the current waveform is the solid wave. The inductor is the other way round: the voltage is the solid wave and the current is the dotted one.

Although reactance in both the C and L circuits is measured in Ω, it cannot be used directly in Ohm's law. A term called *impedance* is used and this is resistance plus reactance. Both the reactive ohms and resistive ohms present in the circuit must be considered and the overall opposition to current flow (the impedance) calculated at the frequency required, taking the phase difference into account. This can be dealt with more rigorously using a mathematical technique called *complex numbers*. Resistors in AC circuits can still use Ohm's law as in the DC case.

## Transformers

A transformer consist of two separate (or more) coils (inductors) normally placed around a iron, or ferrite core. The transformer diagram and circuit diagram is shown in Figure 4.10. The voltage in the *primary* circuit induces magnetic flux in the iron core. The magnetic field to which this flux belongs induces a voltage in the *secondary* coil.

The changing voltage applied to the primary coil causes a changing current flow, which causes a changing magnetic flux in the core. Because of the changing flux, a voltage is induced in the secondary coil, which opposes the direction of the flux change in the core. No direct electrical connection between

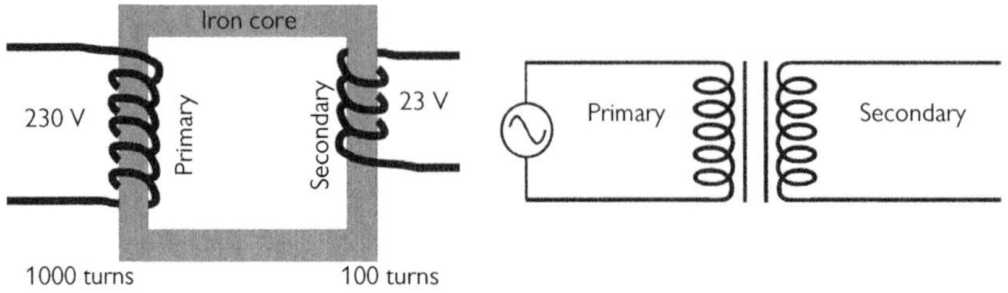


**Fig. 4.10** A diagram of a transformer, showing turns around an iron core. Also shown is the circuit diagram of a voltage supplied to the transformer of 230 V RMS being stepped down to 23 V RMS.

input and output exists or is necessary. Because only changing currents (AC) are involved, the output circuit can be isolated from a DC component at the input.

The coils are usually made of copper to reduce losses and the core is made of steel with a high permeability to minimise hysteresis loss and laminated to minimise other current losses.

Transformers are used for *stepping* down the domestic mains supply to safe voltages, isolating patient circuits and also in electronic filters. The power available on the primary side of the transformer will be similar to the secondary, so if the voltage is stepped down by a certain ratio, then the current is stepped up by a similar amount. The amount of stepping down (or up) is dependent on the ratio of the turns. In Figure 4.10, if the primary has 1000 turns, and the secondary has 100 turns, then the voltage will be reduced 10 times. If the secondary had 10000 turns, then the voltage would be increased 10 times. By adjusting the number of coils on the primary and the secondary winding it is possible to step up or step down the voltage between the input and the output. The equations are simply $V_s/V_p = N_s/N_p$ and $N_pI_p = N_sI_s$, where $V$ is the voltage, $I$ is the current, s is the secondary and p is the primary.

## Other electrical analogies

The water analogy has been already discussed, but there are many well established techniques available for solving electrical circuits by using other analogies. Computer simulations are available that emulate the workings of resistors, capacitors and inductors and so can predict with ease the voltage/current relationship in different parts of the circuit. Many mechanical problems, e.g. in the body or in transducer design, can be made far more understandable if the situation can be made into an electrical analogue and then analysed by a computer An example of this is blood flow.

In a hydraulic system, blood flow is analogous to electrical current, pulsatile blood pressure to (AC) voltage, and vascular resistance to electrical impedance. Parts of the circulation have storage properties and are therefore like capacitors and inductors. The elasticity of the arterial wall acts as *capacitance* and the mass of blood passing through it will behave as an *inductor*. The thin-walled non-elastic venous system will tend to be like *resistors*. As there are reactance elements, flow and pressure will not necessarily be in phase. If the circulation is modelled out in terms of electrical equivalents, then the system can be modelled on a computer to make good estimates of what is happening at various points around the body. The driving force (pressure or voltage) reduces as the distance from the heart is increased. It starts in the left ventricle, with an almost square wave as the aortic valve opens, with pressure leading the flow. But once the blood starts moving its momentum will tend to keep it moving and the flow will start to lead the voltage. But this can reverse again due to interactions between the '*capacitance*' and '*inductance*'. Various electrical analogue models for arterial blood-flow situations have been investigated.

## *Further reading*

**Brown, B. H., Smallwood, R. H., Barber, D. C., Lawford, P. V. and Hose, D. R.** (1999) *Medical Physics and Biomedical Engineering*, Taylor and Francis, New York.

**Horowitz, P. and Hill, W.** (2015, 3rd edition) *The Art of Electronics*, Cambridge University Press, Cambridge.

**McDonald, D. A.** (1974) *Blood Flow in Arteries*, 2nd edn, Camelot Press, Southampton.

**Strackee, J. and Westerhof, N.** (eds) (1993) *The Physics of Heart and Circulation*, IOP Publishing, Bristol.

**Tooley, M. A.** (2023) Electricity, magnetism and circuits, *BJA Educ.*, **23**(2), pp. 61–5.

# Chapter 5 **Electronics and biological signal processing**

This chapter contains: filters; amplifiers, including patient-connected differential amplifiers; signal processing; digital processing; and electrodes and transducers.

The chapter links with: Chapters 1, 2, 3, 4, 10, 12, 15, 18, 19, 20, 21 and 24.

## Introduction

This chapter continues the discussion of electricity but looks at the effect of connecting components together and briefly looks at the *operational amplifier* and *active* circuits (circuits discussed in the previous chapter have been *passive* ones, which involve no electronic circuits). It will then describe how the circuits can be used to process biological signals.

## Filters

### *Simple band-pass filters*

If a resistor, an inductor and a capacitor are joined as in Figure 5.1, the magnitude of the voltage across the resistor ($V_{out}$) will vary as the input frequency, $V_{in}$, changes, because of the properties of the capacitor and inductor. The *resistive* action of inductor and capacitor oppose each other, and at a certain *resonant* frequency (*r* in the figure), the total AC resistance (impedance) will be at a minimum. The graph of reactance against frequency demonstrates this, and shows the minimum reactance at the resonant frequency. As the LC and R are forming a voltage divider, the voltage across R will be maximum at this frequency. At other input frequencies, the output voltage will be low. This simple circuit forms the basics of the passive *band-pass* filter, where the filter passes, or lets through, a certain band of frequencies (around the resonant frequency in this circuit). Frequencies lower or higher than the band-pass will be attenuated. Normally operational amplifiers (discussed in the next section) or digital filters are more effective and are used to achieve the same effect. Resonance is important for the understanding of the behaviour of transducers and this is discussed in Chapter 12.

### *Simple low-pass filters*

If a square wave is applied to the resistor capacitor network as shown in Figure 5.2, the capacitor charges up on the rising edge of the input with a time constant equal to the product of the resistance (Ω) and the capacitance (F), *RC*, and the output voltage will be $V_{ouput} = V_{input}(1 - e^{-t/RC})$. When the square wave is in the *off* state, or zero volts, the voltage will fall exponentially with the same time constant. It can be seen from the diagram that, with the appropriate values of *R* and *C*, the output from the network is a filtered version of the input.

This RC network is a simple *first order* low-pass filter removing the high-frequency components of the square wave and letting the low-frequency parts through. The *cut-off* frequency of this filter is the frequency value where *attenuation* (i.e. the loss in intensity of the signal) characteristics change. Below the cut-off value, the filter lets all frequency values through with no attenuation and above that value the frequencies are attenuated. If the filter had its cut-off frequency low enough, the waveform would appear as a sine wave, as only the fundamental harmonic of the square wave would be let through, which is a sine wave! The cut-off frequency of the filter is $f = 1/2\pi RC$. Above the cut-off frequency, as the

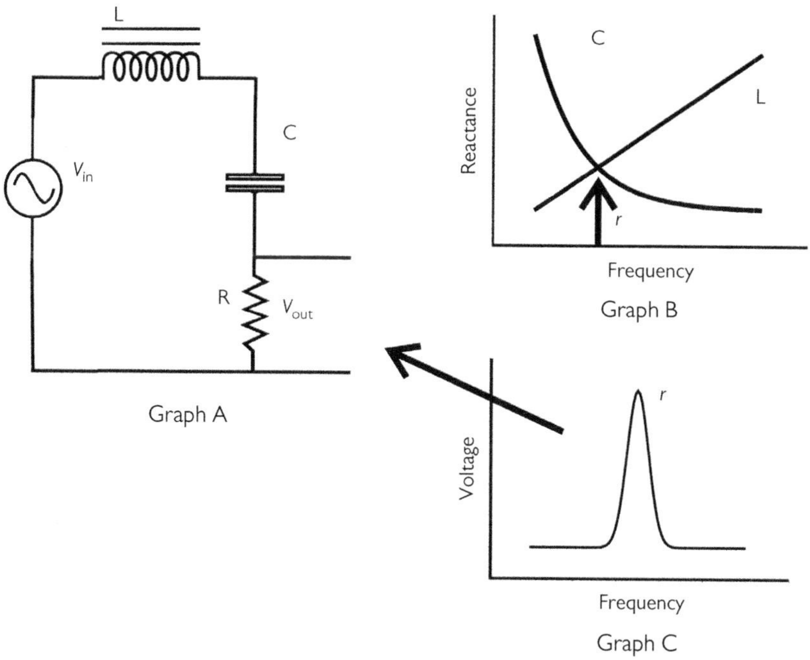


**Fig. 5.1** An RLC circuit (shown in A) being driven by a variable frequency oscillator, $V_{in}$. The frequency response of voltage ($V_{out}$) against frequency across the resistor *R* is shown. The reactances against frequency responses are shown for capacitance (*C*), and inductance (*L*), showing the point (arrowed) in graph B where the combined reactance is a minimum; *r* is the resonant frequency in both graphs.

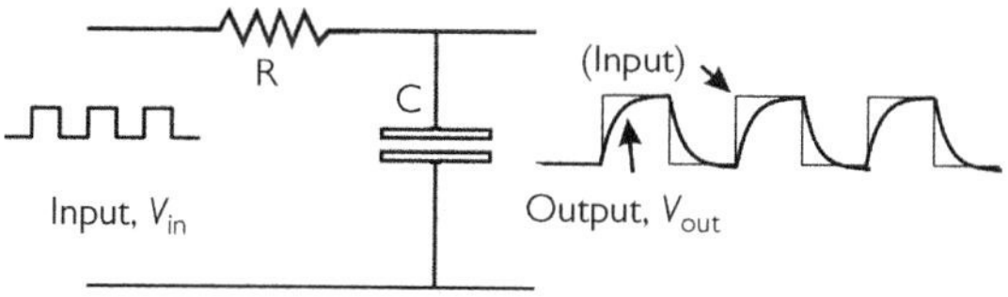


**Fig. 5.2** An R–C circuit, showing a square wave input and resultant output across the capacitor. This circuit also acts as a simple integrator.

input frequency is increased, the output voltage due to the filter action is reduced by half every time the input frequency is doubled. This type of filter could be useful in filtering EEG signals, so that the higher frequency noise, such as muscle signals is prevented from passing through the filter.

This simple RC circuit also acts as a mathematical integrator with certain restrictions. Integration, as discussed in Chapter 1, is the process by which small elements are summed over a period of time.

Now *Q* (charge) = *CV*. If this is differentiated, the left side of this equation will be rate of flow of charge, which is current (*I*), and the right side will become *C* d*V*/d*t*. Therefore *I* = *C* d*V*/d*t* through the capacitor.

The voltage across R is

$$V_{in} - V_{out}, \text{ so } I = Cd\,V_{out}\,/\,dt = \left(V_{in} - V_{out}\right)/\,R$$

If $V_{out}$ is much less than $V_{in}$ over most of the input range, or if the time constant *RC* is large, then $C\,dV_{out}/dt \approx (V_{in})/R$.

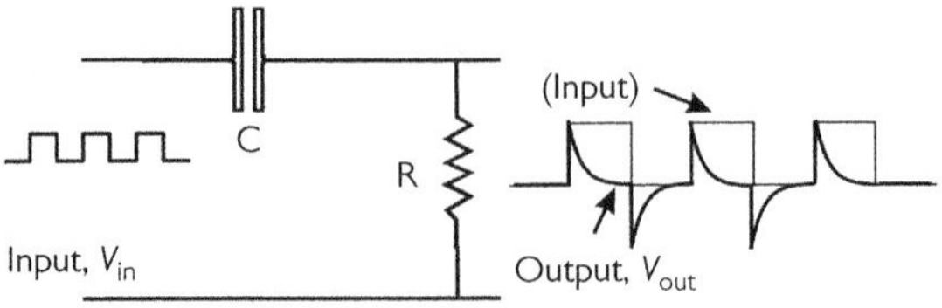


**Fig. 5.3** A C–R circuit, showing a square wave input and resultant output across the resistor. The circuit also acts as a simple differentiator.

This can be written

$$dV_{out} / dt = (V_{in}) / CR.$$

If each side is integrated,

$$V_{out}(t) = 1/RC \int^{t} V_{in}(t)\mathrm{d}t + constant.$$

What this equation indicates is that the RC circuit performs an integral over time for a given input. The restriction is that both the input voltage and the time period must be small compared with the time constant of the circuit (so that $V_{out}$ is much less than $V_{in}$). This restriction can be overcome by using operational amplifiers, as explained later. The integrator is used in analogue computation, control systems, feedback, analogue/digital conversion and waveform generation.

### *Simple high-pass filters*

If the resistor and capacitor are used the other way round, as in Figure 5.3, then this circuit will behave very differently. It will *block* a DC input but will *pass* high frequencies with little attenuation. Again the input frequency at which this situation changes is given by the time constant. This CR combination is called a high-pass filter. The combination has another important property. The voltage across C is $V_{in}$ - $V_{out}$, so in a similar manner to the RC circuit discussion,

$$I = C\,\mathrm{d}(V_{in} - V_{out}) / dt = V_{out} / R.$$

If *R* and *C* are very small (so that $V_{out}$ is much less than $V_{in}$), $V_{out}(t) = RC\ \mathrm{d}/\mathrm{d}t\ V_{in}(t)$. This means that the *RC* combination is acting as a differentiator or producing an output proportional to the rate of change of the input waveform.

Differentiation is used extensively in medicine. For example, left ventricular pressure waveforms can be differentiated and used as a means of estimating myocardial contractility. In practice the maximum value of the differential (max d*P*/d*t*) divided by the left pressure occurring at the same time as the maximum d*P*/d*t* provides a useful index of myocardial contractility.

In order for all these circuits to function, the output $V_{out}$ must not have any additional load or resistance across it. This is impossible in real situations - the circuit must be connected to something! In order to provide *buffering* operational amplifiers are used.

## Amplifiers

### *Operational amplifiers*

Operational amplifiers have replaced the transistor as building blocks in electronics circuits. They can be made to provide amplification (output/input), filtering, oscillators, and many other functions. The symbol for an operational amplifier is shown in Figure 5.4, and these devices are contained typically in an 8 pin (legs), mini dual-in-line package containing hundreds of components. It provides very high amplification on its own (> $10^6$) and has an extremely high input resistance (> $10^6\Omega$), which means it does not load or draw any significant current from the preceding circuit. Its inputs are also differential, i.e. it

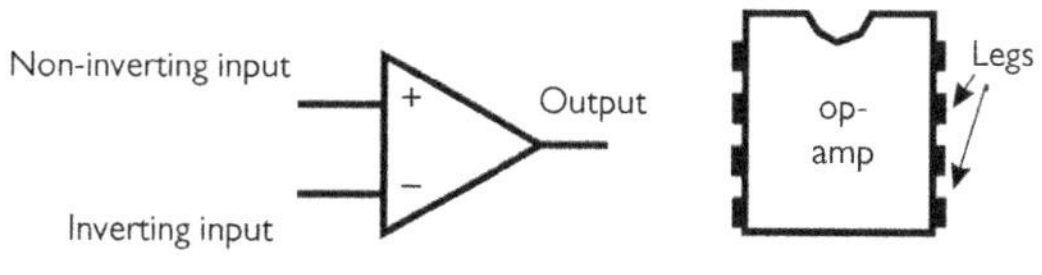


**Fig. 5.4** Symbol of an operational amplifier and a plan of mini dual in-line 8 pin package. The package typically measures 10 mm × 5 mm.

will amplify only a voltage difference and not an absolute voltage. The performance of an operational amplifier is controlled by *feedback*, which is achieved by connecting the output to the input, usually by a resistor or capacitor, which enables the designer to determine the gain and stability of the circuit.

The four basic circuits in which operational amplifiers are used are shown in Figure 5.5(a)–(d). The inverting amplifier circuit is shown in (a), and this has a gain of $-2k/1k = -2$. The non-inverting amplifier (c) has a gain of $1 + R_2/R_1$. The differentiator in (d), and integrator (b) give similar results to the RC and CR circuits described in Figures 5.4 and 5.3, except that the results are much more accurate, and fewer approximations are needed.

The amplifier circuits can be added to the simple RC circuits described earlier to provide practical filtering circuits. However such filters are inefficient because they filter typically only a quarter of the signal amplitude after the signal frequency has been doubled. The ideal filters would totally attenuate the signal amplitude directly after the cut-off frequency. Complicated circuits containing many operational amplifiers are required to produce efficient filters that are near the ideal case.

## *Single-ended amplifiers*

Since biological electrical signals, or signals that originate from transducers (see later), are very small in magnitude, they need to be amplified by an amplifier, which provides voltage *gain* (output voltage/

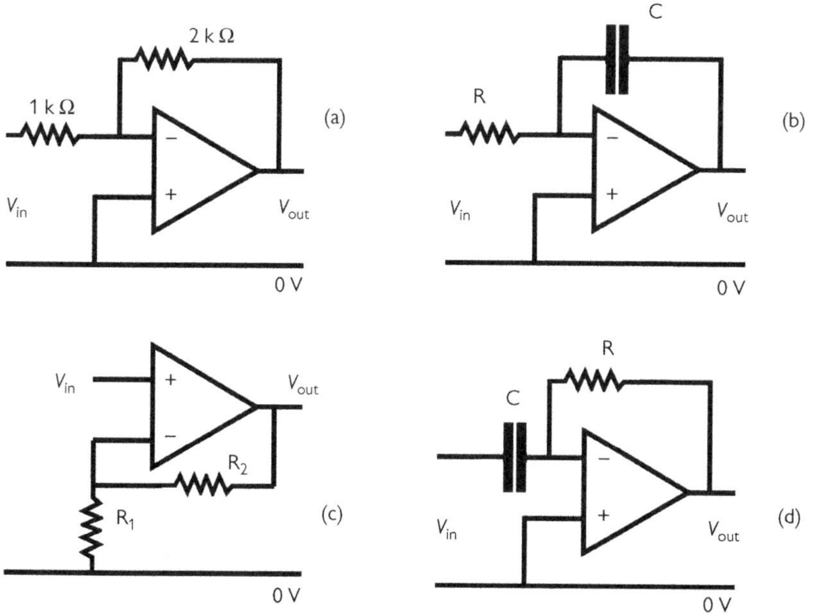


**Fig. 5.5** Basic op amp circuits.

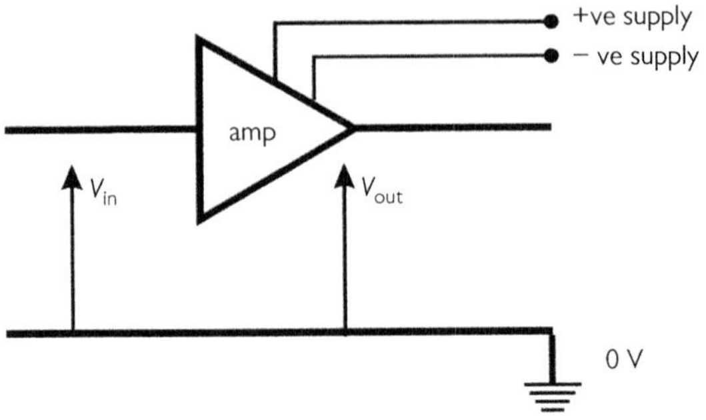


**Fig. 5.6** A single-ended amplifier in which the common ground is both one side of the input and one side of the output.

input voltage). The simplest amplifier is *single ended*, where there is one input terminal and one output terminal with a common to both input and output. A diagram is shown in Figure 5.6.

This form of amplifier is suitable for audio amplification, for example from a microphone, and the output could be connected to a loudspeaker. The gain in this case can be around 1000 times, similar to that required for an *electrocardiogram* (ECG) amplifier. If this amplifier were connected to a patient via two electrodes, then the loudspeaker would only give out mains *hum* and the ECG signal would be submerged in the noise. The mains voltage from lights, etc. (which is much larger than the ECG voltage) appears at the input via a small *natural* capacitance as shown in Figure 5.7. The amplifier will amplify this as well. Also in this situation the patient is earthed, which is not desirable in terms of patient safety, which is described in the next chapter. One solution would be to make the amplifier battery powered and put the patient in a completely screened room, with no mains apparatus near by. Another solution would be to use a patient-isolated differential amplifier.

## *Patient isolated differential amplifier*

The problem in obtaining an ECG signal is that the amplifier must detect the *difference* in potential between the two electrodes applied to the patient whilst ignoring the induced electrical interference signals that appear equally at both electrodes (by capacitance) and are therefore common to both. A differential amplifier does this and has two inputs in addition to the common point. Three electrodes are connected to the patient. For best results the common electrode is ideally placed at a neutral point on the body, and commonly the right leg is used for this in the ECG amplifier. The differential amplifier is shown in Figure 5.8.

If the ECG signal, referenced to the neutral point, is applied between the positive and negative inputs of the amplifier, as shown, then the output of the amplifier will be a magnified version of the ECG. If the ECG signal, or any other signal, is connected to both the active inputs at the same time, then no output will result. The mains signal will thus be appearing at both of the active inputs. At all times throughout the mains voltage cycle, the voltage, with respect to the common input, will be the same value, and so will not be amplified. The facility to ignore signals that are *common* to both input terminals is defined as the *common mode rejection* and the manner in which the amplifier can amplify only the ECG signal and reject the common mains signals is called the *common mode rejection ratio* (CMRR) and is the differential signal gain/common mode signal gain. The common electrode is needed so that the ECG voltages are referred to it and are in the range of the supply of the amplifier. It could be connected to earth, which is undesirable, or it can be *floating* (i.e. not connected to earth). A floating or patient isolated amplifier is shown in Figure 5.9.

The supply for the patient amplifier (and modulator and associated circuits) is obtained from an isolating transformer, which is *rectified* (and smoothed) to produce DC. This provides isolation

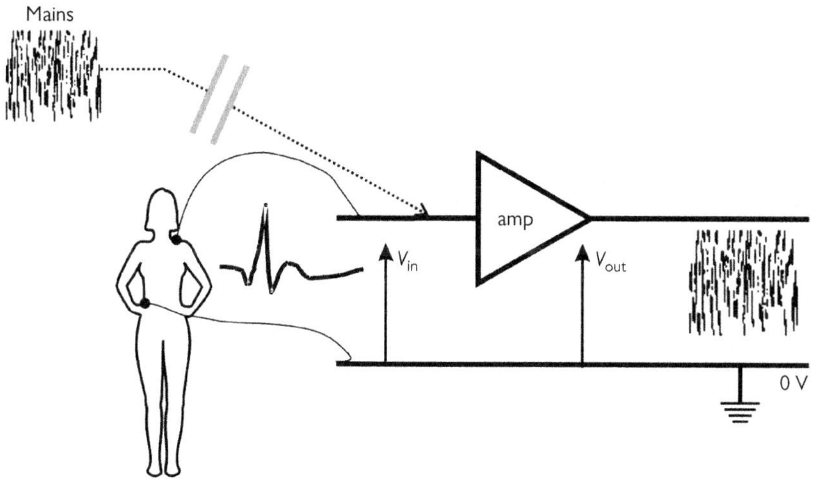


**Fig. 5.7** A single ended electrocardiogram amplifier, showing the system amplifying the domestic mains voltage at the input and output.

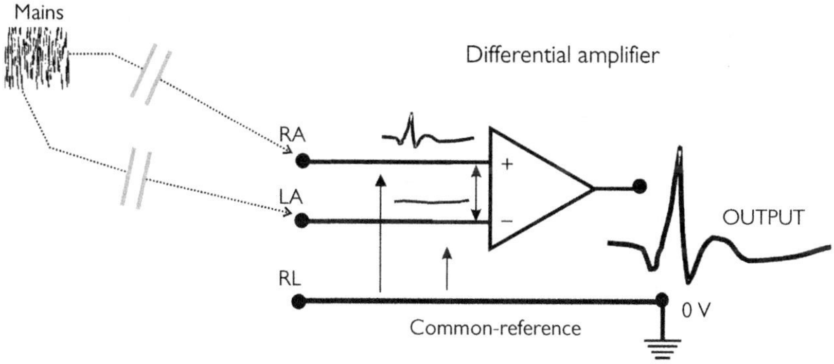


**Fig. 5.8** Patient connected differential amplifier measuring the ECG, showing connection to a patient, RA is right arm, LA is left arm, and RL is right leg.

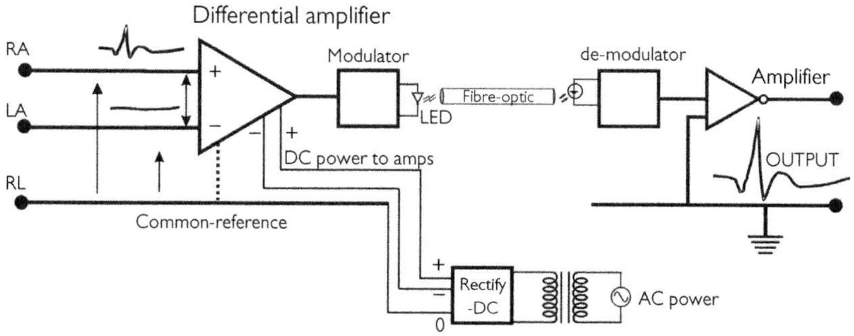


**Fig. 5.9** Patient isolated differential amplifier showing isolation provided by fibre-optics, and the power supply arrangements for the patient amplifier. LED is light-emitting diode.

from the earth and mains supply, as is discussed in the mains safety (Chapter 6). The signal output from the patient amplifier is connected to the main equipment by either an optoisolator (as in the figure) or another signal isolating transformer. In this way the patient side of the equipment is totally separate from the main equipment and not earthed, but floating. The signal output from the patient-connected amplifier first *modulates* a light beam (i.e. the signal fluctuations are impressed on the beam by using a light-emitting diode), and this beam is passed through a fibre-optic cable (this is discussed in Chapter 24). At the end of the cable, the light is converted back to an electrical signal by a photodiode (or similar), and then is *de-modulated* to bring the signal back to its original form. It is then further amplified as necessary. The output now is completely isolated from the patient.

## Signal processing

Signal processing is a broad definition, but it includes the processes involved in taking an analogue signal, processing it in the analogue domain, converting it into a *digital* value (see next section), and then either displaying the results or using the results to perform some other function.

### *Biological signals*

The basic signal processing set-up is shown in Figure 5.10. The biological signals can either come directly from the body via electrodes (e.g. the ECG) or can be electrical signals produced from a transducer (e.g. a blood pressure transducer). The electrical signals are amplified by the patient-connected differential amplifier, whilst the transducer output (normally via a bridge) is amplified via a single-ended amplifier.

The amplifiers used to process these raw signals must have sufficient bandwidth; for example, the ECG has harmonics up to 100 Hz, and so the amplifier must amplify each harmonic equally to maintain the signal accuracy. Also each frequency must be amplified with no time delay or at least each must have the same time delay. If any of these criteria are not met there will be amplitude and phase distortion.

The signals are then manipulated and processed by the electronic circuits (e.g. filtered or differentiated), quantified by the *analogue-to-digital converter* (ADC), and analysed by the computer. If the signal is hidden in the noise, or very noisy, signal processing can often help to improve matters.

## Digital signal processing

The advantages of digital signal processing is that once a signal, such as a voltage, is converted to a series of numbers or *digitised*, the values cannot change, drift or become noisy, as in the analogue processes described previously.

The computer can carry out numerous mathematical tasks on the digital data, which are now just a series of numbers. For example, it can digitally filter them, carry out Fourier transforms on

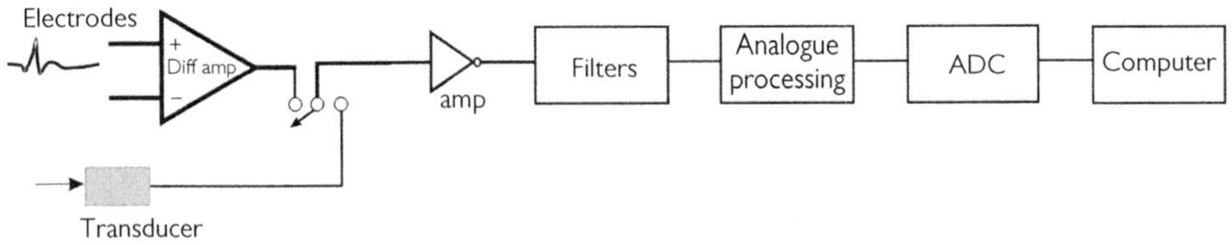


**Fig. 5.10** Signal processing block diagram showing the path from electrodes or transducer, to amplify, filter, process and then convert the signal to digital form. ADC = analogue to digital converter, see text.

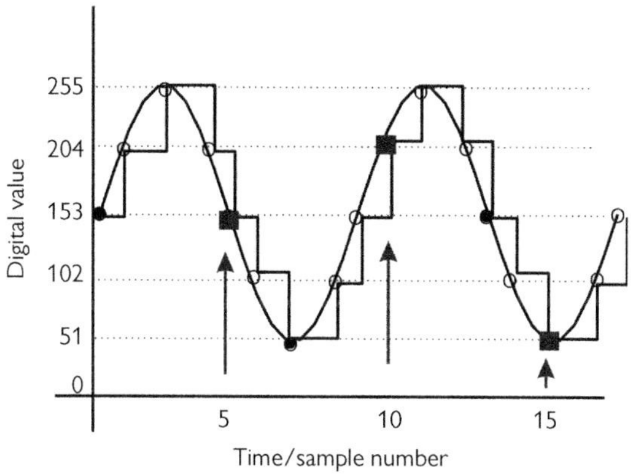


**Fig. 5.11** Conversion of analogue signal to digital values. The diagram shows a sine wave sampled at ten equally spaced in time points. The open circles represent a sample, and these samples will have a corresponding digital value. For example, the 5th sample in the diagram has a value of 153, the 10th 204 and the 15th 51.

them to obtain the power spectrum, or just obtain simple parameters such as the maxima of the signal.

The analogue signal is first converted to a digital value by an analogue-to-digital converter (ADC). This device takes a *snap-shot* or a single *sample* of the waveform at exact time intervals, converts this analogue value to a number and sends it to the computer for storage and processing. The effect of sampling a sine wave is shown in Figure 5.11, and it appears that a staircase waveform is the result. In the reconstruction, this staircase is simply low-pass filtered to give the same sine wave again. For an eight-bit system, as shown in the figure (8 units of memory, each either 0 or 1, giving values of 00000000 to 11111111) the sampled number is between 0 and 255. If the signal ranges from 0 to 5 V, then the digital number produced is the signal multiplied by 255 and divided by 5. For example, 2.5 V would be 128 or 10000000 binary. Systems can have many more bits, which can give higher resolutions. For example, 16 bits will give 0–65536.

There are mathematical rules about how frequently samples need to be taken from a waveform so that the information of the original analogue waveform is preserved. The minimum sample rate is defined as the *Nyquist* rate and this rate is greater than twice the bandwidth (the highest frequency component) of the signal being processed. At this rate, all the frequency information in the original signal will be kept. If it is sampled less, frequency aliasing occurs where low-frequency components suddenly appear that are not really there. This is illustrated in Figure 5.12. If a certain sampling rate is fixed, the signal must be filtered to achieve this criterion. In practice, the signal tends to be sampled at between 3 and 8 times the Nyquist rate. No advantage is gained by sampling the waveform at 10 times or more the Nyquist minimum frequency required.

# Electrodes and transducers

## *Electrodes*

Electrodes, which are applied directly to the human body, are both used for the measurement of bioelectric events and to deliver current to living tissue in the form of stimulation. This section will consider just the measurement aspect. An electrode may have direct contact (via an electrolyte) to the tissue or the mode may be capacitive (the contact is via an air gap or insulator). The most frequent are the direct contact ones.

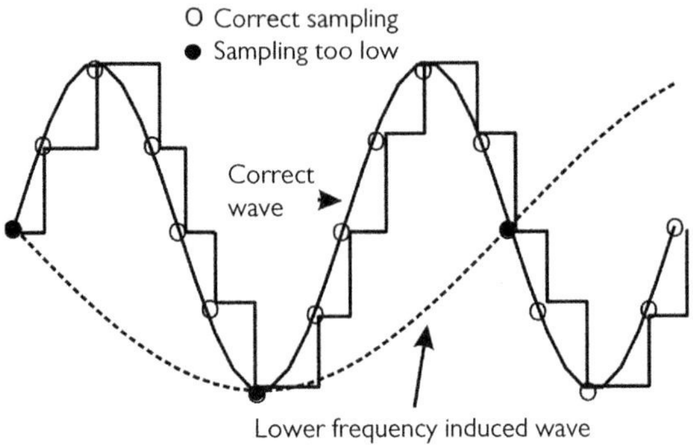


**Fig. 5.12** Diagram showing a sine wave sample at above the Nyquist rate (open circles) and below the rate (closed circles). Aliasing occurs when the sampling is too low and results in an aliased wave – a much lower frequency wave than the sampled sine wave.

When a metallic electrode comes into contact with an electrolyte (a conductive gel), an electrochemical reaction occurs, which in a conceptual sense resembles a voltage source, a capacitor and a resistor. The voltage source developed by this reaction at the electrolyte interface is called the half-cell potential. Different metals have different half-cell potentials and there is a range of values from near zero to ±1.7 V. Table 5.1 gives some half-cell values.

If different metals are used for each of the electrodes then large voltages can be produced (as in batteries). For a pair of electrodes used, which is the minimum number needed to obtain a physiological event, the voltage difference should be the difference between the half-cell voltages. This voltage – the voltage needed to *polarise* – should be zero if the metals are well matched. It has been found [Geddes 1967] that silver (Ag) coated with a chloride layer (AgCl) has a low half-cell potential and also has good stability and low drift voltages between the two electrodes connected to the skin via the electrolyte. The electrical *noise* from the Ag electrode dramatically reduces when the chloride layer is applied. AgCl electrodes are therefore fragile because of this property – the noise increases greatly if the Cl layer is chipped or broken, and are also photosensitive. Light change can affect the half-cell potentials.

**Table 5.1** Some electrode potentials for material used in electrodes (source de Bethune 1964)

| **Metal** | **Potential** (V) |
|---|---|
| Aluminium | −1.7 |
| Zinc | −0.8 |
| Iron | −0.4 |
| Nickel | −0.3 |
| Lead | −0.1 |
| Silver | +0.8 |
| Silver/Silver chloride | +0.2 |
| Copper | +0.3 |
| Platinum | +1.2 |

## Electrodes on humans

The electrodes used on humans must be connected to a suitable biological amplifier as mentioned previously. The total impedance of both the electrode impedance and the electrode-skin impedance must be much lower than the amplifier input impedance in order to maximise the transfer of the physiological signal from the body and to minimise signal distortion. Also low skin-electrode impedance will minimise the pick up of interference, especially domestic mains supply interference. The total electrode impedance (skin plus electrode) can be thought of as a series resistor ($R_{electrode}$) with the physiological signal generator as in Figure 5.13. The combination of the electrode-related impedance and the amplifier input resistance ($R_{amplifier}$) forms a voltage divider. As the electrode resistance becomes lower than the amplifier input resistance, the voltage across the amplifier input will be similar to the signal source voltage. It is also important to make the electrode impedance as low as possible so that the induced interference voltage (normally domestic mains) is as low as possible. As $V = IR$, where $I$ is the induced interference current (transmitted from the mains equipment by capacitance) and $R$ is the electrode impedance, then to get the lowest $V$, $R$ should be as low as possible. Obviously, reducing the mains interference (lowering $I$) by switching off any unused equipment, increasing the distance from mains-powered equipment, or using battery-powered equipment. It is wise to clean the skin (which can decrease the skin-electrode impedance) before applying the electrodes.

## Transducers

A transducer converts one form of energy into another. In biomedical applications transducers are used to convert physiological signals to analogue electrical signals that can then be processed as described previously.

Transducers come in many forms. The majority fall into the following classes: resistive, inductive, capacitive, photoelectric, piezoelectric, thermoelectric and chemical. Examples of each will be discussed briefly here, and then in more detail in the appropriate chapters.

The variation of resistance has been used extensively to convert temperature and mechanical displacement (pressure) to electrical signals. The resistance of a conductor is dependent on the material, the geometric configuration and the temperature. The choice of material is dependent on its linearity or sensitivity for that purpose. The resistance transducers have a wide range of uses in medicine from strain gauges, thermometers, thermistors to pressure (resistive) transducers.

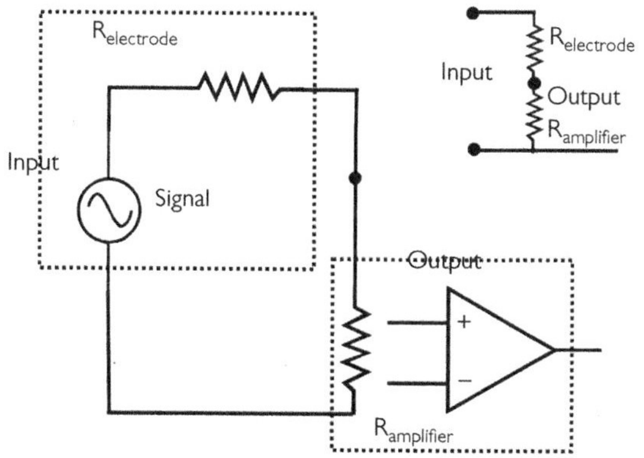


**Fig. 5.13** Diagram of a physiological signal generator plus series electrode resistance ($R_{electrode}$) plus amplifier input resistance ($R_{amplifier}$). The voltage divider is formed by the combination of the two resistances with the signal being the input voltage, and the output voltage being the voltage across the amplifier. This equivalent circuit is also shown in the diagram in the top right.

Inductive transducers are also used in medicine. The inductance of a coil depends on its geometry, the magnetic permeability of the medium in which it is located, and the number of turns of the coil. Changing any of these will give a change in reactance and this can be measured. Only certain changes, however, will have the sensitivity required. An example of its use is the pressure transducer discussed in Chapter 12.

Capacitive transducers are another alternative. These can be very accurate and linear but require complex driving electronics. A capacitor consists of two conducting surfaces separated by an insulator (dielectric), which can be a solid, gas, liquid or a vacuum. They are used in blood pressure transducers (discussed in Chapter 12) and differential capacitive pneumotachographs. Also living tissue can form part of the capacitive transducer.

Photoelectric transducers consist of photovoltaic cells, photoconductive cells, and the phototransistor and they are also used in medicine. The photovoltaic cell typically consists of a thin coating of selenium on an iron backing. Above the selenium is a thin transparent metal film. When this is illuminated a potential difference appears across the barrier. Photoconductive cells consist of a thin film of typically silicon and, when exposed to certain types of radiant energy, its resistance decreases. The phototransistor can have a very fast response time and the collector (the output) amplifies the small current change caused by the light by the same process as transistors do. The most well known use of the phototransistor has been in pulse oximetry, as discussed in Chapter 15. This uses two detectors and each receives different wavelengths of light, obtained by filtering, typically 640 nm and 805 nm.

Piezoelectric transducers rely on the effect of certain materials that develop a voltage difference across them when a pressure is applied or the material is distorted in some way. These transducers are used to detect blood pressure and cardiac sounds, and are used as accelerometers. The piezoelectric transducer can also work in reverse, producing movement when a potential difference is applied. Ultrasound transducers, as discussed in Chapter 10, use both these principles.

Chemical transducers play an important role in the assessment of metabolism. There are two main types: those that measure chemical composition of the blood, tissue and organ fluids, and those that measure the composition of the respiratory gases. Many chemical transducers are electrochemical cells in which the quantity to be measured causes a change in cell potential or a change in current through the cell.

## References

**De Bethune, A. J.** and **Loud, S. N. S.** (1965) Standard aqueous electrode potentials and temperature coefficients at 25oC, *J. Electrochem. Soc.*, **112**(4), 107C–8C.

**Geddes L. A.** and **Baker, L. E.** (1967) Chlorided silver electrodes, *Med. Res. Engng.*, **6**, pp. 33–4.

## Further reading

**Brown, B. H., Smallwood, R. H., Barber, D. C., Lawford, P. V.** and **Hose, D. R.** (1999) *Medical Physics and Biomedical Engineering*, IOP Publishing, Bristol.

**Horowitz, P.** and **Hill, W.** (2015) *The Art of Electronics*, 3rd edn, Cambridge University Press, Cambridge.

**McDonald, D. A.** (1974) *Blood Flow in Arteries*, 2nd edn, Camelot Press, Southampton.

**Strackee, J.** and **Westerhof, N.** (1993) *The Physics and Heart and Circulation*, IOP Publishing, Bristol.

**Togawa, T., Tamura, T.** and **Oberg, P. A.** (1997) *Biomedical Transducers and Instruments*, CRC Press, New York.

**Tooley, M. A.** (2023) Electronics and biological signal processing. *BJA Educ.*, **23**(4), pp. 122–7.

# Chapter 6 **Electrical safety**

This chapter contains: electricity supply; safety features; leakage currents; earth faults; earth-free supplies; microshock; circuit breakers; heating effects of electrical current; electrolysis; static electricity.
The chapter links with: Chapters 4 and 5.

## The electricity supply

Domestic 'mains' systems in the UK use alternating current (AC) at 50 Hz. In the USA (and Canada, western Japan, Brazil, the Philippines), their domestic mains systems use 60 Hz. These frequencies are used as they are efficient frequencies for transmission from power generation to the users and minimise the effect of leakage currents due to capacitance, which is discussed later in this chapter. The mains is initially generated in a power station and the power generated there (volts × amps) is enough to supply a number of hospitals and consumers. The voltage and the potential to do work must be transmitted to the user and this is usually achieved with overhead pylons, or sometimes by underground cables. Both types of cable will be designed to carry current, but the higher the current, the greater power lost to heat ($I^2R$). It is desirable to keep the current as low as possible to reduce this transmission heat *loss*, and this can be done by making the voltage as high as possible. For a given power, ($V \times I$) there can be a high $V$ and low $I$ or vice versa. The transmission voltage is normally greater than 11 kV. It arrives at a domestic substation and is transformed down to (in the UK) 230 V RMS by a transformer (see Chapter 4). At the substation, as illustrated in Figure 6.1, one connection of the transformer is firmly bound to earth at what is called the *star point*, and this forms the start of what is called the *neutral* lead. The earth connection forms a vital part of electrical safety. The connection on the other side of the transformer is called the *live* lead and this is at 230 V RMS. These two leads are taken to the individual outlets or mains sockets, the live carrying the voltage to the load, and the neutral lead carrying the return current back to the source of the supply. The earth connection of the mains socket is connected back to the star point separately, although sometimes in older installations this can be earthed locally. In this way, only one of the socket points is live, and the other is at near zero potential. This is all demonstrated in Figure 6.1. The neutral connection at the equipment is not exactly zero, due to the resistance of the long length cables (see figure) supplying the mains equipment. Although the resistance of this lead is very low, if it is 0.5 Ω and the current flow is (for example) 1 A, then the voltage drop between the transformer and the domestic socket will be 0.5 V. Therefore, the neutral point will be 0.5 V.

## Electrical safety features

### *Class 1 equipment*

The first safety or basic principle ensures that the electrical device has a metal case which is earthed, as shown in Figures 6.1 and 6.2. This is class 1 equipment, such as monitors used in theatre, or simple domestic kettles. The live lead is protected by fuses (or a circuit breaker, which is described later). Any fault that causes a low resistance to appear between live components in the circuit and the metal case, is dealt with by the protective earth pathway which takes the *fault* current to earth. In Figure 6.1, the fault is shown by a fault 'resistance' to the case of 100 kΩ. If the leakage voltage source was assumed to be 100 V (it can be anything from low voltage to 230 V), then the fault current would be 1 mA. Normally this low-resistance path to earth causes an increased live current through the fuse but the fuse would

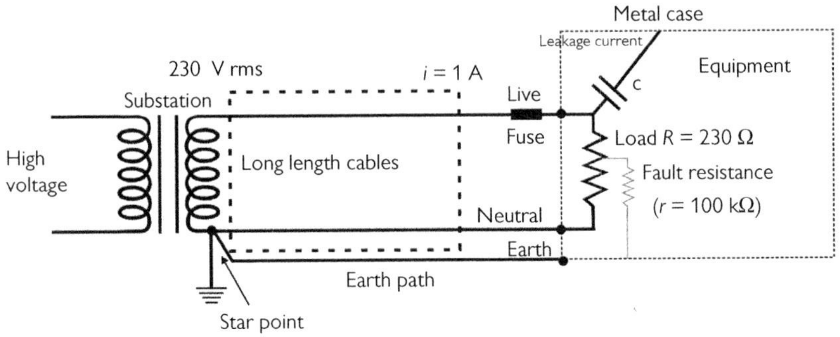


**Fig. 6.1** Diagram of the domestic mains supply, supplying class one equipment. The equipment has a load of 230Ω, and so the normal current would be 1 A. The case of the equipment is earthed. The leakage current by capacitance is shown by C. See text for details.

only melt and *blow*, breaking the circuit, if the fault current was in the order of amps, but in this example nothing would happen to the fuse as the fault current is not high enough.

However, class 1 equipment can only be connected to the patient if there is a separate isolating transformer, as shown in Figure 6.2. The patient must not have a direct path to earth and this is discussed later.

## *Class 2 equipment*

Class 2 equipment has no protective earth. Instead the basic insulation is supplemented by a secondary layer of insulation. This equipment is classified as doubly insulated. The power cable has only live and neutral, and the mains-connected circuitry is then enclosed in a second insulated layer, so that

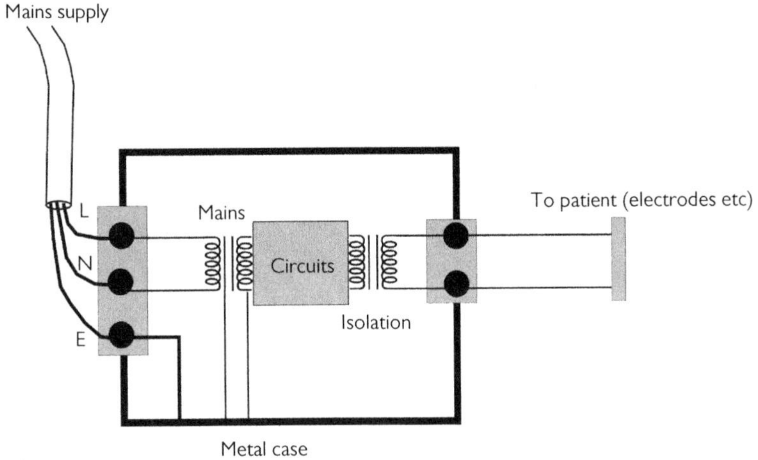


**Fig. 6.2** Diagram of a class I equipment that supplies a patient connected part via an isolation transformer. The mains transformer core and one side of the secondary are earthed for safety.

no conductive exposed parts can be brought into contact with the patient. The case is made of non-conductive plastic.

## *Class 3 equipment*

Class 3 equipment is where the protection is because no voltages are used that exceed safety extra-low voltage (SELV). This equipment can be powered by an external low-voltage transformer not exceeding 25 V RMS AC or batteries less than 60 V DC.

## *Leakage currents*

Apart from inappropriate currents caused by faults, there are normally other 'extra' currents in the system caused by *stray capacitance*. Capacitance exists between all conductors, even if the insulation is intact and adequate, and this is the stray capacitance. The closer the conductors are together, the greater the magnitude of any stray capacitance. As the mains voltage is AC, the stray capacitance between the mains wiring and earth results in 'capacitive' current to earth, because of the capacitive 'resistance' (actually impedance). This occurs both in the supply system and in any equipment connected to it. This current is called leakage current and is illustrated in Figure 6.1. In designing equipment, manufacturers can reduce but not eliminate leakage current. They can keep leakage current within acceptable limits by the careful choice of mains components.

The earthing is vital as it provides a safe, low-resistance path for the leakage current back to the (earthed) neutral point. Every class 1 device has some leakage current passing down the earth wire: this current is called *Earth Leakage Current*. However, an excessive Earth Leakage Current could pose a possible problem for the earthing system and any circuit breakers as described later. There is a maximum allowed limit for Earth Leakage Current of 5 mA in normal conditions and 10 mA in single fault conditions.

*Touch Current* does present a hazard to users and patients, as shown in Figure 6.3(a). Touch Current is the leakage current that can find a path to earth through a user who touches the metal case of the equipment. In normal conditions, if the enclosure is conductive and earthed, then the Touch Current will be, for all practical purposes, zero. If the case of the equipment is not earthed, due to a problem or a fault, such as a broken earth in the diagram, then normal Touch Current will flow through the person. In this condition, where the earth has been disconnected, the upper safe limit is 500 μA.

Apart from the classes 1–3 safety features, if equipment is to be connected to patients (e.g. ECG, etc.), it must be designated type B, BF or CF. Type B may be class 1, 2 and 3 mains-powered equipment. This equipment is not suitable for direct connection to the heart, but must have adequate protection against electric shock with regard to allowable leakage currents. The allowable patient leakage currents are shown in Table 6.1. Single fault conditions are when a single condition such as an earth disconnection occurs. There can be multiple faults, such as earth disconnection and excessive leakage occurring.

Type BF equipment where that part of the equipment is applied to the patient is isolated from all other parts of the equipment to an extent that allowable patient leakage current (under single fault conditions, i.e. only one of the possible faults being present) is not exceeded even when 110% of the mains voltage is applied between the applied part and earth. This degree of isolation is called an F-type isolated floating applied part. This applies to CF as well.

Type CF is class 1 or 2 mains powered with an internal electrical power source. This equipment provides the most stringent protection against shocks and has an F-type isolated floating applied part. This equipment can be connected to a patient's heart.

Some commonly used symbols are shown in Figure 6.4.

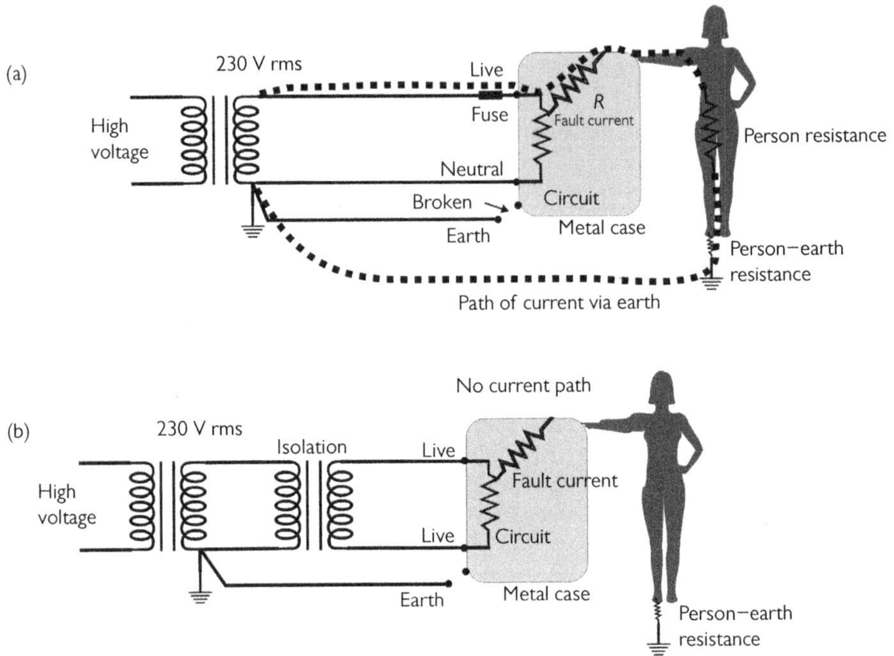


**Fig. 6.3** (a) describes a situation where there is a dual fault. The earth connection to the metal case is broken and there is a fault resistance to the case caused by an internal fault. There will be a flow of current through the person, via earth. The magnitude of the current will be dependent on the person resistance and the person–earth resistance. *R* is the fault resistance. (b) shows a situation where there is an isolation transformer present. In this case, the dual fault situation described in (a) does not give a complete current path, and no current flows through the person.

**Table 6.1** Allowable values of continuous leakage and patient auxiliary currents in μA (international regulations defined by IEC 60601-1)

| | **Type B** | | **Type BF** | | **Type CF** | |
|---|---|---|---|---|---|---|
| **Current** (μA) | **Normal** | **Single fault** | **Normal** | **Single fault** | **Normal** | **Single fault** |
| Patient leakage current and patient auxiliary current DC | 10 | 50 | 10 | 50 | 10 | 50 |
| Patient leakage current and patient auxiliary current AC | 100 | 500 | 100 | 500 | 10 | 50 |
| Patient leakage current with reference supply voltage on applied part | - | - | 5000 | 5000 | 50 | 50 |

## Earth faults

The earth connection can become disconnected due to trauma to the mains cable, for example, if it has been continuously stepped on or rolled on by an anaesthetic machine. The plug can be badly wired and also the connection might be from the socket to an old, corroded water pipe. Hospital maintenance or

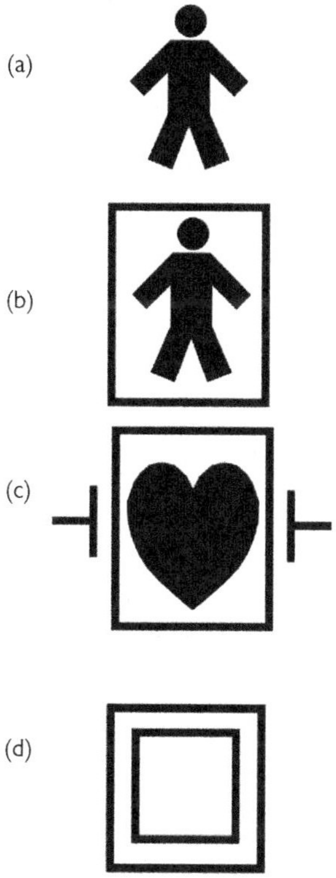


**Fig. 6.4** A selection of commonly used electrical safety symbols. (a) is the sign for type B equipment. (b) is the sign for BF equipment. (c) is for type CF equipment but, in addition, the two symbols outside the square indicate that the equipment is protected from defibrillation damage. (d) is the symbol for class 2 equipment. There are no symbols for classes 1 and 3.

the equipment management service should always check the integrity of the earth connection. If an earth fault develops, normally no one would notice any difference. If a small leakage current develops, then the user would feel that the equipment has a *fuzzy* feel to it. If two or more faults develop, i.e. earth lead breakage and severe leakage fault currents (and the order in which this happens is not important), then this situation is highly dangerous to both clinician and patient. In this dual fault situation, if an anaesthetist touches the instrument case, for example, then a connection to earth can be made via the resistance of the person and the circuit will be completed. This is described in Figure 6.3(a).

There will be current flow through the person and the magnitude of it will be dependent on many factors: humidity, sweating, shoe insulation, etc. These factors will change the resistance to earth (person–earth resistance in the figure) and therefore the amount of current through the person. For example, if the anaesthetist is standing on an antistatic floor with one hand touching the faulty equipment and touching nothing else, then the resistance to earth is in excess of 20 kΩ, so that by Ohm's law the maximum current that can flow is 230/20 = 11.5 mA. Whilst this shock would be painful, it would not kill.

However, if the subject touches the metal equipment with one wet hand while touching an earth conductor, such as a water tap with the other (or standing in a puddle of water or saline with normal footwear), the resistance to earth would be much lower and possibly less than 2000 Ω. In this case the subject would sustain a lethal electric current of 115 mA, which can induce ventricular fibrillation. However, this is still a small current for the circuit, so it is likely that the circuit fuse will remain intact. Table 6.2 gives the physiological effects of different currents through the body.

**Table 6.2** External AC currents through the body, and the physiological effect

| Current | Effect |
|---|---|
| 0.5 mA | Threshold of perception |
| 1 mA | Tingling sensation |
| 5 mA | Pain and threshold of cannot let go current. |
| 15 mA | Severe pain with local muscle spasm. |
| 50 mA | Tonic muscle contraction of respiratory muscles and respiratory arrest |
| 80–100 mA | Ventricular fibrillation |

## Microshock

Table 6.2 shows currents through the external regions of the body. However, the currents needed to do damage within the body are much less, and very small currents around 50 μA are needed through the ventricular endocardium to produce ventricular fibrillation. The effect of these currents is called *microshock*. The frequency is important as well, and low frequencies such as 50 Hz are the most dangerous frequencies. High voltages at high frequencies in the MHz range are used in diathermy, and these do not harm the patient, but they are used for controlled cutting and coagulation, and this is discussed in Chapter 21.

Microshock can occur in a few situations: pacemaker wires, cardiac catheters with incorporated electrodes, a catheter filled with conductive medium, such as a saline-filled cardiac catheter. A fault condition could cause the potential of the catheter or associated devices to rise above zero volts and then any earth path available to the patient would be disastrous. One example of this (Bousvaros *et al.* 1962) was when a patient developed *ventricular fibrillation* (VF) when the motorised syringe pump connected to the cardiac catheter was switched on. There was a double fault on the syringe driver: the motor was poorly insulated (and therefore had high leakage current) and the earth connection to the device was broken. The patient was earthed by a right-leg ECG electrode that was connected to the earthed chassis of a (now not legal) non-isolated ECG machine. Leakage current flowed along the cardiac catheter, through the patient's heart and right-leg electrode to earth. The equivalent circuit of this situation is shown in Figure 6.5. It can be seen that over 400 μA flows, which is well above the hazardous microshock level. To prevent microshock, stringent leakage levels must be applied to all equipment making contact with the patient either directly or via an endocardiac lead. A stringent code must be observed: all electrical equipment in the vicinity of the patient must conform to a leakage specification of less than 10 μA under normal working conditions; wherever possible such equipment should be battery operated and fully isolated from earth; all electrical circuits making contact with the patient must be electrically isolated from earth; all such equipment in the susceptible zone should whenever possible be coated with insulating material; pacemaker leads or catheters must only be handled with gloved hands and a user should never hold the lead in one hand while using an oscilloscope, monitor or other mains powered equipment in the other.

## Circuit breakers

For general protection of equipment, there is a fuse situated in the live line. This will break when a fault situation occurs where the addition of the leakage current to the normal current is high enough to melt the fuse. Automatic electronic circuit breakers that can be reset also exist, and these operate in the same manner as the fuse. These devices (fuse and circuit breaker), however, are not sensitive enough to prevent any shock situation occurring, due to the relatively small currents involved. A *residual current device* (RCD) is a much more sensitive circuit breaker and can break a circuit before a person perceives

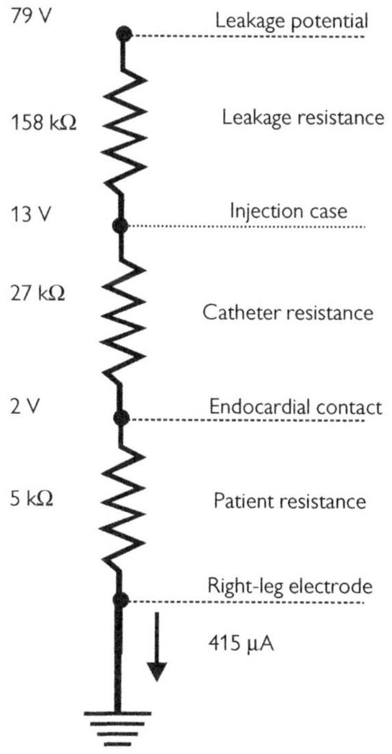


**Fig. 6.5** Circuit of the multiple fault condition described in the text.

any pain. This relies on the principle that normally in a correctly working system there is a balance of current in the live and neutral leads. In a fault situation, there is an imbalance of current and this causes an electrically operated switch to break the circuit. This can be in the form of a transformer solenoid-type switch or a semiconductor type as shown in Figure 6.6. The sensitivity for the RCD can

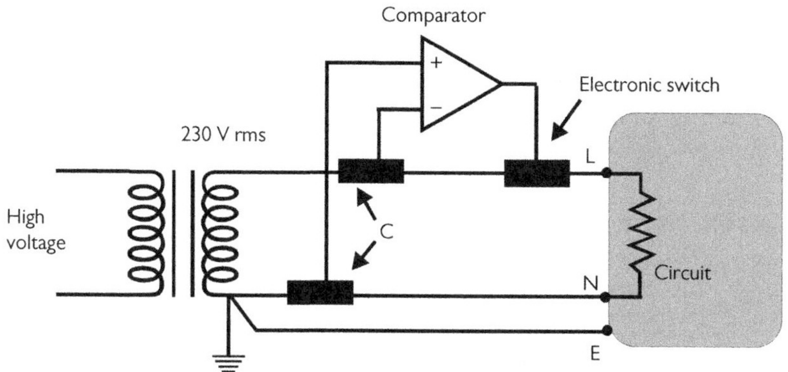


**Fig. 6.6** An example of a sensitive circuit breaker. Cs in the diagram are circuit components that give a voltage output proportional to the current flowing through them. These outputs, one from the live line and the other from the neutral line, are supplied to a comparator circuit. This circuit compares the two inputs and gives an output if they are different by a desired amount. This output will operate an electronic switch and break the circuit.

be an imbalance of 100 mA for the least sensitive and up to 10 mA for the most sensitive. In order for the user not to notice any physiological effects, the RCD must operate within 30 ms. Normally a fuse or automatic circuit breaker would be used in addition to break the circuit if very high currents exist.

One problem with using RCDs is that they rely on disconnecting the supply to provide safety. In some medically used rooms, this is unacceptable. Consider a situation where a mains lead plug that has become wet is plugged in at an intensive care unit (ICU) bed. This results in excessive leakage current and the supply is disconnected to protect the users. In doing so it might also shut off the supply to the monitors and ventilators. A solution to this, but this solution can be used only in strictly controlled situations (such as ICU and theatres), is to use earth-free supplies.

# Earth-free supplies

The conventional live–neutral–earth system has some advantages, especially for domestic use (only one lead is at mains potential; this has advantages, e.g. only one fuse needed), but as discussed, an earth-free mains supply for theatres is possible. A 1:1 isolating transformer is added to the normal system so that no voltage change occurs. The primary winding is connected to the live and neutral and the secondary is not connected to earth and is therefore earth-free. This feeds one or more of the power outlets. The earth can be connected to the case as before. In the situation when either of the two live leads (2 now instead of 1) becomes connected to the case (and the earth connection to the case is not present or is a high resistance), then the current cannot pass through the patient to earth, as shown in Figure 6.3(b).

# Other safety issues of electricity

## *Heating effects of electric currents*

When a current passes through a conductor, work is produced and the energy is converted into heat, in proportion to the resistance. As heat is produced, the temperature of the conductor rises. The rate of heat production is heat energy per unit time, or J $s^{-1}$ = watts. The effect of a given amount of heat on the temperature of the conductor depends upon the *specific heat capacity* (SHC) of the material (kJ $kg^{-1}$ $K^{-1}$). Water has a SHC of 4.128 kJ $kg^{-1}$ $K^{-1}$. Body tissues have a SHC of 3.5 kJ $kg^{-1}$ $K^{-1}$ and for blood it is 3.6 kJ $kg^{-1}$ $K^{-1}$. If a body is heated by a certain amount, then the temperature reached depends on its mass and SHC. The rate of cooling depends on the rate of heat lost by conduction or dissipation, convection and radiation. The body can be thought of as a complex structure composed of multiple elements each with a unique combination of resistance, heat capacity and dissipation. When current passes through these elements, each one produces heat proportional to the square of the current ($I^2R$) and the temperature reached depends on the dissipation. Surface elements will dissipate heat by radiation and convection. But deeper elements depend on their neighbours' heat production and nearness to the surface. The heating effect of the deep elements depends on the heat-dissipating capacity of their neighbours near the surface.

## *The effect of current density*

The current density is the current per unit area, perpendicular to the flow. It is measured in A $m^{-2}$ and sometimes as mA $cm^{-2}$. The pattern of heating in the body depends on current density and dissipation from different zones to deeper zones with high current density becoming hottest, while those nearer the surface with low density remain coldest. In general, though, high current densities generate the greatest heating, all other things being equal. A large mass of tissue (e.g. the forearm) will heat up less than, say, a small finger.

Current densities of less than 1 mA $mm^{-2}$ are unable to cause damage but burns have been produced by currents of 5 mA $mm^{-2}$ for 10 s or more (Hull 1994). In diathermy, where radio-frequency currents are used, there is no stimulation, but heating is limited to the current densities –the high density at the positive tip will cause massive heating, but at the negative indifferent plate, the density is lower, so no heating is produced. Burns in any tissue situation are produced when the heat produced is more than is dissipated. This is discussed in Chapter 21.

## *DC and electrolysis*

Electrolysis will take place when a direct current is passed through any medium that contains free ions. The positive ions will migrate to the negative electrode and negative ions to the positive one. If two electrodes are placed on the skin and 100 μA DC is passed between them for a few minutes, small ulcers will be found beneath the electrodes. IEC601–01 defines 'DC' as being less than 0.1 Hz. Above this, the movement of ions is balanced because the positive and negative electrodes are reversed. The IEC recommendation limits the current to 10 μA.

## *Static electricity*

Static electricity, as discussed in Chapter 4, that builds up on the body can give rise to short-duration shocks. This happens when the body is insulated from the local earth and accumulates a small electric charge. When a person touches something earthed, there is a discharge between the person and earth and this flow of current can be enough to cause an unpleasant jolt. However, static discharges have durations measured in microseconds and, as these are of short duration, there is little risk of inducing a harmful stimulation to the heart. For this reason, the antistatic floor resistance cannot be infinite as there needs to be a resistance path for the static to discharge to earth.

## *References*

**Bousvaros, G. A.**, **Don, C.** and **Hopps, J. A.** (1962) An electrical hazard of selective angio-cardiography, *Can. Med. Association J.*, **87**, pp. 286–8.

**Hull, C. J.** (1994) The electrical hazards of patient monitoring. In Hutton, P. and Prys-Roberts, C. (eds), *Monitoring in Anaesthesia and Intensive Care*, WB Saunders Co. Ltd, London, pp. 56–77.

## *Further reading*

**Al-Shaikh, B.** and **Stacey, S.** (2002) Chapter 3 in *Essentials of Anaesthetic Equipment*, 2nd edn, Churchill Livingstone, London.

**Tooley, M. A.** (2023). Electrical safety, defibrillation and diathermy. *BJA Educ.*, **23**(3), pp. 84–91.

**Wentworth, S.** (ed.) (2009) *Guide to Electrical Safety Testing of Medical Equipment: The Why and the How. IPEM Report Number 97*. Institute of Physics and Engineering in Medicine (IPEM), York.

# Chapter 7 **Behaviour of fluids (liquids and gases, flow and pressure)**

The chapter has links with: Chapters 1, 3, 8, 9, 13, 14 and 22.

## Fluid flow behaviour

A *fluid* can be either a liquid or a gas. Fluids exhibit different flow behaviours depending on their physical properties, in particular viscosity and density. Flow characteristics also depend on the geometry of the pipes or channels through which they flow, and on the driving pressure regimes. These principles can be applied to any fluid, and the complexity of the analysis depends on the flow regimes described in this section (Massey 1970).

Fluid flow is generally described as laminar or turbulent. Laminar flow is flow in which laminae or layers of fluid run parallel to each other. In a circular pipe, such as a blood vessel or a bronchus, velocity within the layers nearest the wall of the pipe is least; in the layer immediately adjacent to the wall, it is theoretically zero. In fully developed laminar flow, the velocity profile across the pipe is parabolic, as shown in Figure 7.1, and as discussed in Chapter 1 (see Figure 1.10). Peak velocity of the fluid occurs in the midline of the pipe, and is twice the average velocity across the pipe at equilibrium, and layers equidistant from the wall have equal velocity. The importance of laminar flow is that there is minimum energy loss in the flow, i.e. it is an efficient transport mode. This is in contrast to turbulent flow, where eddies and vortices (flow in directions other than the predominant one) mean that energy in fluid transport is wasted in production of heat, additional friction and noise. The result is that the pressure drop required to drive a given flow from one end of the pipe to the other is greater in turbulent than in laminar flow.

The shear stress $\tau$, which is the mechanical stress between layers of fluid and between the fluid and the tube wall, is proportional to the velocity gradient across the tube ($dv/dr$) of the fluid layers. The constant of proportionality between these two variables is the *dynamic viscosity, $\eta$*.

Expressed mathematically,

$$\tau = \eta \frac{dv}{dr}.$$

Where dynamic viscosity is constant, the fluid is a *Newtonian fluid* such as air or water. Blood is a suspension of particles in a liquid and is therefore a non-Newtonian fluid, which means that $\eta$ is not constant and depends on the time dependent rate of shear between layers. Dynamic viscosity has units of N s $m^{-2}$ or kg $s^{-1}$ $m^{-1}$. There also exists the property *kinematic viscosity*, $\nu$, where $\nu = \eta/\rho$, where $\rho$ is the fluid density. The flow will decrease as the viscosity ($\eta$) increases. As temperature increases, the viscosity of liquids decreases, while that of gases increases. The reason for this can be thought of as a decrease in the tightness of the intermolecular bonds of liquid, decreasing viscosity, and an increase in the random kinetic energy of gas molecules, increasing intermolecular collisions.

Fluid flow occurs only when there is an appropriate pressure gradient between the two ends of a pipe. At a low-pressure gradient (*low* is a context-sensitive term here, depending on the fluid and the pipes being studied), the flow rate is directly proportional to it and the flow is laminar. At a critical point (*critical flow rate, critical velocity*), the flow becomes turbulent, and the flow rate is subsequently approximately proportional to the square root of the pressure gradient, and to the reciprocal of the square root of the fluid density and to the reciprocal of the square root of the tube length. One of the tools used by

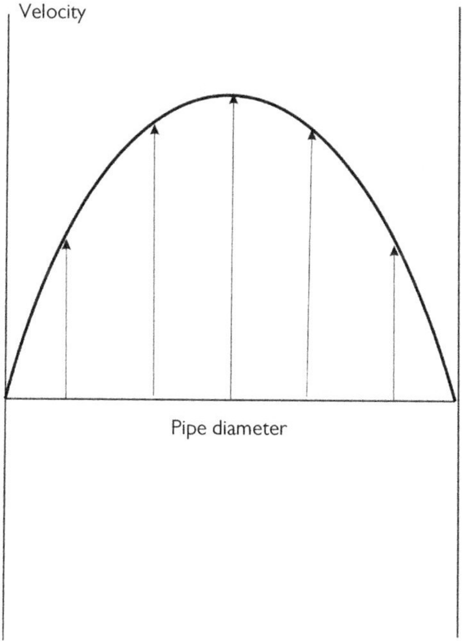


**Fig. 7.1** Fluid velocity profile across a tube in laminar flow.

hydraulic engineers for modelling fluid flow is a series of dimensionless ratios, one of which is *Reynolds' number*, *Re*, where

$$Re = \frac{V\,D\rho}{\eta},$$

and $V$ is a characteristic velocity, and $D$ is a characteristic dimension, usually tube diameter.

Whatever the size of the pipe and whichever fluid is used, in a smooth circular pipe, such as a blood vessel or a bronchus, fluid flow changes from laminar to turbulent when *Re* exceeds approximately 2000. Turbulence may occur intermittently, locally and prematurely at lower values of *Re* if the tube is not smooth or straight locally, for example, at bends, orifices, and changes of diameter. The resistance to fluid flow down a tube can be thought of as

$$\frac{pressure\,gradient(\Delta P)}{flow(Q)},$$

an hydraulic analogy to Ohm's law in electrical terms, $R = V/I$ (see Chapter 4). In laminar flow, this ratio is constant. In thinking about the variables that might govern flow it is intuitive that increasing $\Delta P$ or pipe diameter, or decreasing $\eta$ or pipe length will increase $Q$. The *Hagen–Poiseuille* equation for laminar flow, which can be deduced from first principles, embodies these concepts and states:

$$Q = \frac{\pi r^4 \Delta P}{8\,\eta L},$$

where $r$ and $L$ are pipe radius and length, respectively. (See Chapter 3, where the Hagen–Poiseuille equation has been used to discuss dimensions.) Note the fourth power of radius in the equation, which means that this influences changes in $Q$ to a much greater extent than the other factors. This has clinical importance in relation to the flow of fluids down intravenous cannulae, gas flow down endotracheal tubes, and the significance of bronchospasm. A doubling of the radius multiplies the flow rate by 16. Resistance to turbulent flow is less easily represented mathematically but, as indicated above,

$$Q \propto \frac{\sqrt{\Delta P}}{\sqrt{\rho L}}.$$

These expressions can be used to predict that the velocity at which transition from laminar to turbulent flow occurs is directly proportional to viscosity and inversely proportional to density and to tube diameter. In other words, flow becomes turbulent at a higher velocity (e.g. remains laminar for longer) with more viscous and less dense fluids, and in smaller diameter tubes. As indicated in the Hagen–Poiseuille equation the more the variables change to increase $Q$ ($\uparrow r$, $\uparrow \Delta P$, $\downarrow \eta$, $\downarrow L$), the more likely the flow is to approach turbulence. Turbulent flow also occurs where fluid flow is accelerated or decelerated at changes in diameter or direction of the pipe, such as at entry and exit orifices or bends, and is associated with kinetic energy loss.

# Theory of flow measurement devices

While a pipe can be thought of as having a length many times its diameter, an orifice can be considered as a structure with a length many times shorter than its diameter, and fluid behaviour is correspondingly different. Nevertheless, flow of fluid through an orifice has some uses, not least in the measurement of flow. If a U-tube manometer is placed with the outlets each side of the orifice, as shown in Figure 7.2, the pressure downstream is found to be lower than that upstream by an amount proportional to the flow squared; this confirms incidentally that the flow is turbulent through such an orifice.

If the orifice is turned on its end and the geometry altered slightly, it begins to resemble a flow meter familiar to anaesthetists, the *Rotameter*, shown in Figure 7.3, a device that has its origins in the brewing

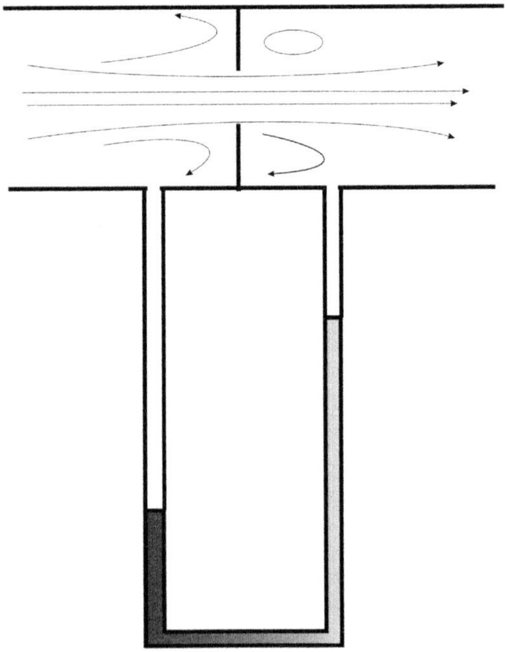

**Fig. 7.2** Orifice meter flow measurement device.

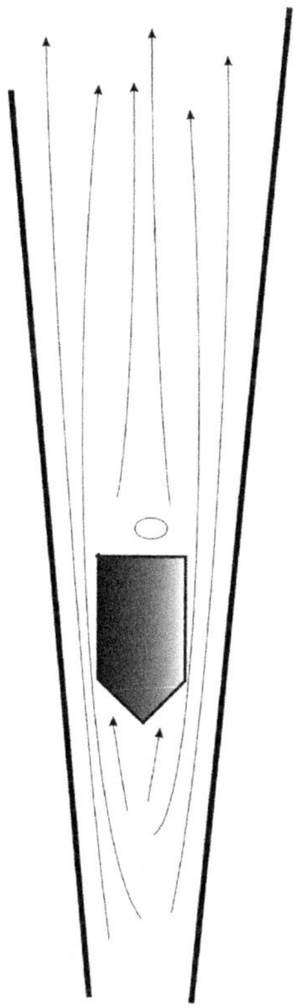

**Fig. 7.3** The Rotameter flow measurement device.

industry. By altering the tube to a tapering section and inserting a float in the tube, the transformation to a *constant pressure, variable orifice flow meter* is complete. In this application, constant pressure caused by the weight of the bobbin is supported by the flowing gas that escapes through the orifice created by the annular gap between the bobbin and the tube wall. An algebraic expression for the upthrust on the bobbin by the gas flow is a function of annular cross-sectional area, gas density, gas viscosity, velocity gradient across the annulus and velocity squared (Hutton and Prys-Roberts 1994). The higher the flow, the higher up the tapered tube the bobbin is supported to allow the gas to escape through the widening annulus. As in an orifice, the flow here is turbulent and fluids of different densities, such as oxygen and helium, flow at different rates. When gas flows are lower and the bobbin sits lower in the tapered tube, the annular gap is more like a pipe than an orifice, and the flow is likely to be laminar. Under these conditions, the fluids with similar viscosities, such as oxygen and helium, will flow at similar rates. Therefore, Rotameter tubes are calibrated for specific gases at specified temperatures over a range of gas flow rates.

If the orifice flowmeter is evolved into a slightly different shape, it becomes a venturi, with a smooth transition in pipe diameter at the throat, as shown in Figure 7.4. The pressure at the throat is lower than the upstream pressure for the following reason: a fixed volume flow rate of fluid has a certain mean velocity upstream of the throat. For continuity, the mean velocity has to increase through the reduced cross-sectional area of the throat in order to maintain the same flow rate. The energy increase associated with that velocity change is kinetic energy, which has a velocity-squared term in it. For conservation of energy, an increase in kinetic energy is accompanied by a loss of potential energy (see Figure 3.9).

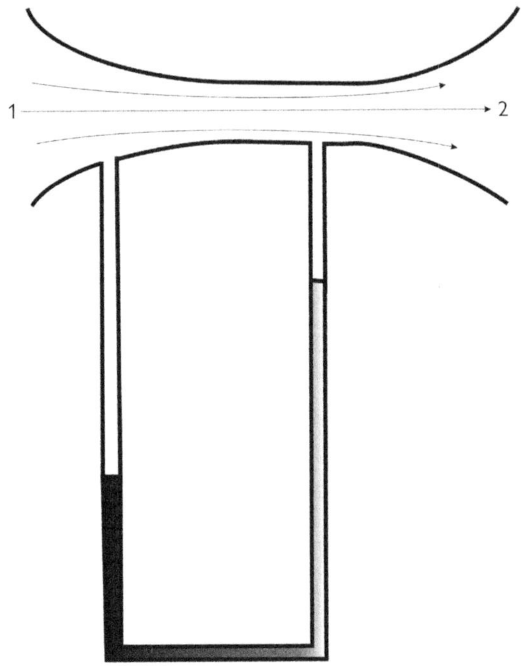


**Fig. 7.4** The Venturi flowmeter.

It was *Bernoulli* who explained that, for fluids, the hydraulic potential energy term is expressed as a pressure term, and because kinetic energy increases, the pressure decreases at the throat of the venturi. Bernoulli's equation, which should be thought of as a way of describing conservation of energy is:

$$\frac{P_1}{\rho}+\frac{v_1^2}{2}=\frac{P_2}{\rho}+\frac{v_2^2}{2}.$$

A venturi can be used as a flow meter like an orifice, but with greater accuracy, because the flow through it is more likely to be laminar with a linear relationship between pressure difference across it and the flow through it as predicted by Hagen–Poiseuille. It can be seen that, if a measurement of $(P_1 - P_2)$ is obtained from a manometer, this gives an equation for the two unknowns $v_1$ and $v_2$; the other equation is the continuity equation for flow rate $Q = A_1v_1 = A_2v_2$, where $v_1$ and $v_2$ are the velocities at cross-sectional areas $A_1$ and $A_2$ respectively of the venturi at 1 (entrance) and 2 (throat) of the venturi in Figure 7.4, giving $Q$. A venturi has other uses too; for example the pressure drop at the throat of a venturi can be used to entrain another fluid. This is the principle behind medical suction devices, or to

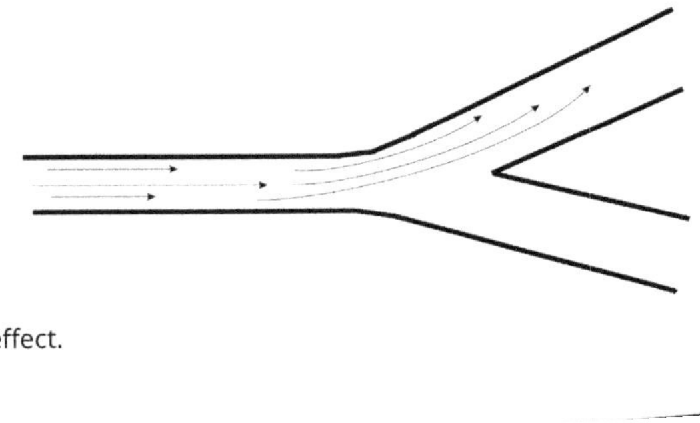

**Fig. 7.5** The Coanda effect.

provide patients with oxygen-enriched air to breathe, or as a means of ventilating a patient through an open bronchoscope. Another related application of the lowering of pressure in a narrowed section of a tube is the Coanda effect, shown in Figure 7.5. Where there is a branching of the tube downstream of the low pressure, the flow will tend to adhere to one wall rather than the other; this might be the reason for some causes of hypoxia, where some downstream alveoli are not supplied with gas; it can also be used as a fluidic valve mechanism to switch flows between inspiratory and expiratory ports in a ventilator (see Chapter 26).

When ultrasound is used to measure cardiac output (see Chapters 10 and 13), the ultrasound apparatus usually also produces a result for aortic gradient. It does this by measuring $v_2$ (the aortic velocity), assuming $v_1$ the mean velocity of blood in the ventricle is zero, and deduces $(P_1 - P_2)$ from Bernoulli's equation. In addition, the principle of a venturi is identical to the one describing lift over the curved surface of an aerofoil.

# Pressure

Atmospheric pressure is the pressure exerted on us by the air around us; the weight of the atmosphere above us, acted on by gravitational acceleration, means that it behaves like a pressurised container. The pressure in a pressurised container can also be stated in numbers of atmospheres. If the pressure in a cylinder is quoted as 5 ATA, this means it is 5 **AT**mospheres **A**bsolute, which means that the pressure inside the cylinder will be 4 atmospheres above atmospheric or 4 atmospheres gauge pressure. If the cylinder pressure is quoted as gauge pressure, then its absolute pressure is gauge pressure plus atmospheric pressure.

The numerical value of atmospheric pressure at mean sea level (m.s.l.) is 1.013 bar, or $1.013 \times 10^5$ Pa, or 101.3 kPa, or 760 mmHg on a mercury column, or about 10 m on a water column. A reasonable approximation of atmospheric pressure at m.s.l. is 100 kPa, which allows convenient calculation of partial pressures of components in gas mixtures from volume percentage concentrations using Dalton's law of partial pressures (see below).

Columns of liquid in closed tubes, with a vacuum above the fluid level (sometimes referred to as a Torricellian vacuum), are sometimes used to measure pressure. To deduce the expression for pressure in such a column, consider a column of fluid of height $h$, cross-sectional area $A$ and density $\rho$ as shown in Figure 7.6.

The volume of this fluid column is $A\,h$, and its mass is $\rho\,A\,h$. The force exerted by the fluid column at its base, is thus $\rho\,g\,A\,h$. As the figure shows, the base of the fluid column coincides with the surface of the surrounding reservoir, which is acted on by ambient pressure. This pressure can be calculated as the force exerted at the base of the column divided by the area of the column:

$$P = \frac{\rho g A h}{A}$$

or $P = \rho\,g\,h$ Nm$^{-2}$ (Pa), which is how we rather loosely refer to pressure as mmHg or cm $H_2O$. If a dimensional analysis is done on this expression (see Chapter 3 for principles), it will be seen that the units are those of pressure. Pressure difference is sometimes as useful a measurement as absolute values are, and this can be measured using a U-tube manometer, as for example in the venturi or orifice flow meters described above. In a manometer mercury is often the fluid used, and $\rho = 13.6 \times 10^3$ kg m$^{-3}$, $g = 9.81$ m s$^{-2}$. At m.s.l., $h = 0.760$ m (760 mm). These days, pressure is usually measured using an electronic transducer.

Therefore,

$$\begin{aligned}\text{pressure at m.s.l.} &= 13.6 \times 10^3 \times 9.81 \times 0.760 \\ &= 1.013 \times 10^5\,\text{Nm}^{-2} \\ &= 101.3\ \text{kPa}.\end{aligned}$$

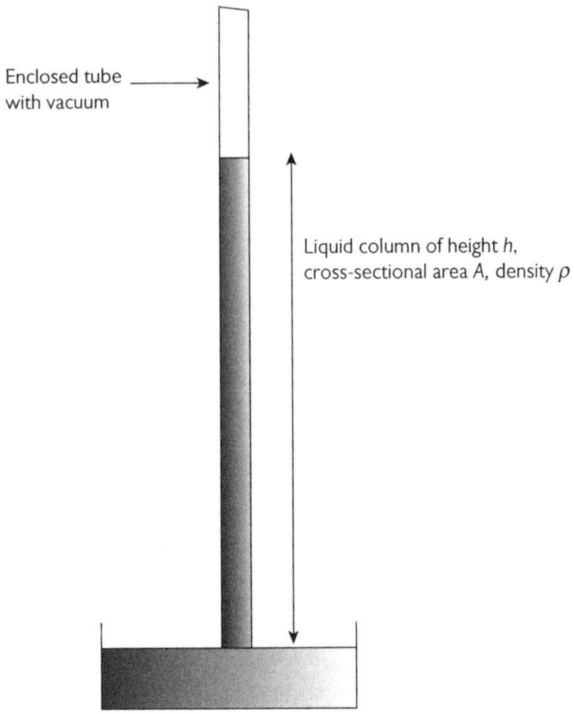


**Fig. 7.6** A column of fluid used to measure pressure.

## *Hypobaric and hyperbaric atmospheres*

To further illustrate concepts of pressure, consider changes in ambient pressure. Air is compressible, and its density diminishes with altitude, making the variation in pressure with altitude a non-linear relationship. The situation is further complicated by the fact that in the troposphere at least (the lowest part of the atmosphere with which we are most familiar), there is a linear temperature change of -6° $C.km^{-1}$ increase in altitude (in aviation this is often quoted as -2°C per 1000 ft of altitude). At the cruising height of commercial aircraft of 10 000 m, the ambient pressure is approximately one quarter that at m.s.l. (25 kPa). The alveolar gas equation (West 1979) states that, to an approximation

$$P_{alveolarO_2} = P_{inspiredO_2} - \frac{P_{CO_2}}{R},$$

where $R$ is the respiratory quotient,

$$P_{inspiredO_2} = F_{iO_2} \cdot (P_{ambientO_2} - S.V.P._{H_2O,37C}),$$

where $S.V.P._{H2O,37C}$ is the saturated vapour pressure of water at body temperature, 6.3 kPa, and does not vary with altitude, only temperature (see Chapters 8 and 9). At 10 000 m altitude,

$$P_{inspiredO_2} = 0.21 \times (25 - 6.3)\text{KPa}$$

$$= 3.7\text{KPa}.$$

Clearly the $P_{CO_2}$ will be driven down by the resulting hypoxaemia, but the physiological situation is one of extreme hypoxia in the alveoli, likely to lead rapidly to loss of consciousness and even death. Furthermore, the ambient temperature at this altitude is -50°C, and is itself a threat to life.

To counteract the possibility of hypoxia, aviators breathe oxygen in increasing fractional concentration with increasing altitude. This continues to be beneficial up to 11 000 m altitude, at which point breathing 100% oxygen at that ambient pressure gives the same alveolar oxygen partial pressure as breathing air at m.s.l. Above this height $P_{alveolarO_2}$ falls further unless the oxygen is breathed through a pressurised mask, a sort of aviators' CPAP (continuous positive airway pressure).

Atmospheric pressure continues to increase below ground level, such that it is 270 mbar greater than that at m.s.l. at the bottom of a 2 km mineshaft. The physiological danger here is one of nitrogen loading, and the dissolving of nitrogen in body tissues rather than hypoxia, and this is discussed in detail in Chapter 9 on solubility.

## Partial pressure

Assume that a container of volume $V$ contains compressed air, which is a mixture by volume of one part oxygen and four parts nitrogen (20% and 80%, respectively), and has a pressure of 5 bar (Figure 7.7). Assume that the $O_2$ and $N_2$ constituents are separated, stored separately, and then put back into the volume $V$ sequentially and separately. If the pressure of each of these components were measured in turn, they would be respectively $P_{O_2} = 1$ bar and $P_{N_2} = 4$ bar, and these are the partial pressures of the constituents of a mixture of gases. In this case $P_{O2} + P_{N2} = P_T$, the total pressure.

*Dalton's law of partial pressures* states that in such a mixture of gases, each gas exerts the same partial pressure within the mixture as if it alone occupied the whole volume of the mixture, and the sum of partial pressures of the constituents equals the total pressure of the mixture. Moreover, the ratio of partial pressures of the constituents to the total pressure in the container equals the ratio of partial volume to total volume. Put algebraically, if a gas mixture consists of gas components a, b, c, ... $n$, then,

$$P_a + P_b + P_c + \dots + P_n = P_{\text{Total}}$$

and, applying Boyle's law (see Chapter 8),

$$\frac{V_i}{V_T} = \frac{P_i}{P_T},$$

where $i$ = a, b, c, ... $n$.

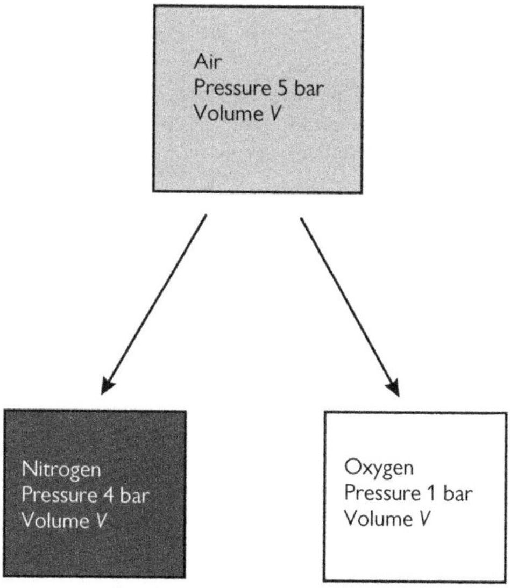


**Fig. 7.7** Dalton's law of partial pressures (see text for explanation).

Thus by Dalton's law of partial pressures, the atmosphere, which is composed of 21% oxygen and 78% nitrogen by volume, therefore contains an oxygen partial pressure of about 21 kPa and a nitrogen partial pressure of about 78 kPa, the difference between the sum of these two partial pressures and atmospheric pressure (101 kPa) being due to the presence of argon.

The concept of partial pressure is important for a number of reasons, not least because the anaesthetic or metabolic effect of a gas depends on its partial pressure rather than its concentration (see Chapter 9, concerning vaporiser output at altitude).

## Diffusion

Molecules in liquids, and to a greater extent those in gases, are sufficiently far apart with enough kinetic energy that they move randomly and widely in the space available. Such motility allows the mixing of two families of molecules (say oxygen and nitrous oxide, or two different concentrations of saline), initially separated by a barrier that may be simply an intervening medium or it may be a semipermeable membrane. The mixing, or diffusion, can occur up to the point where the species are evenly mixed. A molecular transfer process takes place between two gas mixtures or species across an intervening medium or a membrane, such as the alveolar-capillary membrane, or within the alveolus itself. The rate of diffusion depends on the concentration gradient across the medium or the membrane and, as indicated in the previous section, this really means partial pressure difference when a gas is being considered, or concentration gradient in the case of liquid diffusion (see Figure 7.8).

The greater the concentration difference of a substance between two parts of a container, whether or not separated by a membrane, the greater the rate of diffusion per unit area from a higher to lower concentration regions, and this applies even if the membrane separates two different media, e.g. a gas mixture and blood in the case of the alveolar-capillary membrane. This is *Fick's law of diffusion*, which also says that the rate of diffusion is directly proportional to the membrane area and inversely proportional to its thickness. Note that as the molecular species diffuses, the concentration or partial pressure gradient diminishes and so does the rate of diffusion. Clinical examples include oxygen and carbon dioxide diffusion across the alveolar membrane in opposite directions. As discussed in an earlier section, bulk transport of a fluid takes place along a pressure gradient. Diffusion, or molecular transport, can occur without the presence of a global pressure gradient if the concentration gradient or partial pressure gradient of the individual species exists as shown in Figure 7.8. If a semi-permeable membrane

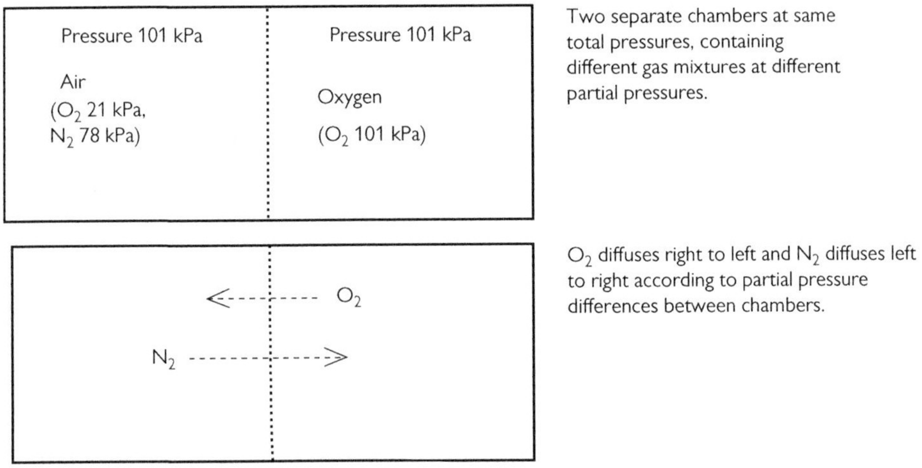


**Fig. 7.8** Diffusion of fluids depends on the partial pressure difference.

separates two different groups of molecules at equal pressures, and the membrane is permeable to both groups, diffusion can occur across the membrane. Such semi-permeable membranes vary in both their absolute permeability to and their rates of diffusion of different substances.

It will be recalled that the diffusion capacity of the lung is tested using carbon monoxide, as the diffusion of this gas across the alveolar-capillary membrane is the rate-limiting step for the uptake of this particular gas. Another clinical example of diffusion is the risk of diffusion hypoxia following an anaesthetic, which includes a significant concentration of nitrous oxide; following a nitrous oxide anaesthetic there is a diffusion gradient for $N_2O$ from the tissues to the lungs; if a patient is breathing air, 78% of which is nitrogen, there is a diffusion gradient for $N_2$ from the lungs into the tissues; however, $N_2$ is less soluble than $N_2O$ in tissues, which means the predominant diffusion is by $N_2O$ from the tissues into the lungs, which displaces $N_2$ from the lungs and its accompanying oxygen. For the same reason, we avoid the use of $N_2O$ in patients with body spaces containing nitrogen (air), such as a pneumothorax. Solubility of gases in liquids is another important topic in relation to the behaviour of gases and liquids, particularly in relation to altering diffusion gradients, and will be discussed in another section.

There is another aspect that governs the rate of diffusion and that is the size of the molecules. Bigger molecules diffuse more slowly than smaller ones. *Graham's law of diffusion* states that the rate of diffusion of a gas is inversely proportional to the square root of either its density or its molecular weight.

## Osmosis

Imagine a semi-permeable membrane separating two families of molecules (perhaps a glucose solution and water), which is permeable to one (say water but not glucose). Water diffuses across the membrane and dilutes the glucose solution until the hydrostatic pressure on that side of the container has risen to a level higher than that on the water side of the membrane, as shown in Figure 7.9. This hydrostatic pressure difference prevents further diffusion of water across the membrane, and is called the osmotic pressure. The process of water diffusion is called osmosis in this context.

The generation of an osmotic pressure depends on the number of particles in a solution, and their size does not matter, assuming the membrane is not permeable to them. An NaCl solution has $Na^+$ and $Cl^-$ ions, two ions in solution per molecule of solute, and therefore has twice the osmotic power of, say, a glucose molecule, which does not dissociate, but is a much larger molecule. A 0.5 molar solution of NaCl has the same osmotic power as a 1 molar solution of glucose. One mole of a substance which does not dissociate, dissolved in 22.4 L of solvent, exerts an osmotic pressure of 1 bar gauge pressure (this is a corollary of Avogadro's hypothesis) (Davis and Kenny 2003). The term 'osmolarity' is used to describe the potential for exerting osmotic pressure because of the different types of molecules that exist in the body fluid compartments, each with a different degree of osmotic potential. The osmolarity of the plasma, the interstitium and most other body fluids is around 300 milliosmol $L^{-1}$, and we give intravenous fluids that are isotonic (with equal osmolarity) to avoid fluid shifts by diffusion between, say, the circulation and the extracellular or intracellular space. The plasma also contains large molecule proteins; these contribute only a small proportion of the osmotic pressure of the plasma, the majority being due to electrolytes; the capillary membrane is impermeable to protein but not to electrolytes, so protein molecules form the osmotic pressure to drive water molecules into the plasma, sometimes referred to as 'oncotic pressure'. At the arteriolar end of the tissue microcirculation the intravascular hydrostatic pressure usually exceeds oncotic pressure so that fluid loss to the tissues occurs; at the venular end of the tissue microcirculation, the intravascular hydrostatic pressure is exceeded by the oncotic pressure, and tissue fluid returns to the circulation. Osmotic pressure within the renal tubules governs the way the kidney handles water and electrolytes.

The term *osmolality* is often used rather than osmolarity, and is defined as millimol solute per kg of solvent (rather than millimol per litre of solution); this is preferred because it avoids the need to consider volume changes in solutions due to temperature change. When icy roads are gritted, the presence of particles in the water lowers the freezing point of water by 1.86°C for each milliosmol per kg of water. Osmolality, usually of urine or plasma, is measured using the same principle of freezing point

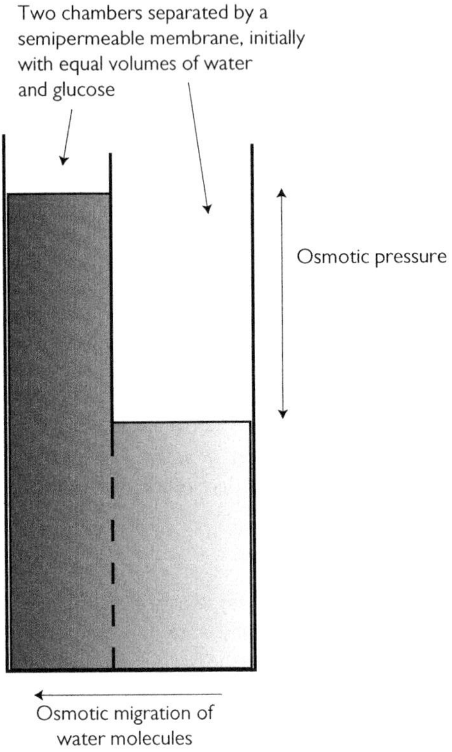


**Fig. 7.9** Osmosis and osmotic pressure.

depression in an osmometer. This device allows a few ml of solution to be collected in a container while being cooled and stirred; initially, the temperature falls below the freezing point (supercooling) until the freezing process starts in the water of one part of the solution; stirring allows the freezing process to spread throughout the solution, during which the temperature rises to the value that is the freezing point for the solution.

Dissolving such a solute in a solvent and raising its osmotic pressure also reduces the vapour pressure of the solvent, and this is *Raoult's law*. This is thought to be because the presence of the solute molecules reduces the surface area of the solvent at its surface to allow them to vaporise, thereby reducing the vapour pressure (Davis and Kenny 2003) (see Chapter 9); the corollary of this is that the boiling point of the solution is raised.

## *References*

**Davis, P. D.** and **Kenny, G. N. C.** (2003) *Basic Physics and Measurement in Anaesthesia*, 5th edn, Butterworth Heinemann, Edinburgh, pp. 75–85.

**Hutton, P.** and **Prys-Roberts, C.** (eds) (1994) *Monitoring in Anaesthesia and Intensive Care*, WB Saunders, London, p. 186.

**Massey, B. S.** (1970) *Mechanics of Fluids*, 2nd edn, Van Nostrand Reinhold, London.

**West, J. B.** (1979) *Respiratory Physiology, the Essentials*, 2nd edn, Williams and Wilkins, Baltimore, p. 67.

# Chapter 8 **Thermodynamics: heat, temperature and humidification**

The chapter links with: Chapters 1, 7, 9 and 14.

## Introduction

In continuing the concepts of energy and work, heat is a form of energy, and heat and work are related by the laws of thermodynamics. The first law states that the amount of mechanical work achievable out of a thermodynamic system going through a cyclic process is proportional to the amount of heat put into it. The second law states that the amount of work gained from the system is always less than the amount of heat put into it; in other words there is some energy wasted. Heating a substance gives its constituent molecules increased kinetic energy, which can be put to mechanical use, for example, in driving a turbine. Such an increase in energy either raises the temperature of the substance or changes its state. Its increasing energy causes the increasing velocity of movement of molecules and eventually breaks intermolecular bonds, giving the molecules more freedom of movement. As characteristic temperatures are reached, e.g. melting point or boiling point, the energy increase goes into changing the substance's state into a more energetic one, e.g. solid to liquid, or liquid to gas, without any associated temperature change. Loss of heat from a substance involves the reverse processes. The gas laws have their origin in this concept of the kinetic theory of gases, and are an inherent part of consideration of the effects of heating and cooling, compression and expansion of gases.

## The gas laws

Pressure has been defined in Chapter 7, but to understand the concept, one that is taken for granted, it is necessary to start with the idea of molecules of matter undergoing a change in momentum (for the definition of momentum, see Chapter 3). It is unnecessary here to deduce the following equation, but the proof can be found in any physics or engineering text (e.g. Dorrington 1989)

$$PV = \frac{Nmv^2}{3}$$

is the equation based on the molecular theory of gases from which a concept of pressure $P$ (force/area) is derived. $V$ is the gas volume, $N$ is a constant referring to the number of molecules of gas, and all other terms are as used previously; a constant mass of gas is assumed. Notice that both sides of this equation contain energy terms: pressure × volume on the left-hand side, and a kinetic energy term on the right-hand side. This expression suggests that pressure is inversely proportional to gas volume, directly proportional to total mass and to the square of molecular velocity. Conceptually, doubling the velocity doubles the momentum changes, but it also doubles the number of intermolecular collisions, hence the squared relationship to pressure. Molecular kinetic energy is a function of temperature (absolute temperature, measured in Kelvin). Thus, at constant temperature: $PV$ = constant, and this is Boyle's law.

Each $P$–$V$ curve corresponds to a constant value of $T$ (an isotherm) for a fixed temperature and two points on the same curve can be thought of as being governed by the same rectangular hyperbola, i.e. $P_1V_1 = P_2V_2$; these changes are isothermal (constant temperature) by definition. The graphical relationship between $P$ and $V$ is shown in Figure 8.1(a). Under these conditions the equation may be used to work out the volume of gas released ($V_2$) at atmospheric pressure ($P_2$ = 1 bar) from a cylinder of known

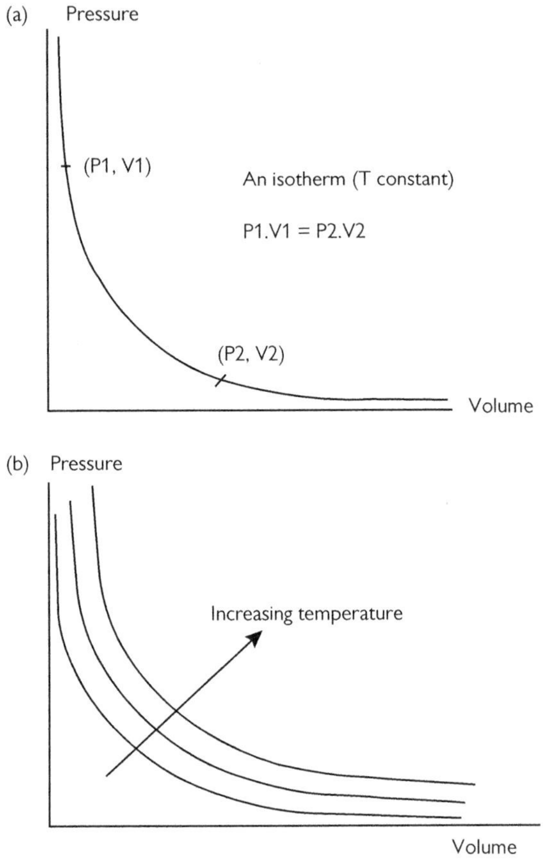


**Fig. 8.1** $PV = nRT$: (a) showing a single isotherm ($T$ constant). (b) showing several curves, each corresponding to a value of $T$.

size (size $E$, $V_1 = 5$ L), whose contents are stored at known pressure ($P_1 = 138$ bar absolute). A family of $P$-$V$ curves for different values of $T$ may be drawn and usefully used to illustrate the gas's behaviour for a range of temperatures and this is shown in Figure 8.1(b). It can be seen that, for increasing temperature, the curves become shifted upwards to the right, suggesting increased thermal energy as indicated by increased area under the $P$-$V$ curves. Under these conditions the combined gas law is sometimes written as $PV = nRT$, with each curve corresponding to a different value of $T$, where $n$ is the number of moles of gas, $R$ is the universal gas constant and $T$ is the temperature in Kelvin.

Just as Boyle's law assumes constant temperature, there are other conditions that can be preset, and the gas law can be expressed differently. For example:

at constant pressure, $V = \text{constant}_1 \times T$ and this is Charles' law;

at constant volume, $P = \text{constant}_2 \times T$ and this is Gay-Lussac's law.

Each of these represents a straight line relationship between temperature and either volume or pressure, and these are shown in Figures 8.2(a) and 8.2(b). It is noted that the lines indicate zero values of volume and pressure at a temperature of −273°C, where the gas is presumed to have no kinetic energy. This was when the concept of *absolute zero* of temperature was first recognised and from which the Kelvin temperature scale evolved.

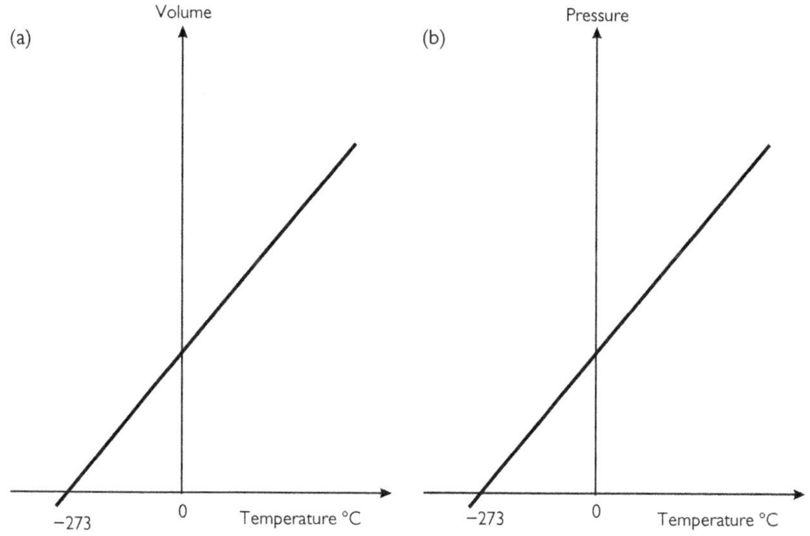


**Fig. 8.2** Graphical representations of (a) Charles' law and (b) Gay–Lussac's law.

As indicated above, the combined gas law is often expressed as $PV = nRT$, and another way of expressing this is:

$$\frac{P_1V_1}{T_1} = \frac{P_2V_2}{T_2}.$$

This equation is used to calculate changes in conditions of a perfect gas when heated or cooled, or expanded or compressed. We usually think of such changes as being isothermal, when $T_1 = T_2$. It must be remembered that temperature is calculated in K (Kelvin) (K = °C + 273) when the gas laws are being utilised. Gases can have energy applied to them in different ways. Rapid compression of a gas results in molecules being forced together without adequate time for heat exchange to occur, and they are unable to move adequately fast for their particular level of energy, and so the energy is converted into thermal energy as a temperature rise; such compression is termed *adiabatic*. If the compression is applied slowly enough, the excess thermal energy is dissipated to the environment outside the container, the temperature rise is minimal or zero, and the compression is isothermal.

If, instead of compressing the gas, heat is applied, then if the volume of the container is kept constant the pressure will rise. Alternatively, the volume of the container may be allowed to increase by way of a piston, such that the pressure remains constant. Under these different scenarios, the pathway of pressure and volume that a gas follows will differ depending on the circumstances indicated.

A perfect gas is one that is assumed to behave in a way described above, with perfectly elastic collisions between molecules and container walls, with no intermolecular forces of attraction, and the size of molecules being negligible. However, a real gas is not a perfect gas under all circumstances, but there are, for example, times when a vapour behaves like a gas. Deviations start to occur from the rectangular hyperbolic relationship between $P$ and $V$ of a perfect gas towards the bottom left hand corner of the curve, close to where the axes meet as shown in Figure 8.3; in other words, at low volumes, low pressures and low temperatures (these are context sensitive terms depending on the substance being considered), where cool, slow moving gas molecules are compressed initially into a vapour, then into a liquid, when the volume shrinks dramatically as the molecules coalesce, then becomes incompressible as a liquid, when the pressure rises rapidly.

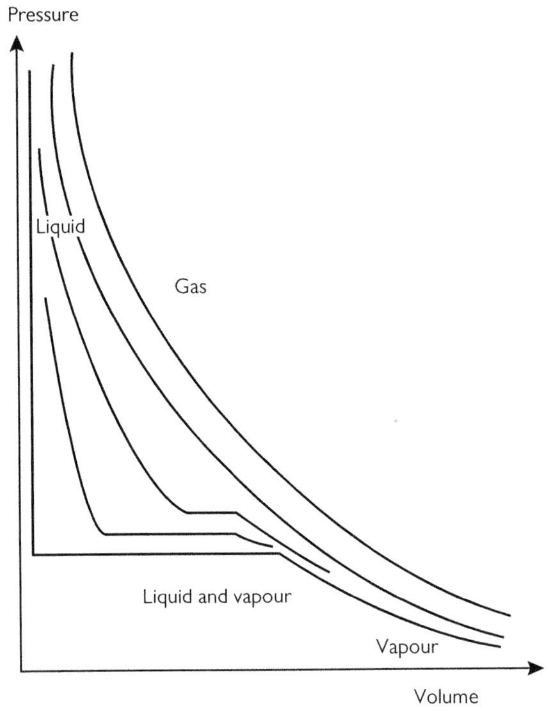


**Fig. 8.3** The extreme bottom left-hand corner of the pressure–volume curve of Figure 8.1.

From this position, if the substance is heated to a higher temperature and the volume is allowed to expand, it is still possible to subsequently re-compress the molecules into a liquid. However, if the temperature of the substance is raised beyond a particular point, called the *critical temperature* for that substance, i.e. to a *P–V* curve displaced upwards and to the right, then no matter how much compression occurs, it cannot be re-liquefied. The substance has too much thermal energy for compression to result in the coalescence of fast-moving molecules into a liquid. The substance can be considered to be a gas rather than a vapour above this critical temperature. Oxygen is thought of as a gas under most circumstances because its critical temperature is low, –116°C. Water, on the other hand, has a critical temperature of 374.1°C, so it is difficult to experience water in its high-energy state as anything other than steam (a vapour, not a gas). Nitrous oxide has a critical temperature of 36.5°C, which may be close to room temperature in some climates. The *critical pressure* is the pressure needed to liquefy a substance at just below its critical temperature.

*Sublimation* occurs when a substance goes straight from the solid state to the vapour state without going through the liquid state. This can occur, for example, with water under very low pressures, and is used to carry metabolic heat from an astronaut's life support system to the ambient vacuum. The *triple point* of a substance occurs when solid, liquid and vapour states of a substance are in equilibrium, as discussed below in relation to water.

## Specific heat capacity

The specific heat of a substance in J $kg^{-1}{}^{\circ}C^{-1}$, is the quantity of heat required to raise 1 kg of the substance through a temperature rise of 1°C. Different substances have different specific heats and in general solids and liquids have higher specific heats than gases, which means they need more heat energy to raise their temperature by a given amount.

Another way of thinking about specific heat is the amount of work done on 1 kg of a substance to raise its temperature by 1°C. Since work can be done on a gas, either by keeping pressure constant or volume constant, specific heats for gases are quoted under these two conditions respectively and are known as $C_p$ and $C_v$. While the gas law *P.V = constant* for isothermal processes is usually used, the law $PV^{\gamma} = constant$, where $\gamma = C_p/C_v$ is used under less well defined thermodynamic processes. For air $C_p = 1.00$ J kg$^{-1}$ °C$^{-1}$, $C_v = 0.714$ J kg$^{-1}$ °C$^{-1}$.

# Latent heats of vaporisation and of crystallisation

The amount of heat required to increase the energy of a fluid to change its state from liquid to vapour without any temperature change is called the *latent heat of vaporisation*. At the other end of the spectrum, involving a change of state, latent *heat of crystallisation* is liberated with no temperature change when a substance crystallises or freezes from a liquid to a solid state. Likewise, the same heat has to be supplied to ensure melting from solid to liquid state with no temperature change.

# Temperature

Temperature is that property by which we may quantify the heat energy of a substance. Heating up a solid, liquid or gas gives their molecules increased kinetic energy, and this results in a temperature rise. Thus, a temperature change is the effect of heating or cooling a body. The section on the gas laws above has already described how temperature change can occur due to pressure and volume changes under *adiabatic* conditions, where no additional heat is exchanged with the gas, and under *isothermal* conditions, where the process occurs slowly enough that temperature remains constant. The same pressure and volume changes can be achieved by heat supply. The S.I. unit of heat is the same as that of energy, namely J, although the kilocal or Calorie is still sometimes used, where 1 Calorie = 4.186 kJ.

The temperature scale used almost everywhere except USA is °C (after Anders Celsius, 1742, or the centigrade scale), chosen because under standard conditions water freezes at 0°C and boils at 100°C. However, gas law calculations require the use of the Kelvin scale of temperature (after Lord Kelvin, 1848), where 0 K= –273°C, *absolute zero*, and one degree change Kelvin equals one degree change Celsius. This can be deduced by plotting volume against temperature (Charles' law), or pressure against temperature (Gay-Lussac's law), as shown in Figure 8.2, and extrapolating to where volume or pressure reach zero. The Kelvin scale was adopted as an international temperature scale in 1954, and used to be defined on a fixed point of physical equilibrium of the triple point of water (where the triple point is defined as the conditions under which solid, liquid and vapour phases are all in equilibrium). This definition changed in 2019, since when the Kelvin temperature scale has been based on the value of the Boltzmann constant, which relates the amount of thermodynamic energy in a substance to its temperature. The Kelvin is defined as the SI unit of temperature with the Boltzmann constant fixed at exactly $1.380649 \times 10^{-23}$ J K$^{-1}$ (Sullivan and Spencer 2022).

The difference in temperature between the ice point for water and the steam point is still 100 units, which makes the range almost identical with the previous empirical Celsius scale. Almost identical but not precisely, because this scale has its datum at 273.15 K, i.e. 0.01 K below the triple point of water. It is usual to denote 273.15 K as 0°C.

The temperature at which human metabolic processes work most efficiently is 37°C. If an anaesthetist allows the patient's temperature to fall intraoperatively, there are physiological consequences.

## Thermometry

Traditionally temperature was measured by the mercury in a glass thermometer, where mercury expands with heating and rises in a glass column on a linear scale, with a maximum operational range of −39°C (the freezing point of mercury) to 250°C (Machin *et al.* 2021). The use of mercury is no longer permitted due to toxicity. An alternative liquid is alcohol, with a maximum operational range between −117°C and 78°C. Mercury is very dense and covers a wide range of temperatures, while alcohol is less dense and expands the scale of measurement over a small range of temperatures.

The thermistor is a semiconductor device whose electrical resistance (or other measurable electrical property) usually decreases with temperature rise, more or less linearly (when it forms one arm of a Wheatstone bridge) over a reasonable temperature range. It is certainly adequate for measuring body temperature, and forms the functional basis of the tympanic membrane thermometer and can be used for measuring naso-pharyngeal temperature (Roth and Braitman 2008).

The thermocouple is a device consisting of two strips of dissimilar metals, connected together at both ends, each end being immersed in a fluid at a different temperature; one is likely to be a reference temperature of 0°C. This arrangement forms an electrolytic cell, and the *Seebeck effect*, important in the thermocouple function, is the induction of a voltage (and subsequently a current), proportional to the difference in temperature between the two junctions; the relationship between temperature difference and induced voltage is a nonlinear one.

Other eponymous effects in relation to heat include:

*Joule effect*: the heating effect of an electrical conductor when current flows through it.

*Peltier effect*: when electrical current is passed through a single junction of two dissimilar metals, heat is released or absorbed, depending on the direction of current flow.

*Thompson effect*: the liberation or absorption of heat caused by the passage of electrical current along a conductor with a temperature gradient.

## Heat transfer

Patients gain and lose heat by convection, conduction, radiation, vaporisation in the respiratory tract and in sweat (Allan 1995).

### *Convection*

Convection is heat transfer through a fluid medium such as air or water. This occurs because the warmer molecules change their position within the fluid, for example, by floating to the top while cooler ones sink.

### *Conduction*

Conduction is heat transfer through a solid medium. If a metal object is heated at one end, this heat is transferred towards the other end as a result of the temperature gradient between the ends. This occurs because thermal energy is transferred between neighbouring atoms.

### *Radiative heat loss*

Radiation from bodies, to different extents emit, absorb, reflect or refract electromagnetic energy, depending on temperature and the nature of their surface. Such energy includes light waves and also heat as infrared waves. The human loses between 40% and 70% of body heat by radiation.

### *Vaporisation*

In the respiratory tract body heat is given up to body water as latent heat of vaporisation, which results in vaporisation of respiratory tract water, which carries heat away. The same applies when sweat is produced and vaporised by surface body heat.

# Keeping patients warm

Operative surgery and anaesthesia usually involves heat loss from the patient, through exposed tissue, vasodilatation, cold intravenous fluid administration, and cold anaesthetic gas ventilation. Anaesthesia also attenuates the efficiency of the patient's thermoregulatory system mediated through the hypothalamus. Therefore it is important that conductive heat loss is not made worse by laying the patient on a highly conducting surface, or convective heat loss is not worsened by placing the patient in a circulation of cold air. Since the patient's physiological well-being depends on maintaining a core temperature of 37°C, active steps have to be taken to keep the patient warm, particularly the critically ill (Faulds and Meekings 2013).

Forced warm air blankets are now used to cover the patient as far as surgical access will allow. The air temperature is maintained between 32 and 38°C and it is pumped into channels in a thin-walled plastic blanket. This reduces the convective temperature gradient and accompanying heat loss, and also acts as a radiative reflective surface. The blankets have proved to be a very efficient means of warming the patient (Stanger *et al.* 2009). A conductive heat pad has also been re-introduced as an intraoperative heating device, but has been found to be less effective than forced air warming (Leung *et al.* 2007).

Intravenous fluids are warmed by passing the fluid giving set through some form of heat exchanger. This can be achieved by wrapping the coils of an extension of the giving set around a heater or putting them inside a heating device. Alternatively, the giving set extension is formed as a coaxial pair of tubes, through the inner one of which passes the fluid intended for intravenous administration, and through the outer one of which circulates warmed water. It is also possible to use a conductive heat exchanger that applies a heating element directly to the fluid channels (Turner *et al.* 2006).

As indicated in the section on low-flow breathing systems (Chapter 25), breathing gas can be warmed and humidified by the use of a heat and moisture exchanger, described next. Furthermore, the use of low anaesthetic gas flows reduces the heat loss through that route and the chemical process of $CO_2$ absorption by 'Soda Lime' is exothermic.

## *Humidity and humidification*

Air that is totally saturated with water vapour at a given temperature is said to be fully saturated, or to have a relative humidity of 100%. The absolute humidity is the number of gram of water per cubic metre of air, or mg $l^{-1}$. At 37°C a fully saturated sample of air (100% humidity) has an absolute humidity of 44 mg $l^{-1}$. This mass of saturated water vapour can be shown by the gas laws to have an associated vapour pressure (its SVP) of 6.3 kPa (47mmHg). A relative humidity (r.h.) of 50% implies half of this mass of water vapour and also a partial pressure of water vapour at this temperature of half the SVP, so relative humidity can also be described as the ratio of the vapour pressure of the sample to the SVP at that temperature. As air cools, the SVP of the water vapour falls. This means the air is able to contain less water vapour, so the relative humidity increases for a given water content. It also means that water condenses out of the air as its temperature falls. As the air is reheated, the SVP of water rises and the water evaporates again.

The wet and dry bulb hygrometer, which can be used to measure humidity, consists of a pair of thermometers, the bulb of one of which is covered in water-soaked cloth. Evaporation of the water results in a fall in temperature of the said thermometer, at a rate that depends on the humidity of the surrounding air, being greater at lower humidity. The difference between the temperature readings of the two thermometers is related to the relative humidity and is read off a table.

Natural humidification occurs when inspired air or gas is heated by the respiratory tract itself. The heating of the air gives greater water vapour carrying capacity. At the same time evaporation of water from the mucosal surface of the respiratory tract increasingly humidifies the air, increasing the water vapour pressure until the SVP for water is reached at body temperature $P_s$, namely 6.3 kPa (47 mmHg) at 37°C. The air is now fully saturated (100% humidity) at that temperature.

Where the ambient pressure $P_{amb}$ is 101 kPa, the fractional concentration of water vapour is:

$$\frac{P_s}{P_{amb}} = \frac{6.3}{101} = 6.2\%, \text{ equivalent to 44 mg l}^{-1}.$$

At 21°C, fully saturated air contains water vapour at 2.5 kPa (19 mmHg), equivalent to 2.4% or 18 mg $l^{-1}$.

Humidification is important in the operating room; a minimum of 50% r.h. is required to ensure electrical antistatic precautions. Within the respiratory tract, it is important to have adequate humidification to avoid drying of secretions, particularly in the small airways of small patients. Secretions can also block the endotracheal tube. There is also considerable heat loss from the patient in breathing in cold, dry gas. Body heat can be lost at the rate of 18 W if high-flow breathing systems are used, delivering cold, dry respiratory gas to the patient. It is therefore highly desirable to heat the gas to body temperature or slightly above, and to humidify it to 100%.

## *Humidification systems*

Older systems were designed to pass a proportion of the breathing gas over the surface of warm water. In the inspiratory tube, the humidified gas cools, and some of the water vapour condenses, releasing the heat of condensation; this minimises the heat loss from the inspired gas. The system was relatively complex and needed different design constraints for small bore or longer tubing, or different gas flow rates if inefficiency or scalding were to be avoided (Harrison *et al.* 1993).

The importance of humidification is recognised as important for almost every patient nowadays (McNulty and Eyre 2015). Modern devices are simple heat and moisture exchangers (HME), in which porous material absorbs heat from the exhaled gas, allowing water to condense out and be stored in or adjacent to the porous material. When the patient inhales, the heat is returned to the incoming gas, and the condensate evaporates. The work of breathing in some of them can be increased when they are wet (Hedley and Allt-Graham 1994), the need for an HME is less in low flow anaesthesia than in high flow (Henriksson *et al.* 1997) and the presence of an HME can hinder anaesthetic gas flow (Da Fonseca *et al.* 2000). It has been found that the use of an HME during surgery can maintain the patient's humidity, but not necessarily prevent a fall in body temperature, even at low fresh gas flows (Johansson *et al.* 2003). Indeed, all intubated patients should have an HME at all times except for minimal fresh gas flows (Braz *et al.* 2017).

Nebulisers are used to produce small liquid droplets, either to humidify or to deliver medication to the respiratory tract. They can be of three types:

- gas-driven nebulisers consist of a gas jet delivered through a venturi, which draws water from a capillary in the low-pressure region just beyond the venturi. The droplets then hit an anvil, which breaks them up into microdroplets of 2–4 μm diameter;
- spinning disc nebulisers allow microdroplets to be formed from larger droplets being broken up by the centrifugal force of a spinning disc;
- an ultrasonic nebuliser allows water to be dropped on to an ultrasonic transducer head, vibrating at, say, 3 MHz, producing 1–2 m droplets (Al-Shaikh and Stacey 2002).

## *References*

**Allan, J. R.** (1995) The thermal environment and human heat exchange, Chapter 16 in *Aviation Medicine*, 2nd edn, Butterworth Heinemann, Oxford, pp. 219–34.

**Al-Shaikh, B.** and **Stacey, S.** (2002) *Essentials of Anaesthetic Equipment*, 2nd edn, Churchill Livingstone, London, pp. 106–7.

**Braz, J. R. C., Braz, M. G., Hayashi, Y.** ***et al.*** (2017) The effect of different fresh gas flows, with and without a heat and moisture exchanger on inhaled gas humidity in adults undergoing general anaesthesia; a systematic review and meta-analysis of randomized controlled trials. *Eur. J. Anaesthesiol.*, **34**(8), pp. 515–25.

**Da Fonseca, J. M. G., Wheeler, D. W.** and **Pook, J. A. R.** (2000) The effect of a heat and moisture exchanger on gas flow in a Mapleson F breathing system during inhalational induction, *Anaesthesia*, **55**, pp. 571–73.

**Dorrington, K. L.** (1989) *Anaesthetic and Extracorporeal Gas Transfer*, Medical Engineering Series, Oxford Science Publications, Oxford, pp. 4–7.

**Faulds, M.**, and **Meekings, T.** (2013) Temperature management in critically ill patients, *BJA CEACCP*, **13**(3), pp. 75–9.

**Harrison, D. A., Breen, D. P., Harris, N. D.** and **Gerrish, S. P.** (1993) Performance of two IC humidifiers at high gas flows, *Anaesthesia*, **48**, pp. 902–5.

**Hedley, R. M.** and **Allt-Graham, J.** (1994) Heat and moisture exchangers and breathing filters, *Br. J. Anaesth.*, **73**, pp. 227–36.

**Henriksson, B-Å., Sundling, J.** and **Hellman, A.** (1997) The effect of a heat and moisture exchanger on humidity in low flow anaesthesia, *Anaesthesia*, **52**, pp. 144–9.

**Johansson, A., Lundberg, D., and Luttrop, H. H.** (2003) The effect of a heat and moisture exchanger on humidity and body temperature in a low-flow anaesthesia system, *Acta Anaesthesiol. Scand.*, **47**, pp. 564–8.

**Leung, K. K., Lai, A. and Wu, A.** (2007) A randomized controlled trial of the electric heating pad vs. forced air warming for preventing hypothermia during laparotomy, *Anaesthesia*, **62**, pp. 605–8.

**Machin, G., Brettle, D., Fleming, S. *et al.*** (2021) Is current body temperature measurement fit for purpose? *J. Med. Eng & Technol.*, **45**(2), pp. 136–44.

**McNulty, G.** and **Eyre, L.** (2015) Humidification in anaesthesia and critical care, *BJA Educ.*, **15**(3), pp. 131–5.

**Roth, J. V. and Braitman, L. E.** (2008) Nasal temperature can be used as a reliable surrogate measure of core temperature, *J. Clin. Monit. Comput.*, **22**, pp. 309–314.

**Stanger, R.** *et al.* (2009) Predicting the efficacy of convection warming in anaesthetised children, *Br. J. Anaes.*, **103**, pp. 275–82.

**Sullivan, G. and Spencer, M.** (2022) Heat and temperature, *BJA Educ.*, **22**(9), pp. 350–6.

**Turner, M., Hodzovic, I. and Mapleson, W. W.** (2006) Simulated clinical evaluation of four fluid warming devices, *Anaesthesia*, **61**, pp. 571–5.

# Chapter 9 Solubility, vaporisation and vaporisers

The chapter links with: Chapters 7 and 8.

## Introduction

In discussing humidity in the preceding chapter, the concept of equilibrium between water and its vapour has been introduced as a thermodynamic concept. The concept of vaporisation of other liquids such as volatile anaesthetic agents follows on naturally from that, but first of all it will be worth taking a detour through a discussion on solubility of gases and vapours in their own and other liquids (Davis and Kenny 2003).

## Solubility of molecules in liquids

To maintain simplicity in the discussion on humidity, no mention was made of the presence of air or other gas above the surface of the water, only the water vapour. Depending on the solubility of the gas in the liquid, a variable amount of the gas dissolves in the liquid, whether that be air in water or carbon dioxide in blood. As will be discussed in the section on vaporisation, some molecules of gas enter the liquid and some leave it, depending on their individual kinetic energies, until equilibrium is reached. If the pressure inside the container with the gas or vapour and liquid is increased, then the partial pressure of the gas above the liquid surface increases, resulting in more of the gas molecules dissolving in the liquid. *Henry's Law* states that for a fixed temperature the solubility of a gas in a liquid is proportional to its partial pressure in equilibrium with the liquid. Note the condition of constant temperature because, in addition, solubility decreases with increased temperature. This occurs because an increase in the thermal energy of the dissolved gas molecules increases the partial pressure of the dissolved gas and encourages it to come out of solution. Thus gas bubbles are more apparent in liquids that are heated.

Historically, the relevance of ambient pressure and nitrogen solubility in body tissues was in decompression sickness associated with tunnel workers. Modern examples include underwater diving and, to a lesser extent, aviators and spacewalking astronauts. Nitrogen is a compressible gas and goes into solution in body tissue spaces under compression if the miner, tunnel worker, or diver is breathing ambient air. The longer they work under increased ambient pressure, the more nitrogen becomes dissolved in body tissues, according to Henry's law. The danger lies in coming to the surface, when the nitrogen is decompressed and forms bubbles in those tissues, exactly analogous to opening a bottle of carbonated drink. The collated pathological effects of such bubble formation in tissues are known as decompression sickness, known colloquially as 'the bends'. The same problem occurs in aviators whose cockpits explosively decompress above 7500 m or in a space walking astronaut who has been breathing air at 101 kPa in the space station and has to step into a 30 kPa space suit ventilated with oxygen at $F_{\mathrm{iO_2}} = 1.0$; without an appropriate prebreathing protocol to denitrogenate the body, decompression sickness could result. The problem of decompression sickness is more highly accentuated in diving, where for every 10 m increase in depth in water, the diver's ambient pressure increases by 1 atm. Therefore, for a depth of 30 m, the diver is required to breathe gas at 4 ATA. If the diver is breathing air, and stays at depth beyond the time recommended in diving tables (guidance tables to help divers avoid decompression sickness), significantly hazardous nitrogen loading occurs. Failure to unload the nitrogen bubbles through the lungs adequately slowly by a slow or staged ascent to the surface will result in decompression sickness. This is usually treated by repressurising the victim in a hyperbaric chamber, thus redissolving the nitrogen in the tissues and having the diver breathe oxygen for a number of hours, then slowly decompressing until the nitrogen bubbles have been safely excreted from the lungs. Furthermore, pressurised nitrogen has anaesthetic properties, pressurised oxygen has toxic effects on the central nervous system and the lungs, and an increase in the density of the breathing air leads to an increase in respiratory work. All these factors make air less than ideal as a breathing gas for diving at depths greater than 50 m. Instead a helium/oxygen mix is preferred, and it is also preferred clinically where upper airway obstruction exists.

As already mentioned, different gases dissolve in liquids to different extents. Nitrous oxide is much more soluble in all liquids than nitrogen, which is why its use may cause diffusion hypoxia postoperatively and why its use is avoided in patients with pneumothoraces. For example, at ambient pressure and body temperature, one litre of water dissolves 0.14 L of nitrogen, but 0.39 L of nitrous oxide; one litre of blood dissolves even more nitrous oxide under the same conditions, 0.47 L.

There are two measures of solubility. One is the *Bunsen* solubility coefficient, which is the volume of gas dissolved per litre of liquid at 1 atm pressure and at the relevant temperature, where the partial pressure of the gas is corrected to standard temperature and pressure (STP). A more useful measure is the *Ostwald* solubility coefficient, which is the volume of gas dissolved per litre of liquid at the relevant temperature, uncorrected. This is therefore independent of partial pressure, although it is necessary to state the temperature and pressure being used.

This brings the discussion to the concept of the *partition coefficient*, which is the ratio of the amount of a substance in one phase (e.g. a vapour), dissolved in another substance, usually in another phase (e.g. a liquid, although it can also describe the solution of one liquid in another), when the two phase samples are of equal volume and in equilibrium with each other. For example, the blood–gas partition coefficient for nitrous oxide at body temperature is 0.47, because, given one litre of nitrous oxide in equilibrium with one litre of blood, 0.47 litre of $N_2O$ dissolves in the blood. The concept of equilibrium is important, because this means that the partial pressure of the vapour or gas above the liquid is the same as its partial pressure in the dissolved state in the liquid. The word *tension* is sometimes used synonymously with partial pressure when a gas or vapour is in solution in a liquid. If the partial pressure of the vapour or gas above the liquid is raised, Henry's law dictates that the amount dissolved in the liquid will increase until the tensions are in equilibrium. For a relatively insoluble substance this tension equilibrium will be reached more quickly. Hence, for an anaesthetic agent that is relatively insoluble in blood, such as $N_2O$, tension equilibrium is reached quickly, and this is reflected in the fact that the alveolar partial pressure rapidly reaches the inspired partial pressure. For anaesthetic agents that are highly soluble in blood, such as isoflurane or historically halothane, the high blood solubility (1.4 and 2.5, respectively) means that more of it is transported by the circulation away from the alveolus to the effector site and the partial pressure or tension of the agent in the alveolus only slowly approaches the inspired partial pressure.

Another important partition coefficient for anaesthetic agents is the oil–gas partition coefficient. Because the solubility in oil is similar to the solubility in nervous tissue, and the anaesthetic action appears to depend on this, a high oil–gas partition coefficient is an indicator of anaesthetic potency. For example, $N_2O$ is not a potent agent and has an oil–gas partition coefficient of 1.4, whereas sevoflurane is and has a coefficient of 53. The *Overton–Meyer hypothesis* suggests a near-linear relationship between the logarithm of lipid solubility and anaesthetic potency.

## Solubility of gases in gases

As already indicated in Chapter 7, gases and liquids are simply variants of fluids, so it is possible therefore for gases to dissolve in gases if pressure and temperature are appropriate. A clinical example of this is *Entonox*, a 50:50% mixture of oxygen and nitrous oxide. It is normally a gas mixture unless its temperature falls below -6°C, when the mixture separates (see Chapter 22).

# Vaporisation

A liquid can be thought of as incompressible; at a molecular level it is because the molecules are so close together that very little further approximation of them is possible. If these molecules are given sufficient energy in the form of heat, they acquire more kinetic energy as shown by an increase in temperature. The molecules near the surface of the liquid are thus able to loosen themselves from the attractive forces of neighbouring molecules and leave the liquid surface with their excess kinetic energy. These molecules are considered to form a vapour, with an increased distance between them, compared with those in the liquid state. This allows the vapour to be thought of as compressible. If the liquid is in a closed container, a state of saturated equilibrium exists, with as many molecules leaving the liquid state as re-entering it. Within this closed container, the kinetic energy of the vapour molecules creates a pressure within it. This is called the *Saturated Vapour Pressure* (*SVP*), which increases with increasing kinetic energy (temperature), and represents the pressure at which a vapour and its associated liquid can coexist in equilibrium in a closed container at that temperature. Applying external pressure to a vapour will compress those molecules together and re-form them into a liquid (as well as increase the amount of vapour dissolved in the liquid as described above). As the temperature of a vapour (which is not necessarily in association with a liquid) is raised, there comes a point where, no matter how much pressure is applied to it, it is no longer possible to liquefy it; the molecules have too much kinetic energy to allow this. The temperature at which this occurs is known as the *Critical Temperature.* A vapour at a temperature above its critical temperature is considered to be a gas in terms of its physical behaviour at a molecular level. For oxygen the critical temperature is –116˚C (157 K), and hence it is a gas at all imaginable terrestrial ambient temperatures, even at pressures of gases stored in cylinders. In contrast, the critical temperature of nitrous oxide is 36.5˚C (309.5 K), and the pressure required to liquefy it is 74 bar just below this critical temperature. Thus in temperate or cold climates, $N_2O$ exists in liquid form in cylinders. Water has a critical temperature of 374.1˚C (647 K), which means that it is a vapour under conditions met by an anaesthetist, when most vapours behave very much like gases.

Just as pressurising a vapour below its critical temperature results in liquefaction of the vapour, sufficient depressurisation of a liquid results in vaporisation. The energy required for this process, the *Latent Heat of Vaporisation*, in the absence of another energy source, is taken from the heat contained in the liquid itself, its container and surroundings. Hence, a cylinder containing nitrous oxide that is suddenly opened to allow rapid depressurisation and consequent outflow of $N_2O$ will become cold; water vapour on the cylinder surface will turn to ice. Note that the latent heat of vaporisation results only in a change of state, not in a temperature change. The heat of vaporisation is non-linearly related to the temperature of the liquid, being greater at lower temperatures and falling as temperature rises. Once the critical temperature is reached, the heat of vaporisation is zero since, by definition, the substance can exist as a vapour without the addition of any further heat. Figure 9.1 shows this relationship for nitrous oxide. Hence a cylinder containing nitrous oxide liquid at 20˚C, which is slowly emptied, will have less heat removed initially for the vaporisation process than later on when the liquid is cooler. The astronaut's life support system uses the process of depressurisation of ice and water to a vacuum to remove metabolic heat from a spacesuit.

Figure 9.2 shows (a) a simple vaporiser without any device to regulate its output and (b) a graphical representation of its output of volatile agent with time. A stream of gas is made to pass over the surface of the volatile liquid. As the output switch is turned on, the initial output is due to the saturated vapour pressure of the vapour in the container (1). As the gas flow continues, only a small proportion of it comes into saturation contact with the liquid, and the average output falls rapidly (2). The subsequent gradual fall in output is because of the fall in temperature of the liquid due to the heat of vaporisation and results in a diminishing amount of vaporisation of the liquid (3) (Nielsen *et al.* 1993). As the temperature falls further and approaches that of the surroundings from which the heat of vaporisation is drawn, it becomes the constant temperature that determines the vapour pressure, and hence the output from the vaporiser (4) (White and Strunin 1996). It is clear that the output from the vaporiser also depends on

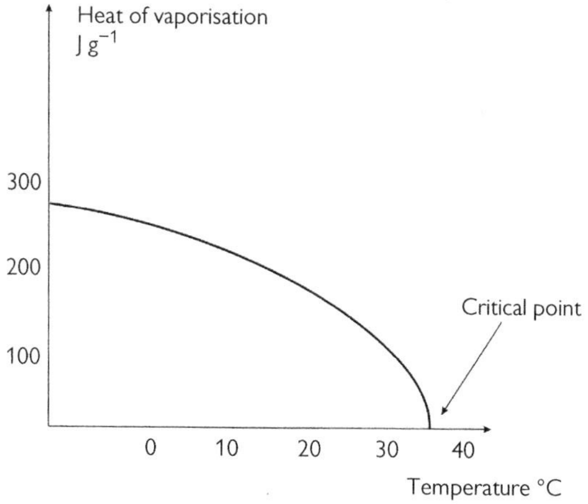


**Fig. 9.1** Variation of heat of vaporisation with temperature for nitrous oxide.

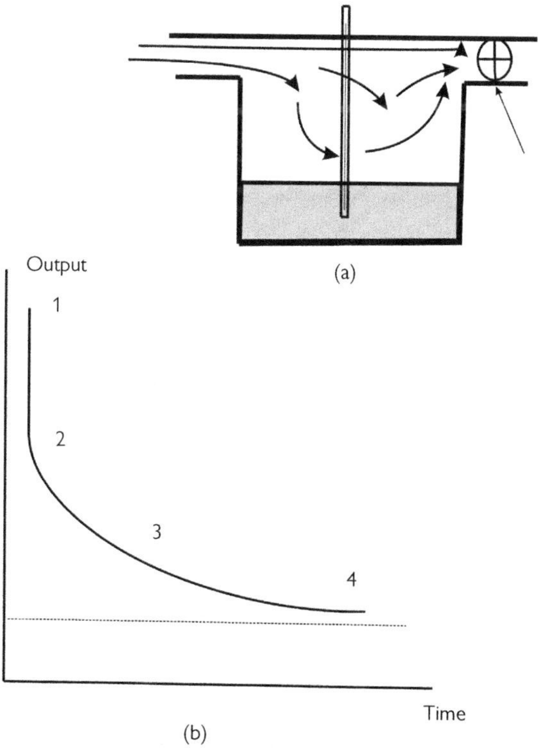


**Fig. 9.2** (a) An uncompensated anaesthetic vaporiser. (b) Vaporiser output with time.

the flowrate of carrier gas over the liquid surface in the chamber; a very low carrier gas flowrate might well be expected to give a lower output than a high flowrate, all other things being equal.

## The basis of vapour production by a vaporiser

Figure 9.3 shows a vaporiser in an ambient pressure of $P_{amb}$ (101 kPa), containing a volatile liquid whose saturated vapour pressure (SVP) is $P_s$. If the vaporiser is efficient and there is maximum access to the liquid by the gas, then the maximum fractional output concentration in the vaporising chamber is

$$\frac{P_s}{P_{amb}}.$$

If the vaporiser dial is set to a small fraction *f* of this output by increasing the bypass flow, then the fractional output from the vaporiser becomes

$$\frac{fP_s}{P_{amb}}.$$

Thus if *f* is a factor that constitutes, say, a 1% concentration setting on a vaporiser calibrated at sea level, then at sea level

$$\frac{fP_s}{101} = 0.01 \quad (1\%) \text{ by calibration,}$$

of 101 kPa or 0.01 × 101 kPa = 1.01 kPa by Dalton's law of partial pressures.

If the same vaporiser is taken to Salt Lake City at an altitude is 2000 m, where the ambient pressure is 80 kPa, with the same setting *f* on the vaporiser of '1%' the fractional output is in fact

$$\frac{fp_s}{80},$$

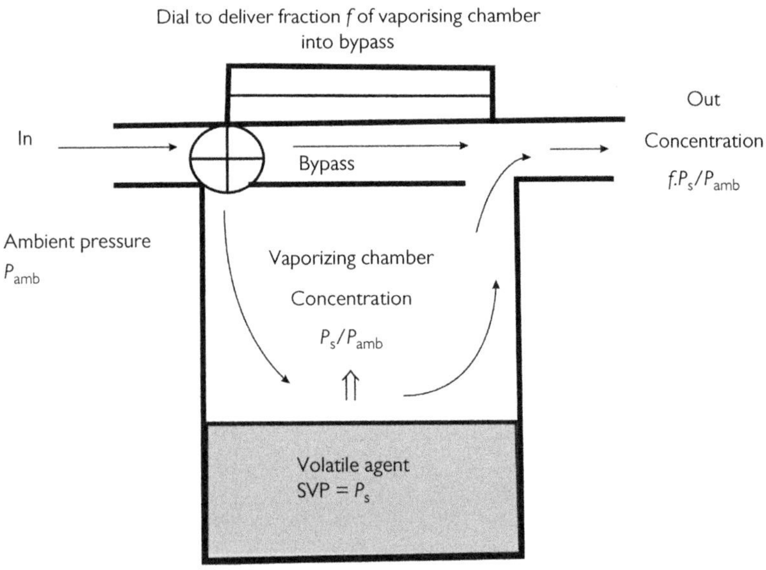


**Fig. 9.3** A vaporiser and its output in relation to ambient pressure $P_{amb}$, SVP of the agent $P_s$, and dial setting fraction *f*.

somewhat greater than the output at sea level. The partial pressure of the volatile agent delivered from the vaporiser output, however, is still $fP_s$, the same as at sea level, assuming no ambient temperature change. Since it is the partial pressure of the volatile agent that is important for pharmacological and anaesthetic purposes, the vaporiser does not need recalibrating at altitude.

It has been stated that the saturated vapour pressure is the pressure at which a vapour is in equilibrium with its associated liquid at a given temperature in a closed container. If the container is opened and the temperature of the liquid/vapour complex is raised, then eventually bubbles of vapour appear in the liquid itself. The liquid body itself can be considered to have started to vaporise. The vapour pressure has risen with temperature until it equals ambient pressure, and the liquid is said to be *boiling*.

Water has an SVP of 101 kPa at 100°C, and oxygen has the same SVP at −183°C (90 K). Therefore, at normal ambient temperatures of between 0 to 30° C (273 to 303 K), the SVP of oxygen greatly exceeds 101 kPa, and the oxygen rapidly boils away as a gas. A vacuum-insulated flask is used in hospitals and other settings to provide a stable liquid source of oxygen, to keep the temperature and the SVP as low as possible to minimise boiling and wastage (see Chapter 22). At 20°C the SVP of water is less than 3 kPa, and at 37°C it is 6.3 kPa (see Chapter 8).

Figure 9.4 shows how SVP varies with temperature for a number of commonly used volatile anaesthetic agents. Although desflurane use has been discontinued, it is illustrative to note that it has a higher SVP than most volatile anaesthetic agents, reaching 101 kPa at 23°C. This means that, to be clinically useful, a specially designed vaporiser is required to prevent uncontrolled vapour output (Graham 1994; Weiskopf *et al.* 1994). The desflurane vaporiser incorporates a heater that ensures that the liquid vaporises fully and is released to the rest of the vaporiser in a controlled fashion (see below).

As an experiment to demonstrate the nature of vapour pressure, it is known that atmospheric pressure is supported by a column of mercury 760 mm high with a vacuum above it (see Figure 7.6). If some water is introduced into the base of the mercury column, it rises to the top, vaporises in the vacuum above the mercury, and depresses the mercury column to, say, 742 mmHg. Thus water vapour at this temperature is 18 mmHg (Macintosh *et al.* 1987).

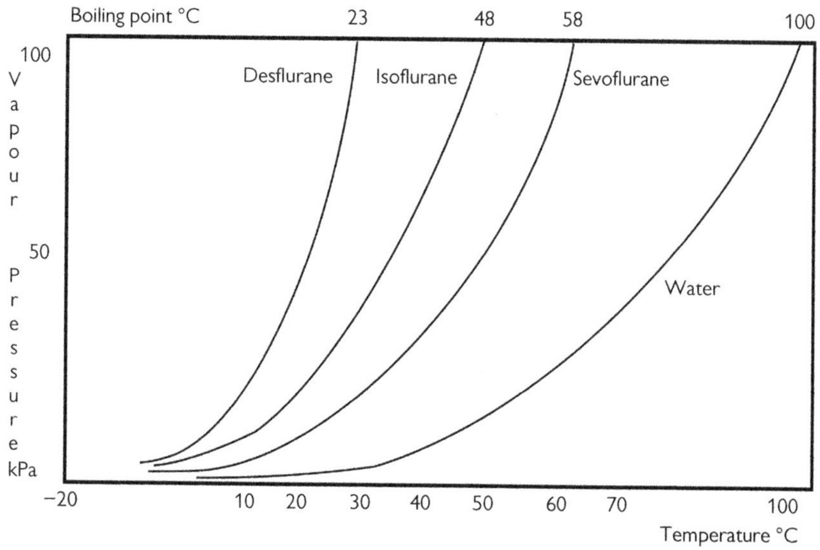


**Fig. 9.4** Vapour pressure and boiling point.

# Vaporisers

The principle of SVP and vaporisation has been discussed and the predicted output from a simple, uncompensated plenum vaporiser was used to demonstrate it (Boumphrey and Marshall 2011). In order to accurately deliver a few per cent of a volatile agent in a gas stream, either a well-designed vaporiser or reliable volatile agent monitoring is required, and these days both are often incorporated together. Not all anaesthetic workstations have agent monitoring, but most modern vaporisers are engineered to a high standard to ensure a controlled output, unlike that shown in Figure 9.2.

In order to provide a controlled output, most vaporisers include some specific design features. The first change made to the simple plenum shown above (the plenum is the vaporiser's main chamber) is to provide two routes for the gas supply: one to the vaporisation chamber, the other as a bypass route; the ratio between these two flows – the *splitting ratio* – is what the control knob dictates. The maximum amount of volatile agent vaporised depends on the SVP of the agent, its temperature and that of the gases passing through the chamber, the gas flow rate, the amount of contact between the gases and the liquid, and the geometry of the vaporisation chamber. To a small extent it also depends on the gas components because of differences in density and viscosity, and because, for example, nitrous oxide is more soluble in the liquid agent than air is; there is also a small variation with altitude, again because of density change in the carrier gases. If the vaporiser is switched off, all the gas passes through the bypass; if it is switched on to maximum output, a maximum gas flow passes through the vaporisation chamber. At other dialled concentrations, a variable proportion passes through both pathways.

The second design change is to provide a means of maximising contact between the carrier gas and the liquid. The principles of these are shown in Figure 9.5 and include wicking, multiple baffles and a nebuliser, and elongating the gas pathway to maximise exposure.

The third design change is the provision of temperature compensation to prevent a fall in output that would otherwise occur, such as that shown in Figure 9.2. The earliest method was to attach the vaporiser to a material with a large heat capacity to minimise the temperature fall during the vaporisation process, such as a large mass of metal or water (Zuck 1988). Figure 9.6 shows two later temperature compensation designs. One is a bimetallic strip, acting as a cap over the gas entry port to either the bypass chamber or the vaporising chamber; as the chamber temperature falls during vaporisation, the bimetallic strip bends and either restricts the flow to the bypass chamber or allows more gas to enter the

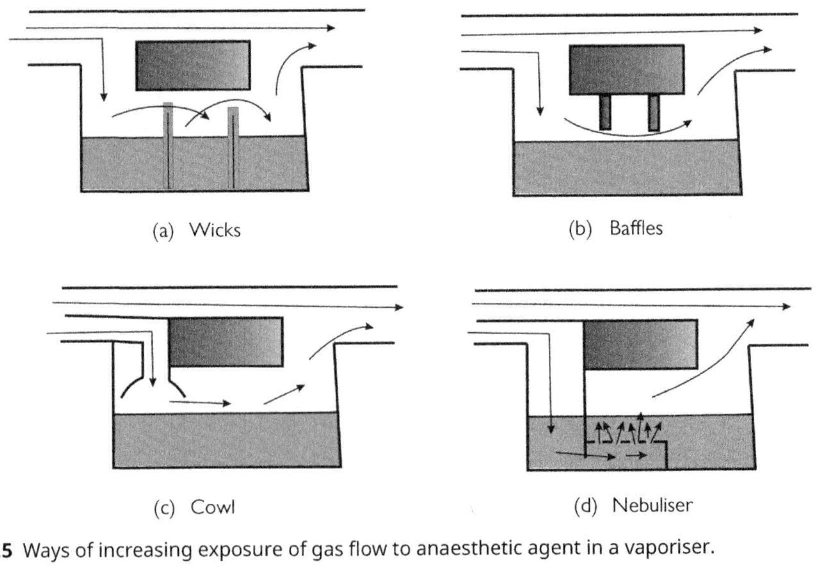


**Fig. 9.5** Ways of increasing exposure of gas flow to anaesthetic agent in a vaporiser.

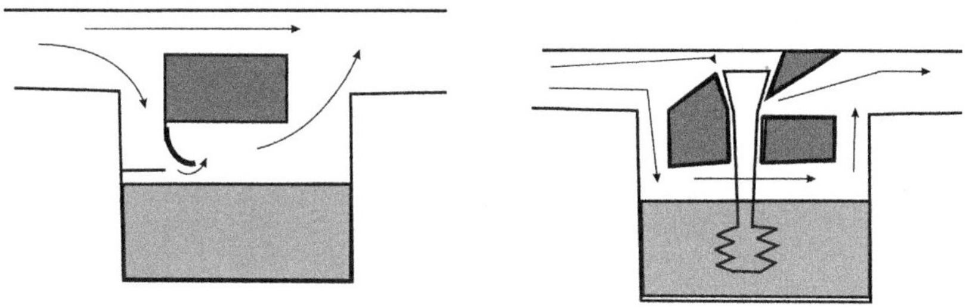

(a) The bimetallic strip (b) The ether bellows and cone

**Fig. 9.6** Two designs for temperature compensation in vaporisers.

vaporisation chamber, thus compensating for reduced temperature. Another design uses an aneroid bellows, which sits in the vaporisation chamber and is connected by a rod to a cone in an orifice in the bypass chamber; as the temperature falls in the vaporisation chamber, the bellows contracts, reducing the bypass flow, thereby increasing the splitting ratio.

If the pressure of the gas downstream of the vaporiser increases intermittently, for example due to the presence of a positive-pressure ventilator, some of this downstream gas, which contains volatile agent, can re-enter the vaporising chamber retrogradely, to be discharged again with an additional, unmetered vapour load. This is a hazardous anomaly, which needs a compensation device. It can take the form of either a one-way valve downstream of the vaporiser, or an additional length of tubing between the vaporiser and the ventilator to prevent the *pumping effect* of retrograde movement of gas into the vaporiser. The apparently complex design of modern vaporisers aims to achieve all of these properties and also to maintain the output constant across a wide range of carrier gas flowrates.

Figure 9.7 shows a relatively modern *Tec5* vaporiser and the following features are noted: the bypass chamber (7) passes underneath the vaporising chamber (4); there is an elongated, coiled inlet passage (2) upstream of the vaporising chamber to prevent the pumping effect described above; there is a helical wick (3) to maximise carrier gas contact with liquid agent; the temperature compensation mechanism is a bimetallic strip (8) that restricts flow through the bypass chamber. Figure 9.8 shows a modern *Dräger Vapor* and it has similar features to the Tec. A series of baffles (2) in the upstream inflow tube (1) counteracts the pumping effect. A spiral wick (3) with a sleeve dips into the liquid agent and the wick is made of a synthetic material that has a high capillarity, but does not absorb the agent. The concentration control valve (6) is directly linked to the control knob (7), and the mixing chamber (9) is where the vapour is mixed with the bypass gas. The bimetallic temperature compensation device consists of an inner rod (8) made of a relatively non-expansile material, coated in brass, and the combined structure dips into the liquid; as the temperature of the liquid falls, the brass coating contracts, pulling the inner rod up to constrict the bypass flow.

On acquisition of any vaporiser, the information presented to the user includes calibration curves or the equivalent for output against temperature and gas flow rate, and for these two vaporisers, there is a relatively constant vapour output for a given dial setting, no matter what the fresh gas flow rate or the environmental temperature is (between 15 and 35°C). Output from vaporisers has been shown to vary by more than ±15% (Nielsen *et al.* 1993). Note also that modern vaporisers have a keyed filling port to prevent the chamber from being filled with the wrong agent, but should still not be overfilled (Palayiwa and Hahn 1991).

In recent years, with anaesthetic machines incorporating integral agent monitoring, including modern electronics, new vaporisers are becoming less mechanically engineered, the vaporiser instead incorporating solenoid flow control valves, electronic control and a closed loop feedback mechanism. The vaporiser output is measured by the agent analyser and, if there is any discrepancy with the set value, a servo-control mechanism changes the splitting ratio appropriately. Such

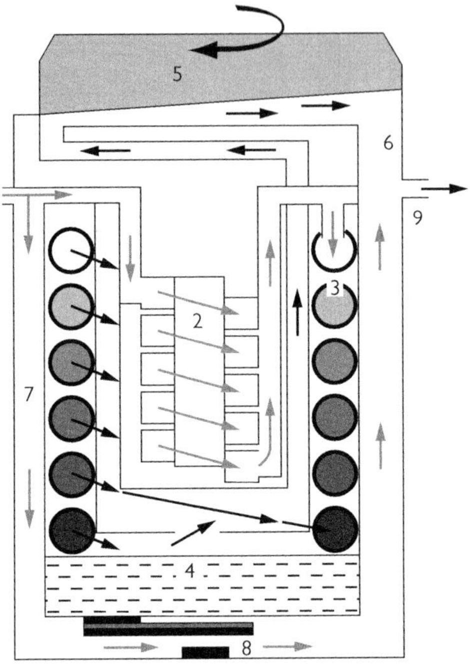


**Fig. 9.7** A cross-sectional view of the Tec5 vaporiser.

Reproduced with permission from Davey, A.J., & Diba, A. (2011). *Ward's Anaesthetic Equipment (6th ed.)* Elsevier.

a vaporiser, shown in Figure 9.9, is used on the modern *Datex-Ohmeda* anaesthetic machine. The vaporising chamber is now a cassette, which contains lamellae made of a synthetic material that behaves like a wick, with metal plates between them to make the gas pathway more convoluted in order to aid vapour contact. At the back, where the cassette interfaces with the anaesthetic machine backbar, there are inflow and outflow valves and a temperature sensor. The filling port is at the front, and there is a valve to the main cassette that closes when the cassette is full. There are magnets on the front that help the control unit identify which agent is in use. The cassette control unit, which is part of the anaesthetic machine, has additional inflow and outflow check valves, a bypass flow measurement device and an agent flow measurement device. When a certain concentration is dialled up by the user, the fresh gas flow is split in a calculated ratio. The small proportion that is diverted to the cassette passes through the one-way valves and into the cassette, where it picks up vapour. It then exits the cassette, whereupon it passes through a flow control valve to a flow measurement device and rejoins the bypass flow, which is also measured. A microprocessor uses the information from these flow measurements and the temperature sensor to calculate the amount of agent to be added to the bypass flow to achieve the dialled concentration and alters the flow control valve accordingly.

Although desflurane has fallen out of use, it is useful to mention in passing, in case a volatile agent with similar physical properties comes into use. Because it has such a low boiling point, special measures have to be taken in the design of the vaporiser to achieve a reliable vapour output. The chamber containing the liquid contains a heater which maintains the agent temperature at 39°C, at which temperature the SVP of the agent is 194 kPa. When an output concentration is dialled up, a shut-off valve downstream of the exit from the vaporising chamber opens and admits vapour under pressure into the downstream pipework. An electronically controlled pressure regulator reduces the pressure of the aliquot of vapour to that which normally exists in a plenum vaporiser (1–2 kPa). The vapour then passes to

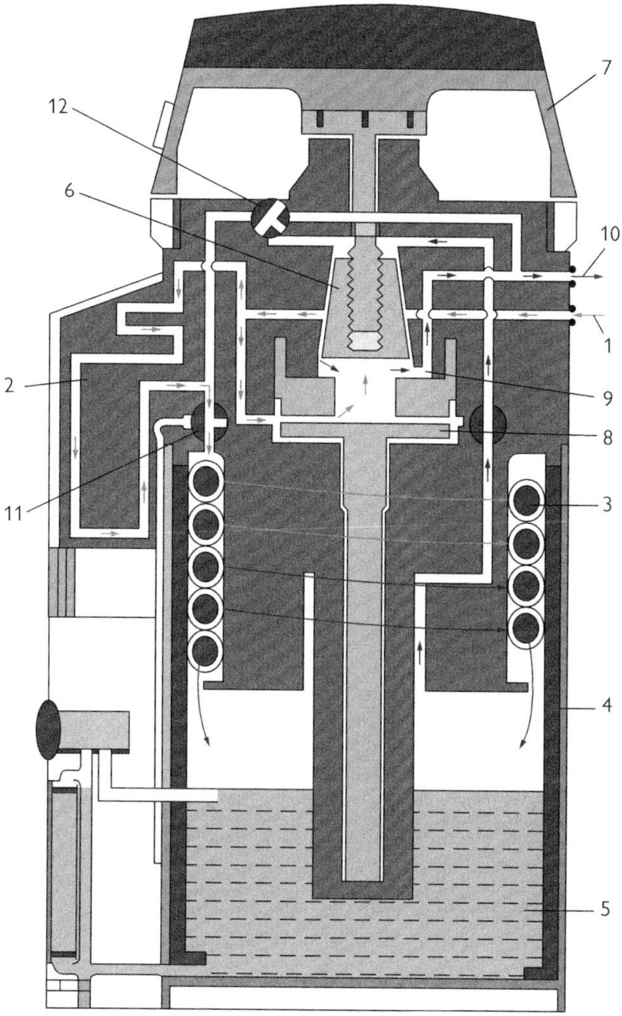


**Fig. 9.8** Cross-sectional view of the Draeger Vapor vaporiser.

Reproduced with permission from Davey, A.J., & Diba, A. (2011). *Ward's Anaesthetic Equipment (6th ed.)* Elsevier.

a variable flow restrictor linked to the concentration control knob, whence it joins the bypass gas flow and leaves the vaporiser. The pressure of the vapour corresponds to the required concentration of the agent. There is a differential pressure sensor in the pipework that compares the pressure coming out of the vaporising chamber with the dialled concentration and acts on the control valve appropriately.

There are also devices for injecting liquid agent directly into the gas stream. This overcomes the problem of the temperature dependence of the SVP of the vapour.

This description thus far of plenum vaporisers refers to those mounted on continuous flow anaesthetic machines with a pressurised gas supply, in which the relatively high resistance to gas flow from plenum vaporisers is not a limiting design consideration. When used with a circle breathing system, a plenum vaporiser is normally used outside the circle breathing system itself, but it is possible to place the vaporiser inside the circle system instead, when its output is very different. Under these circumstances a vaporiser through which the patient breathes air spontaneously needs to be of low resistance

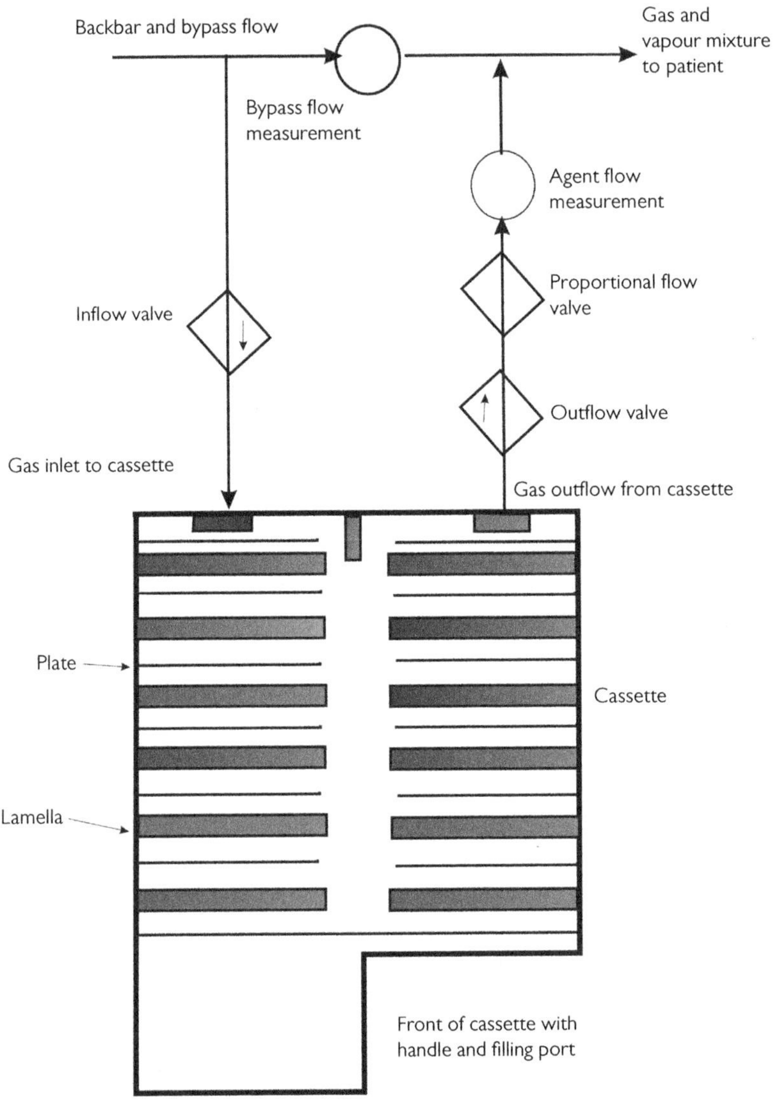


**Fig. 9.9** The Datex Ohmeda cassette vaporiser and backbar connections, plan view.

and is called a *draw-over* vaporiser (Young *et al.* 2000). They are often also used with simpler to-and-fro circuits in military or field anaesthesia situations, or in countries where sources of pressurised medical gases are unavailable. While they are not designed to be as accurate as other devices, they are certainly adequate for clinical use. Several types are in use (English *et al.* 2009) and, given their flexibility, care must be taken in the way they are used (Donovan and Perndt 2007).

It should also be remembered that, despite accurate output from a vaporiser, some of the volatile agent is absorbed by anaesthetic tubing, although this is less true of modern agents and modern tubing material than formerly (Smith *et al.* 2002).

## References

**Boumphrey, S.** and **Marshall, N.** (2011) Understanding vaporizers, *CEACCP*, **11**(6), pp. 199–203

**Davis, P. D.** and **Kenny, G. N. C.** (2003) *Basic Physics and Measurement in Anaesthesia*, 5th edn, Butterworth-Heinemann, Edinburgh, pp. 65–74.

**Donovan, A.** and **Perndt, H.** (2007) Oxford miniature vaporiser output with reversed gas flows, *Anaesthesia*, **62**, pp. 609–614.

**English, W. A. *et al.*** (2009) The Diamedica drawover vaporiser: a comparison of a new vaporiser with the Oxford miniature vaporiser, *Anaesthesia*, **64**, pp. 84–92.

**Graham, S. G.** (1994) The Tec 6 vaporizer, *Br. J. Anaesth.*, **72**, pp. 470–73.

**MacIntosh, Mushin** and **Epstein** (1987) *Physics for the Anaesthetist*, 4th edn, Revised Mushin M. W. and Jones P. L., Blackwell Scientific Publications, Oxford, pp. 101–24.

**Nielsen, J. *et al.*** (1993) Accuracy of 94 anaesthetic agent vaporisers in clinical use, *Br. J. Anaesth.*, **71**, pp. 453–57.

**Palayiwa, E.** and **Hahn, C. E. W.** (1991) Overfill testing of anaesthetic vaporizers, *Br. J. Anaesth.*, **74**, pp. 100–103.

**Smith, C. *et al.*** (2002) Leakage and absorption of isoflurane by different types of anaesthetic circuit and monitoring tubing, *Anaesthesia*, **57**, pp. 686–89.

**Weiskopf, R. B.**, **Sampson, D.** and **Moore, M. A.** (1994) The desflurane (Tec6) vaporizer, *Br. J. Anaesth.*, **72**, pp. 474–79.

**White, S. A.** and **Strunin, L.** (1996) Anaesthesia with the Boyle's bottle vaporizer, *Anaesthesia*, **51**, pp. 939–42.

**Young, D. A.**, **Brosnan, S. G.** and **White, D. C.** (2000) A semiquantitative analysis of the dynamics of a Goldman type vaporizer, *Anaesthesia*, **55**, pp. 557–70.

**Zuck, D.** (1988) The Alcock chloroform vaporiser. An early calibrated, temperature compensated plenum apparatus in its historical context, *Anaesthesia*, **43**, pp. 972–80.

## Further reading

**Davey, A.** (2012) Vaporizers. Chapter 3 in *Ward's Anaesthetic Equipment*, 6th edn, WB Saunders Co. Ltd, pp. 41–64.

# Chapter 10 **Ultrasound and Doppler**

This chapter contains: properties of ultrasound; visualisation of needle positioning; Doppler (continuous wave, pulsed, frequency shift spectrum, blood flow); measurement of absolute blood flow; high power ultrasound. The chapter links with: Chapters 4, 5 and 13.

## Introduction

Ultrasound has many uses in areas of medicine associated with anaesthesia. It is used for imaging, visualisation of needle and catheter positioning, therapy and, together with the Doppler effect, for measurement of flow velocity. Real-time information of tissue movement can be obtained with ease, and with the low energies used, diagnostic equipment exposures are not thought to be a safety issue, either for the operator or the patient.

## Properties of ultrasound

Ultrasound is a form of mechanical energy that consists of high-frequency vibrations at frequencies above human hearing range (>20 kHz). Medical applications lie in the frequency range of 1–20 MHz. The frequencies selected are a compromise between penetration and resolution required. Low-intensity ultrasound passes through living tissue without altering tissue properties. Higher energy can produce heating and mechanical effects, both of which can alter cell well-being.

Ultrasound is generated by electrically inducing a deformation in a piezoelectric material (typically a ceramic material such as lead zirconate titanate), which compresses and decompresses the medium to which it is coupled (see Figure 10.1(a)) at a rate equal to the frequency of the driving voltage. The pressure changes travel through the medium in a longitudinal direction and the distance between the points of maximum pressure, or compression, is known as the wavelength. Figure 10.2 shows the relationship between the period of the wave and the wavelength. This distance is dependent on the *elasticity* (compressibility), the density of the medium, and the speed of sound. As shown in the figure, the wavelength ($\lambda$) and the transmission frequency ($f$) are related to the propagation velocity $c$ by $c = f\lambda$. The magnitude of the wave is the difference between the maximum and minimum pressure values. The wave propagates by the movement of particles: it cannot travel in a vacuum and it does not *ionise* (see Chapter 29) the medium through which it travels.

The propagation speed of an ultrasound wave is not constant throughout the body. Various tissues allow the passage of the wave at different velocities. Also the wave is attenuated differently by the various tissue types. For example, in soft tissues the ultrasound wave has a velocity of between 1460 and 1630 m $s^{-1}$ whereas in bone it is 2700–4100 m $s^{-1}$. Bone attenuates the wave about ten times more than soft tissue.

The wavelength of the beam determines the resolution. The intensity of the beam determines the sensitivity of the instrument and governs the size of echoes recorded. Attenuation increases approximately linearly with frequency in soft tissues but in air and water increases with the square of the frequency. The greatest penetration is achieved with the lowest frequency but because the wavelength is long, the resolution is poor. A compromise is to use the highest frequency that will ensure adequate penetration of the tissues or organs being investigated. For example, a transmission frequency of 3 MHz is normally used to image the kidneys, 10 MHz is used for ophthalmic investigations, and 20 MHz is used for catheter tip intravascular devices. The absorption of ultrasound by the tissues results in the generation of heat that, in the case of diagnostic work, can cause temperature increases of the order of

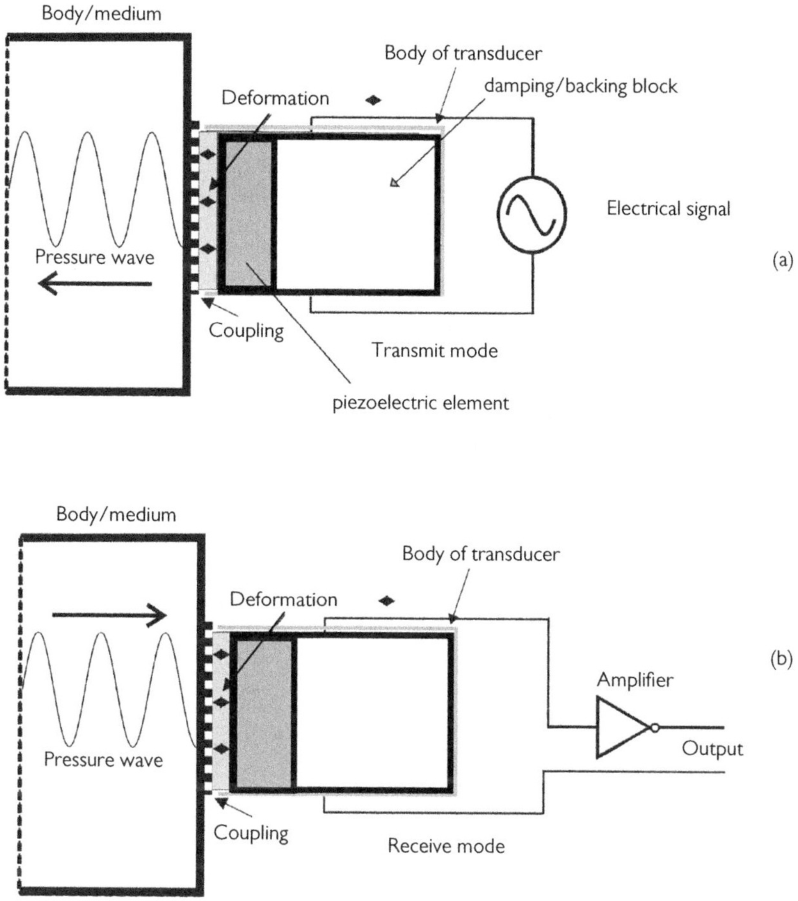


**Fig. 10.1** Production of ultrasound from a piezo-electric material. The piezo-electric element has a damping/backing block behind it, and is surrounded typically by a metal shell (body of transducer), except on the left-hand side. An electrical signal input causes the material to deform (a), and this creates a pressure wave into the body with which it is mechanically coupled. Coupling requires the use of a special gel to transfer the movement of the transducer to the body as the movement is not transmitted by air. In (b) the piezo-electric crystal also allows the reverse process to occur, and a pressure wave on to the crystal causes an electrical signal to be induced, which is further amplified.

1°C. It is the reflection and scattering of the ultrasound beam from the interfaces between two tissues or from tissue–fluid or tissue–air interfaces that forms the principle of the majority of diagnostic techniques. The same piezo-electric element is usually used as the receiver for ultrasound. The pressure changes coupled to the transducer will induce electrical signals proportional to the acoustic pressure (see Figure 10.1(b)).

Imaging is carried out using pulse-echo ultrasound to produce a real-time two-dimensional B scan. In this scanning method, many transducers are used, either in an angular sector scanner way or in a linear array. The sector probe (Figure 10.3(a)) has fewer transducers and the rotation is mechanical, whereas the linear array type (shown in Figure 10.3(b)) has typically over 300 elements and the beam *movement* is carried out electronically. Mechanical devices are not used now, but they are included in the text to discuss the principles involved. Figure 10.3(a) demonstrates the concepts of how

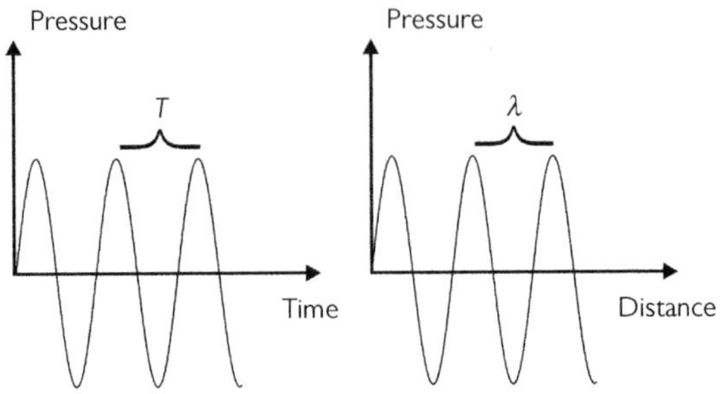


**Fig. 10.2** Diagram showing the period and wavelength of ultrasound pressure waves. *T* is the period of the waveform (the time for one complete oscillation), and is the reciprocal of the frequency, $T = 1/f$. The wavelength λ, is the distance occupied by one oscillation. λ is related to the speed of the wave in the medium c, and the frequency by $c = f\lambda$.

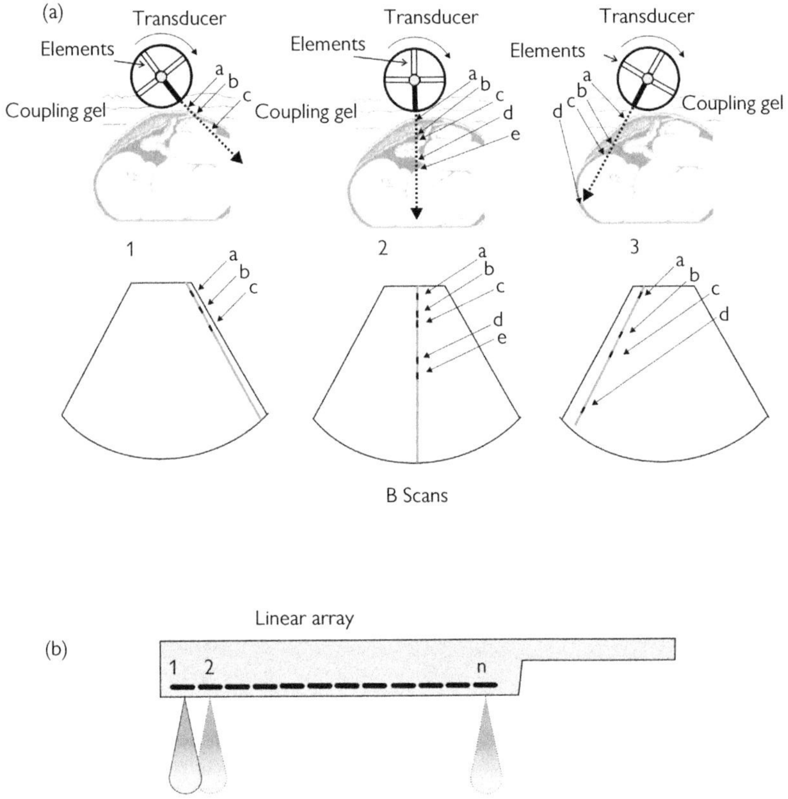


**Fig. 10.3** The use of two-dimensional B-scanning transducers, using (a) a four-sector mechanical transducer, and (b) an *n* element linear array. In (a) the same transducer scans the same anatomical site, only in each case the elements of the transducer have rotated through 45°. The sectors 1–3 show the build-up of the received image showing the interface boundary echoes produced from a, b, c as appropriate. (b) shows a linear array of *n* elements. First element 1 is made to transmit and then receive by an electronic switch, and then element 2, and so on until element *n*.

a mechanical sector scanner functions, and Figure 10.3(b) shows the linear array transducer. The pulse echo transducer is shown at three different paths, although many paths in reality make up the complete sector (the complete sector is shown in the figure as position 1 to position 3). At each position, the transducer sends out ultrasound pulses and the return of these echoes from the various boundaries gives depth information. The position of the transducer in the arc is known and linked to the display, so the echoes will have the correct position. The brightness of each echo point will be related to its strength. A schematic version of this two-dimensional scan is shown at the bottom of the diagram. The real-time display often uses at least 100 scan lines (vertically) that are *refreshed* 30 times per second to appear as a flicker-free picture to the observer.

Other scanners can be miniaturised and inserted into the body to provide images. Successful imaging has been carried out of most parts of the body but, for the anaesthetist, the most important areas are now visualisation of needle positioning, echocardiography, carotid artery and internal jugular vein visualisations, and foetal imaging.

## Visualisation of needle positioning

Historically ultrasound has been used by radiologists to guide needle, catheters and guide-wire placement, but it is now being increasingly used by anaesthetists for vascular access, nerve blockade, drainage of plural or ascitic fluid collections and percutaneous tracheostomy. Ultrasound allows identification of the target structures and gives real-time guidance to place needles and catheters precisely (Chapman *et al.* 2006). Probably the largest use of ultrasound with anaesthetists is with regional anaesthesia, and for central venous cannulation.

The key to success with using ultrasound-guided techniques is acquiring considerable real-time scanning experience. Useful practice can be gained by using water baths and phantoms (inert structure with ultrasound-sensitive recognisable structures buried in it). One of the important areas is in the assessment of needle position. There are a number of factors that influence needle visualisation (Schafhalter-Zoppoth *et al.* 2004). Larger needles are more easily seen than smaller ones, particularly in cross-section, but smaller ones may produce fewer artefacts. Needles placed perpendicular to the ultrasound beam are the easiest to see, and the tip can often be seen due to its irregular surface, when the shaft can not. The introduction of the needle in a short in–out or side-to-side motion can help with visualisation. Also when the needle shaft crosses the beam, an acoustic shadow will be seen, and this can help. The injection of fluid has also been shown to enhance needle and catheter tip visualisation, which is helpful in nerve blockade to confirm the site and spread of the anaesthetic. When small bubbles are in a solution (as is often the case when using a small syringe) and this solution is injected into a fluid filled vessel, then the visualisation is enhanced. This is one of the principles of the use of ultrasound contrast media, where bubbles can enhance the images. The bubbles can be increased by agitation or repeated injection between two syringes with a nearly closed three-way tap. However, injection of air or microbubbles in solid tissues is not helpful because the acoustic shadow that they produce spoils underlying deeper structures. This may be relevant for regional anaesthesia, so pre-warming local anaesthetic solutions may help reduce bubbles.

## Doppler

When an ultrasound beam encounters a stationary target, it is partially reflected back towards the transmitter and the carrier frequency of the wave remains the same. When the reflector, which can be a group of moving blood cells in a vessel, is moved towards the transmitter, however, it encounters more oscillations per unit time than its stationary equivalent, so the frequency is apparently increased. This is demonstrated in Figure 10.4.

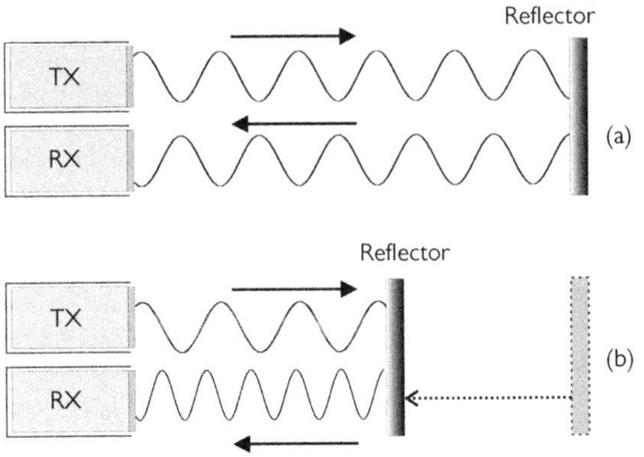


**Fig. 10.4** This figure demonstrates the Doppler effect. In (a) the transducer (TX) transmits an ultrasound wave and it is reflected by a reflector to be received by the receiving (RX) transducer. In (b) the reflector has moved from its initial position to a position nearer the transducer and on the return path the waveform is compressed, which means the frequency increases.

Doppler velocimetry is a non-invasive technique for the detection and potentially the measurement of blood velocity, from which flow can be calcuated within the body. For a transmitted frequency of $f_t$, a wavelength $\lambda$, and the velocity of sound in the medium $c$, $f_t = c/\lambda$.

If the beam hits an object that is moving directly towards the transmitter at velocity $v$, the frequency of the waves arriving at the reflector ($f_r$) will now be:

$$f_r = (c+v)/\lambda.$$

The reflector will now act as a source that is moving towards the transmitter, the actual frequency sensed by the transmitter (in receiver mode) will be $f_r = (c + 2v)/\lambda$.

The apparent increase in frequency is given by:

$$f_r - f_t = (c+2v)/\lambda - c/\lambda = 2v/\lambda = 2v\ f_t/c.$$

Putting some numbers into this equation, in tissue, $c = 1500$ m s$^{-1}$, $f_t = 2$ MHz, $v = 0.1$ m s$^{-1}$, the difference frequency will be 267 Hz. This difference signal is audible and therefore the Doppler output could be amplified and delivered to a loudspeaker or earphones. The *sound* pattern of pulsatile blood flow in different disease conditions can be very descriptive and a trained operator can recognise these changes. Quantification of the Doppler waveform will be discussed later.

Normally the Doppler beam is applied at an angle to the blood vessel from the body surface as shown in Figure 10.5. The resulting frequency shift is now multiplied by cos $\theta$. For the maximum frequency shift, the transmitter/receiver must be aligned with the direction of flow (cos $\theta = 1$). If the beam is perpendicular to the flow, then no signal will be produced (cos $\theta = 0$). Unless the angle is known, the speed of blood cannot be determined using Doppler methods.

## Pulsed Doppler

Ultrasound scanning and Doppler can be combined enabling the user to visualise the cross-sectional anatomy of interest by using the grey-scale image, and by placing a cursor over the particular vessel to be measured. This cursor identifies the position on the image of a range-gate of Doppler ultrasound (the position at which Doppler signals will be detected). The user switches over to the Doppler mode, which normally freezes the image and then blood flow calculations can be made from the desired site. The angle between the flow lines and the beam can also be measured.

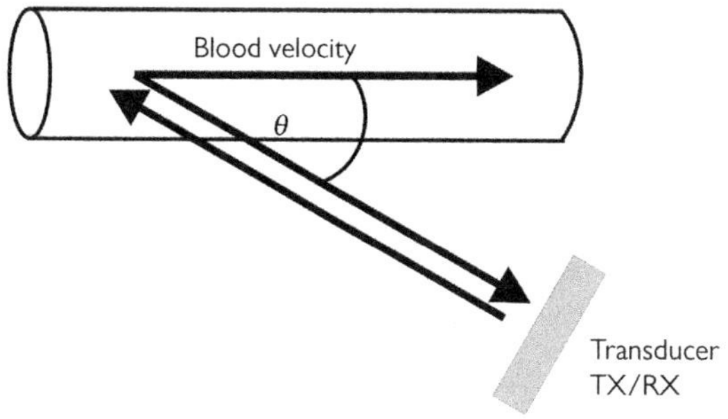


**Fig. 10.5** This figure illustrates the angle $\theta$ between the ultrasound beam and the moving blood.

A more advanced technique is colour flow (Doppler) imaging. This technique uses a conventional black and white ultrasound image, and a real-time colour image, which represents motion detected by Doppler in the same scan plane. They are combined to create a composite image.

## *The use of the Doppler frequency shift spectrum*

A more efficient and quantitative method of analysing the Doppler signal is to produce the Doppler power spectrum or frequency shift spectrum of the audio signal. The Doppler shift frequency is proportional to the velocity, and the power in a particular frequency band is proportional to the number of blood cells moving with velocities that produce frequencies in that band. The Doppler power spectrum should have the same shape as a velocity distribution plot for the flow in the vessel. An example of this is shown in Figure 10.6. The horizontal axis represents time, the vertical axis is the Doppler frequency shifts at that time and the grey scales give the power at that frequency or the number of blood cells moving.

The *shape* of the maximum (peak) frequency shift curve with time can give information that a simple mean flow measurement, which may also be obtained by other clinical methods, cannot. In the assessment of arterial disease, the pulsatile components of a flow waveform are much more sensitive to

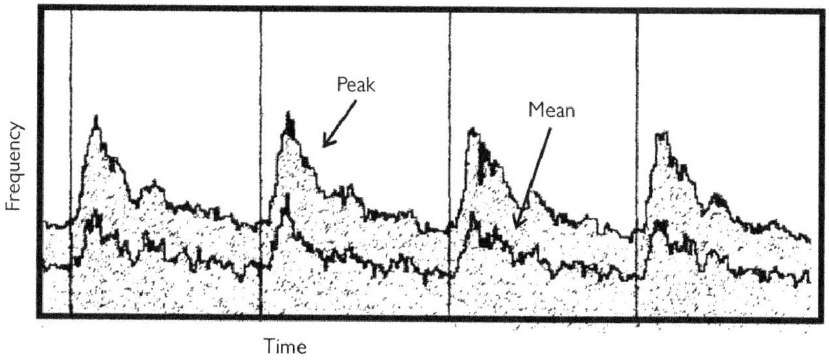


**Fig. 10.6** A frequency shift Doppler power spectrum produced from a Doppler spectrum analyser connected to a Doppler probe. The vertical axis is the positive frequency shift spectrum (it can be negative as well for, for example, the opposite direction of flow). The vertical lines are where the analyser calculates that the new cardiac cycle has begun. The peak is the peak frequency shift spectrum and the mean is the mean frequency shift spectrum.

proximal stenosis than mean flow (Lee *et al.* 1978; Farrar *et al.* 1979), and allow a quantification of the severity of the disease.

Figure 10.7 shows two waveform shapes from a femoral artery, one from a normal artery (a) and the other showing a high impedance downstream (b), found in a stenosed artery. It would be convenient for the quantification of disease state if each different waveform shape could be represented by a single number or series of numbers. In the cardiac cycle, the maximum frequency shift waveform comprises two parts, the systolic and diastolic parts, having different frequency characteristics. The systolic component has a fast rise of frequency with respect to time, whereas the diastolic part has lower frequency components. A stenosed artery has different frequency-dependent characteristics from a normal artery. The two sections will change in differing proportions depending on which type of artery is being examined. In the absence of a pulsatile waveform, a downstream stenosis would result in a decrease in both flow and the amplitude of the spectrum throughout the cycle (i.e. the same reduction in both sections).

Two popular indexes for giving an *index* of upstream resistance or impedance are the *pulsatility index* (*PI*) and the *resistive index* (*RI*). The PI is calculated as $(S - D)/mean$ as shown in Figure 10.7. The RI is calculated as $(S - D)/S$, where $S$ is the maximum frequency shift during systole and $D$ is the maximum shift during diastole. $D$ can also be negative for reverse flow situations.

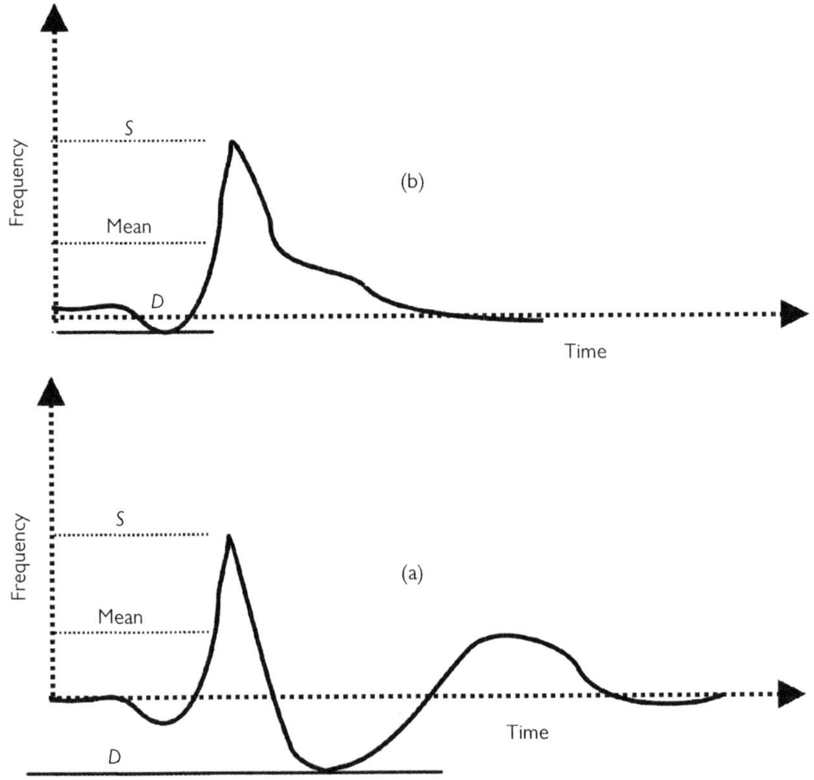


**Fig. 10.7** This diagram shows typical waveforms taken from frequency shift plots from a common femoral arteries from a normal subject (a), and (b) a patient with peripheral disease. In (a) the frequency goes negative, indicating reverse flow. The horizontal axis is time and the vertical axis is the positive and negative frequency shift spectrum. $S$ is the maximum frequency shift during systole, $D$ is the shift during diastole, and the mean is the mean shift over the whole cycle.

There are many applications of Doppler velocimetry of interest to anaesthetists, for example renal blood flow, uteroplacental artery flow, transcranial middle cerebral artery, hepatic blood flow, cardiac output and many others. Doppler velocimetry can be used as a non-invasive measure of renal blood flow and impedance, allowing measurement of the effects of certain drugs on the renal circulation (Stevens *et al.* 1989; Tooley *et al.* 1994; Munn *et al.* 1993).

## Measurement of absolute blood flow

The measurement of the blood flow requires the measurement of the angle between the ultrasound beam and the vessel, estimation of the mean diameter of the vessel, and estimation of the mean velocity of the flow in the direction of the ultrasound beam. The simplest formula involves converting the beam parallel to the vessel axis, by knowing the angle, and multiplying this by the vessel cross-sectional area to give mean flow. Deciding which is the mean velocity can create problems as the blood velocity profile in arteries is complex. For example, near the aortic valve it resembles plug flow but downstream the flow has a more parabolic profile. Even with so many causes of error, a reasonable estimation of volumetric blood flow can be made by using the formula:

$$Mean\ flow = kA\ f_d c / (2 f_t cos\theta),$$

where $k$ is a factor to convert the velocity to its mean value and must depend on where the blood flow is in the body. For parabolic flow $k = 0.5$. $A$ is the cross-sectional area of the vessel and is usually calculated using the internal diameter of the vessel ($d$) and the formula $\pi$ d2 /4$f_d$ is the Doppler shift, $f_t$ is the transmission frequency, $c$ is the velocity of sound and $\theta$ is the angle of the ultrasound beam to the flow line.

This formula has been used in real-time standalone Doppler instruments, such as the sternal notch device (Donovan *et al.* 1987) and trachea device (Hausen *et al.* 1992). One of the problems associated with these devices is the assumption about the angle. If this is near zero, as in the case of the sternal notch device, this is not so much a problem, but in the other instrument mentioned the angle is assumed to be near 54° and the errors associated with variations to this angle are much higher and this may be why the device is very inaccurate.

## High-power ultrasound

Much higher levels of ultrasound, however, can be used in a practical way. Lithotripsy is one of these and it often proves to be the best method for the removal of kidney, uretonic and gall bladder stones. No invasive surgery is required, but general anaesthesia is used. The technique usually employs shock waves created by the rapid vaporisation of fluid that surrounds a spark gap, the wave being focused by an elliptical reflector such that maximum intensity coincides with the position of the stone. Alignment of the focus can be performed using ultrasound imaging. The stone fragmentation typically requires about 4000 shocks.

## Conclusions and future directions

Four-dimensional ultrasound (real-time 3D scans with Doppler flow information) is used in specialist clinics and in anaesthetic domains. The equipment for general scanning is becoming much smaller and portable. This has enabled ultrasound technology to be used in operating theatres, intensive care units and pain clinics.

### *References*

**Chapman, G. A., Johnson, D.** and **Bodenham, A. R.** (2006) Review article: Visualisation of needle position using ultrasonography, *Anaesthesia*, **61**, pp. 148–58.

**Donovan, F. D., Dobb, G. J., Newman, M. A. *et al.*** (1987) Comparison of pulsed Doppler and thermodilution methods for measuring cardiac output in critically ill patients, *Crit. Care Med.*, **15**, pp. 853–7.

**Farrar, D. J., Green, H. D.** and **Peterson, D. W.** (1979) Noninvasively and invasively measured pulsatile haemodynamics with graded arterial stenosis, *Cardiovasc. Res.*, **13**, pp. 45–7.

**Hausen, B., Schafers, H., Rohde, R. *et al.*** (1992) Clinical evaluation of transtracheal Doppler for continuous cardiac output estimation, *Anesth Analg.*, **74**, pp. 800–4.

**Lee, B. Y., Assadi, C.** and **Madden, J. L.** (1978) Haemodynamics of arterial stenosis, *World J. Surg.*, **2**, pp. 621–9.

**Munn, J., Tooley, M., Bolsin, S., Hronex, I., Lowson, S.** and **Wilcox, J.** (1993) The effect of metoclopramide on renal vascular resistance and renal function in patients receiving a low-dose infusion of dopamine, *Br. J. Anaesth.*, **71**, pp. 379–82.

**Schafhalter-Zoppoth, I., Mcculloch, C. E.** and **Gray, A. T.** (2004) Ultrasound visibility of needles for regional nerve block: An in vitro study, *Reg. Anesth. Pain Med.*, **29**, pp. 480–9.

**Stevens, P. E., Gwyther, S. J., Boultbee, J. E.** *et al.* (1989) Practical use of duplex Doppler analysis of the renal vasculature in critical ill patients, *Lancet*, **1**, pp. 240–2.

**Tooley, M., Greenslade, G., Halliwell, M.** and **Bolsin, S.** (1994) A pilot study to assess the validity of Doppler pulsatility and resistance indices as correlates of renal blood flow changes produced by dopamine in normal subjects, *Br. J. Radiol.*, **67**(799), pp. 733–4.

## *Further reading*

**Evans, D. H., McDicken, W. N., Skidmore R.** and **Woodcock, J. P.** (1989) Waveform analysis and pattern recognition. In *Doppler Ultrasound, Physics, Instrumentation, and Clinical Applications*, John Wiley & Sons Ltd, Chichester, pp. 163–87.

**Wells, P. N. T. (ed.)** (1993) *Advances in Ultrasound Techniques and Instrumentation*, Churchill Livingstone, New York.

# Chapter 11 **Principles and standards of anaesthetic monitoring**

The chapter links with: Chapters 12, 13, 14, 15, 16, 18 and 19.

## Introduction

The World Federation of Societies of Anaesthesiology (WFSA) adopted standards relating to the safe practice of anaesthesia in 1992 in order to cut the morbidity due to anaesthesia itself, and these standards have been continually reviewed and updated (Gelb *et al.* 2018). In the last ten years, safety in the operating theatre has also included the implementation of a WHO safety checklist prior to the start of an operating list, not least to flatten the hierarchy within the operating team, as well as to check that equipment and processes are in place. This is apart from safety checks an anaesthetist might do on drugs and equipment before the operating list starts and before each case (AAGBI, Checking Anaesthetic Equipment 2012). In modern times, it is easy to forget that historically anaesthesia and surgery did indeed have associated morbidity and mortality and there was very little assistance from technology to monitor patients.

Clearly, technological monitoring has played its part in improving patient safety (Checketts *et al.* 2016), and the evolution of safety standards includes two main requirements of monitoring. The first is to record anticipated deviations from normal values, which require accurate measurement to ensure patient safety. The second is to warn of unexpected, life-threatening events that, by definition, occur without warning, and could affect the fit, young patient as easily as the old and infirm. All international standards stress the importance of the continual presence of a fully trained and accredited anaesthetic person. Central to the maintenance of these standards is the quality of persons entering the specialty, the quality of training programmes, and the continuing education of specialists throughout a professional lifetime (Sykes 1992), even if local circumstances require the use of non-physicians in the administration of anaesthesia.

It is difficult to determine with certainty the effect that additional technological monitoring has on safety. One clear example is the inability of the trained human eye to detect cyanosis, this human failure occurring maximally at 81–85% oxygen saturation. Clearly, the pulse oximeter has improved the quality of cyanosis detection, and efforts have been made to ensure the worldwide availability of this monitor (Walker *et al.* 2009).

Numerous worldwide studies have shown that mortality due to anaesthesia itself fell significantly between the 1950s and the 1980s, by which time extensive technological monitoring was being introduced, and training programmes had been greatly improved.

Utting (1987) reviewed 750 cases of death and cerebral damage reported to the British General Medical Council between 1970 and 1982 that were thought to be the result of errors in technique. Of these, 37% were thought to be accidental, therefore not correctable, and 63% due to error, and therefore correctable. Two-thirds of these were concerned with problems of the airway, endotracheal tube, ventilation or hypoxia. A number of these incidents, especially those concerned with airway obstruction, occur in the immediate postoperative period. It is also true that by far the greatest proportion of incidents, including death, are due to human error (Cooper *et al.* 1978) and, of the critical incidents reported, problems with airway control and inspired gas composition constituted the majority. It is not incidental that human factors studies in anaesthesia are subject to scrutiny these days in order to try to minimize such errors (Lomax *et al.* 2024)

It is probably true that the market availability of monitoring has driven clinical standards, rather than the other way around. Nevertheless, it is hard to prove that monitoring standards improve safety in anaesthesia, but it has long been agreed that the controlled trials required for this purpose would be unethical (Eichorn 1989). Runciman *et al.* (1993) concluded that the problems that give the most risk to patients have been identified as those relating to hypoxic gas mixtures, gas flows, breathing systems, endotracheal tubes, the airway, and ventilation; that most of these problems can be avoided following guidelines outlined below; and that, in many countries, the expense of this additional monitoring is far less than the medico-legal consequences of failing to provide them.

Other studies also concluded (Webb *et al.* 1993; Holland *et al.* 1993) that more than 70% of the anaesthetic incidents which occur during induction, maintenance and recovery from anaesthesia, are detectable by monitor and that, of these, over 80% would be detectable by the correct use of a pulse oximeter. When used in conjunction with a capnometer, over 90% of monitor-detectable incidents are detectable, and this argues strongly in favour of the combined use of these two monitors. It has been shown that increasing the amount of physiological monitoring to a level above that of modern standard critical care monitoring (Watkinson *et al.* 2006) does not improve adverse outcomes or mortality. On the other hand, novel ways of automatically integrating patients' physiological information (Tarassenko *et al.* 2006) can lead to earlier detection of untoward physiological events, particularly in the immediate postoperative period, when one-on-one patient care may not be available (Michard *et al.* 2020; Webster *et al.* 2022).

Given the plethora of monitoring data available to the modern anaesthetist, it is possible to be overwhelmed with information to the extent that a suboptimal response to a critical incident is affected. Work has been carried out to try to determine the best way to present data to the anaesthetist, and although reaction times to graphical displays are more rapid, it is appropriate to have a mixed graphical–numerical display (Chakrabati *et al.* 2009; Kennedy *et al.* 2009), and the evolution of optimal graphical displays continues (Görges and Staggers 2008).

With regard to anaesthesia on a worldwide basis, however, it is reasonable to say that safe anaesthesia does not require a mass of complex equipment and the greatest degree of safety for the available resources is achievable by a careful, conscientious anaesthetist who balances risk, benefit and cost in the context in which he or she works.

Before outlining current international monitoring standards, it is worth discussing alarm systems. Because monitors have vastly increased the amount of information available to anaesthetists, alarm noise has made the use of alarms unpopular thus risking their non-use, or the possibility that the anaesthetist's attention will be directed towards the alarm itself rather than to the patient's problem (Edworthy and Hellier 2006; Tarassenko *et al.* 2006; Roche *et al.* 2021; Foley *et al.* 2023). The current international standard on alarms is IEC 60601–1, parts 1 to 8, which has been developed with cooperation between clinicians, engineers and psychologists. It is important that alarm design is appropriate for the intended users, and that the alarm device is appropriately positioned so as not to be useless.

The anatomy of a critical incident, shown in Figure 11.1, forms a sound basis on which to design alarm systems.

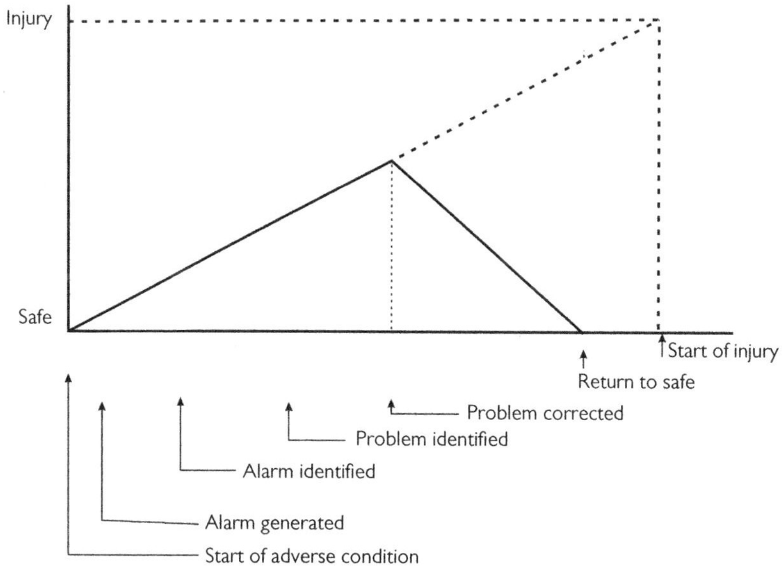


**Fig. 11.1** Development of a critical incident in relation to detection, alarms and safety (Schreiber and Schreiber 1987).

## Recommendations for standards of monitoring

The Association of Anaesthetists of Great Britain and Ireland (AAGBI) issues a short summary of its recommendations for standards of monitoring during anaesthesia and recovery, which it regularly reviews and updates (Klein *et al.* 2021). A more detailed outline of monitoring requirements is given below to enhance the reader's understanding of these requirements.

### *Oxygenation*

#### *Oxygen supply*

Supplemental oxygen is usually given to patients. The anaesthetist should ensure the integrity of the oxygen supply and, when nitrous oxide or other supplemental gases are used, the concentration of oxygen in the inspired gas should be monitored throughout each anaesthetic with a monitor fitted with a low oxygen concentration alarm. There should also be an oxygen supply failure alarm and a device to protect the patient against the delivery of a hypoxic gas mixture. In addition, a system should be in place to prevent the misconnection of gas sources. Ensuring the integrity of the oxygen supply means ensuring that pipeline connections are intact, that oxygen pipeline pressure is adequate, that there are no cross-connections, and that at least one spare oxygen cylinder with adequate contents is present and connected, with a means available of turning it on immediately. Therefore, pipeline and cylinder should both have a pressure gauge, and pressure is usually an indication of contents. An oxygen meter, of the fuel cell, polarographic or paramagnetic analyser type should be used (see Chapter 16) to ensure that the oxygen supply is uncontaminated, and if other gases are used, that the rotameters give a reasonable indication of the fractional oxygen in the mixture. Note that if very low fresh gas flow is used in a circle system, the fractional oxygen delivered from the anaesthetic machine outlet is not the same as the concentration delivered to the patient's lungs, since oxygen consumption by the patient is a significant proportion of the recirculated gas. Therefore, the oxygen meter should be placed close to the patient's airway rather than close to the anaesthetic machine. The human condition is such that the presence of the monitor itself may provide an unwarranted feeling of security, and a low oxygen concentration alarm should be fitted. In case of oxygen supply failure, a supply failure alarm should be fitted, and ideally, the rotameters should be fitted with a device to prevent the delivery of a hypoxic mixture, either as a chain-linked device on Ohmeda machines, or as hydraulic linkage as on Draeger machines (see Chapter 22). All pipelines and cylinders should be pin-indexed to prevent misconnection of gas sources.

### *Oxygenation of the patient*

As suggested earlier, the human eye is particularly bad at detecting the adequacy of tissue oxygenation. This is no excuse for not looking at the patient, and keeping adequate parts of the patient exposed to do so where surgical conditions permit. However, there is no doubt that continuous pulse oximetry is highly desirable, and its function is described in Chapter 15.

## ***Airway and ventilation***

The adequacy of the airway and ventilation should be continuously monitored by observation and auscultation of the patient whenever practicable, and the use of a precordial, pretracheal, or oesophageal stethoscope has the advantage of keeping the anaesthetist in clinical and physical contact with the patient, even if such is rarely used these days. The correct placement of the endotracheal tube is confirmed initially by observation of equal bilateral chest movements (difficult in the obese patient) and subsequently with a stethoscope by the presence of bilateral axillary breath sounds and an absence of gastric sounds. Its correct placement or indeed the placement of a laryngeal mask and the adequacy of ventilation may be initially confirmed by the feel and quality of manual ventilation, and subsequently by continuous measurement and display of the carbon dioxide waveform and concentration. The continual presence of carbon dioxide monitoring, with both numerical and waveform output, warns of changes to the airway, the ventilation and circulation. Most commonly available devices are of the infrared variety, described in Chapter 16. Other devices include mass spectrometry and Raman spectrometry. Since many cases of adverse events in anaesthesia, ICU and emergency departments involve failure to secure the airway, the absolute need for capnography in all such situations cannot be overemphasised (Cook *et al.* 2011; Russotto and Cook 2021). Furthermore, all clinicians should be fully conversant with the full value of capnography, particularly in ICU (Kerslake and Kelly 2017). As well as indicating airway integrity and respiratory pathology, capnography has also been used successfully as an indicator of cardiac output change in response to fluid challenge (Lakhal *et al.* 2017).

When mechanical ventilation is employed, a disconnection alarm should also be used continuously, as should measurement of the inspiratory and/or expired gas volumes. A disconnection alarm is highly desirable, and can take the form of detection of low volume, flow or pressure, or lack of a $CO_2$ trace. Volume detectors used to be of the Wright's respirometer type, but are these days manifested by electronic integration of the flow signal, which itself is measured by a differential U-tube manometer.

The continual presence of the anaesthetist is emphasised because it is only the anaesthetist or the designated, trained anaesthetic staff who have the training and experience to detect an inadequate airway; untrained staff do not have this skill or experience. The basic clinical skills of observation of a patient's breathing, of the reservoir bag, are crucial; auscultation is a reassuring adjunct, especially if an endotracheal tube is involved.

## ***Circulation***

### *Cardiac rate and rhythm*

The circulation should be monitored by continuous palpation or registration of the pulse and/or auscultation of the heart sounds. There should be continuous monitoring and display of the heart rate with a plethysmograph (usually incorporated into a pulse oximeter), or with an electrocardiograph (see Chapters 5 and 18). Continuity of observation is stressed here and again the basic clinical skills of palpation and auscultation are very adequate monitors, which should not be neglected. The oesophageal/ precordial stethoscope is also useful, and gives a qualitative measure of the force of cardiac contraction. A plethysmographic device, such as the one on a pulse oximeter (see Chapter 15), can also be useful to detect rate and rhythm. The ECG has remained an important rate monitor, despite the introduction of pulse oximeters; it is still the most sensitive detector of rhythm change. These days, software for automatic ST segment analysis is available for intraoperative cardiac ischaemia monitoring; it should be remembered, however, that ECG changes usually represent very late changes in a hypoxic episode (see Figure 11.1).

### *Tissue perfusion*

The adequacy of tissue perfusion should be monitored continually by clinical examination and continuous monitoring with a plethysmograph or capnograph (see Chapter 16) is highly recommended. This is another example of a variable that needs the continual presence of the trained eye. A plethysmographic signal can also be useful, but that on the pulse oximeter is electronically amplified or attenuated to within certain limits, so it may only be a crude guide as a monitor of inadequate perfusion. The experienced clinician looks for changes in all monitors to come to a decision about a clinical situation. For example, there may be no change in the blood pressure or oxygen saturation where tissue perfusion is impaired but, in the absence of any other relevant changes, a reduction in end tidal $CO_2$ levels on the capnograph may be an indicator of changes in blood flow to the lungs, which can be a reflection of cardiac output or of pulmonary embolus.

### *Blood pressure*

Arterial blood pressure should be determined at appropriate intervals (see Chapter 12), usually at least every 5 minutes, and more frequently if indicated by clinical circumstances. Continuous registration of arterial blood pressure is encouraged in appropriate cases. While cardiac output is the important variable that we want to know about, historically it has not been as easy to measure as, for example, blood pressure.

Contemporary methods of cardiac output measurement are relatively non-invasive compared to earlier times (see Chapter 13). However, there is a much longer history of blood pressure measurement, which represents an easily measured, clinically established variable that is directly related to cardiac output. Traditionally, it was measured manually with a double cuff device every 3 or 5 minutes; these days, there are automatically cycling single cuff devices that have a degree of accuracy that is perfectly acceptable when compared against intra-arterial devices, except at very low pressures. The need for intra-arterial blood pressure monitoring as opposed to non-invasive cuff monitoring is usually a matter for clinical judgement.

No technique is without morbidity, and intra-arterial monitoring is no exception. Where continuous monitoring is required, then it is desirable; preconditions for this might include: poor cardiac condition, predicted large blood loss, hypotensive surgery, cardiac or vascular surgery, neurosurgery, prolonged surgery; but each case should be judged on its own merits. The requirement of the device is accurate reproduction of all the harmonics of the blood pressure waveform, with no signal distortion from inappropriate damping or phase distortion (see Chapter 12). Note also that no guideline is given on the need for central venous or pulmonary artery pressure measurement, these being a matter for clinical judgement, such as anticipated large blood loss, or a poorly functioning left ventricle. The use of the pulmonary artery catheter to measure cardiac output has all but disappeared from clinical practice (van Doorn *et al.* 1994) by the emergence of the less invasive echocardiography (see Chapters 10 and 13), which uses the Doppler principle to measure blood velocity and, by deduction, the cardiac output.

### ***Temperature***

Due to attenuation of the function of the autonomic nervous system during anaesthesia, patients can become very cold in the operating theatre, with cold air-conditioning, cold respiratory gases, and cold intravenous fluids, with a subsequent prolongation in recovery. The use of low gas flows, recirculated through a carbon dioxide absorber, heated fluids and blankets has improved this, but hypothermia is a potential problem during long operations. More dangerous is malignant hyperthermia, and patients having operations for the first time are an unknown quantity here. There are very adequate and inexpensive thermistor temperature probes for oesophageal, tympanic or rectal use. In any case temperature should be measured pre-induction and half hourly thereafter.

## *Depth of anaesthesia*

Clinical assessment of anaesthetic depth is not easy, since all the clinical indicators are indirect, i.e. blood pressure, pulse rate. The gas analysers that measure $CO_2$ also measure volatile agents and a continual measure of inspired and expired vapour can be made; with a knowledge of MAC values for each agent, the expired value can be used as a measure of the adequacy of anaesthetic depth. This is particularly important where low fresh gas flows are being used, since what is dialled up on the vaporiser bears little relationship to what is in the breathing system until equilibrium is reached; the patient's absorption of the agent, especially early on in the anaesthesia, forms a large proportion of the amount of agent in the breathing system. Later on, absorption diminishes as the patient becomes saturated, and the amount in the breathing system increases with no change to the vaporiser setting. The *BIS monitor*, which looks at changes in the EEG that are characteristic of the changing depth of anaesthesia, is now recommended and more widely used, particularly as nitrous oxide is less often used with a volatile agent than formerly. This, and other depth of anaesthesia monitors, are described in Chapter 19. AAGBI guidelines strongly recommend the use of such a monitor where total intravenous anaesthesia is used in conjunction with neuro-muscular blockade.

## *Neuromuscular function*

When neuromuscular blocking drugs are given, the use of a peripheral nerve stimulator is recommended. This recommendation is given a relatively low priority but, equally, this monitor is useful to determine the contribution of residual neuromuscular blockade in the patient who fails to resume spontaneous respiration at the end of the operation. This monitor is almost more important where the older neuromuscular blockers are used than it is where newer, shorter-acting agents are used (McGrath and Hunter 2006).

## *Postanaesthesia care*

All patients should be observed and monitored in a manner appropriate to the state of their nervous system function, vital signs, and medical condition, with emphasis on oxygenation, ventilation and circulation. Supplementation of clinical monitoring with quantitative methods described above for intra-anaesthetic patient care is recommended. Pulse oximetry is highly recommended. When patients are sent to general wards postoperatively, where one-on-one nursing staff are not always available, continued technological monitoring is recommended as appropriate.

## *References*

**Association of Anaesthetists of Great Britain and Ireland** (2012) Checking anaesthetic equipment 2012, *Anaesthesia.*, 67, pp. 660–8.

**Chakrabati, S. *et al.*** (2009) Comparison of four different display designs of a novel anaesthetic monitoring system, the 'integrated monitor of anaesthesia (IMA)', *Br. J. Anaes.*, **103**, pp. 670–7.

**Checketts, M. R., Alladi, R.** and **Ferguson, K.** (2016) Recommendations for standards of monitoring during anaesthesia and recovery 2015: Association of Anaesthetists of Great Britain and Ireland, *Anaesthesia.*, **71**, pp. 85–93.

**Cook T., Woodall N., Harper J.** and **Benger J.** (2011) Major complications of airway management in UK: results of NAP4 of the Royal College of Anaesthetists and the Difficult Airway Society: Part 2: intensive care and emergency departments. *B.J.A.*, **106**(5), pp. 632–42.

**Cooper, J. B., Newbower, R. S.** and **Kitz, R. J.** (1978) An analysis of major errors and equipment, failures in anesthesia management: considerations for prevention and detection, *Anesthesiology*, **60**, pp. 34–42.

**Edworthy, J.** and **Hellier, E.** (2006) Alarms and human behaviour: implications for medical alarms, Postgraduate Educational Issue – Clinical Monitoring, *Br. J. Anaes.*, 97, pp. 12–17.

**Eichorn, J. H.** (1989) Prevention of intraoperative anesthesia accidents and related severe injury through safety monitoring, *Anesthesiology*, 70, pp. 572–7.

**Foley, L., Schlesinger, J. J. and Schultz, M.** (2023) Improving detectability of auditory interfaces for medical alarms through temporal variation in amplitude envelope, *B.J.A.*, **130**(3), pp. 351–9.

**Gelb, A. W., Morriss, W. W.**, Johnson, **W. *et al.*** (2018) World Health Organization-World Federation of Societies of Anaesthesiologists (WHO-WFSA) International Standards for a Safe Practice of Anesthesia, *Can. J. Anaesthesia*, **65**, pp. 698–708.

**Görges, M.** and **Staggers, N.** (2008) Evaluations of physiological monitoring displays: a systematic review, *J. Clin. Monit. Comput.*, 22, pp. 45–66.

**Holland, R., Webb, R. K.** and **Runciman, W. B.** (1993) Oesophageal intubation. The first 2000 AIMS reports, *Anaes. Int. Care*, 21, pp. 608–10.

**Kennedy, R. R. *et al.*** (2009) The influence of various graphical and numeric trend display formats on the detection of simulated changes, *Anaesthesia*, 64, pp. 1186–9.

**Kerslake, I.** and **Kelly, F.** (2017) Use of capnography in the Critical Care Unit, *B.J.A. Educ.*, **17**(5), pp. 178–83.

**Klein, A. A., Meek, T., Allcock, E. *et al.*** (2021) Association of Anaesthetists of Great Britain and Ireland. Recommendations for Standards of Monitoring during Anaesthesia and Recovery, Guideline from the Association of Anaesthetists. *Anaesthesia*, **76**(9), pp. 1212–23.

**Lakhal, K., Nay, M. A., Kamel, T. *et al.*** (2017) Change in end-tidal CO2 outperforms other surrogates for change in cardiac output during fluid challenge, *Br. J. Anaesth.*, **118**(3), pp. 365–82.

**Lomax, S., Catchpole, K.** and **Sutcliffe, J.** (2024) Human factors in anaesthetic practice, part 2: Clinical implications, *B.J.A. Educ.*, **24** (2), pp. 68–74.

**McGrath, C. D.** and **Hunter, J. M.** (2006) Monitoring of neuromuscular blockade. Continuing education in anaesthesia, *Crit. Care & Pain*, 6, pp. 7–12.

**Michard, F., Scheeren, T. W. L.** and **Saugl, B. (**2020) A glimpse into the future of postoperative arterial blood pressure monitoring, *Br. J. Anaesth.*, **125**(2), pp. 113–15.

**Roche, T. R., Braun, J., Ganter, M. T. *et al.*** (2021) Voice alerting as a medical alarm modality for the next generation of patient monitoring: a randomised international multi-centre trial, *Br. J. Anaesth.*, **127**(5), pp. 769–77.

**Runciman, W. B., Webb, R. K., Barker, L.** and **Currie, M.** (1993) The pulse oximeter: applications and limitations. first 2000 AIMS reports, *Anaesth. Intensive Care*, 21, pp. 543–50.

**Russotto, V.** and **Cook, T.** (2021) Capnography use in critical care setting: why do clinicians fail to implement this safety measure? *Br. J. Anaesth.*, **127**(5), pp. 661–4.

**Schreiber, P.** and **Schreiber, J.** (1987) *Anesthesia Systems Risk Analysis and Risk Reduction*, North American Draeger.

**Sykes, M. K.** (1992) Clinical measurement and clinical practice, *Anaesthesia*, 47, pp. 425–32.

**Tarassenko, L., Hann, A.** and **Young, D.** (2006) Integrated monitoring and analysis for early warning of patient deterioration, Postgraduate Educational Issue – Clinical Monitoring, *Br. J. Anaes.*, 97, pp. 64–8.

**The International Task Force** (1993) The International Task Force on Anaesthesia Safety: International Standards for a Safe Practice of Anaesthesia, *Eur. J. Anaesthesiol.*, 10(suppl 7), pp. 12–15.

**Utting, J. E.** (1987) Pitfalls in anaesthetic practice, *Br. J. Anaes.*, 59, 877–90.

**van Doorn, C. A. M., Lyons, G., Swindells, S.** and **Unnikrishnan Nair, R.** (1994) Perforation of the right ventricle and cardiac tamponade; the use of a pulmonary artery catheter, *Br. J. of Intensive Care*, **4**(Feb), pp. 66–7.

**Walker, I. A., Merry, A. F., Wilson, I. H. *et al.*** (2009) Global oximetry: an international anaesthesia quality improvement project, *Anaesthesia*, 64, pp. 1051–60.

**Watkinson, P. J. *et al.*** (2006) A randomised controlled trial of the effect of continuous electronic physiological monitoring on adverse event rate in high risk medical and surgical patients, *Anaesthesia*, 61, pp. 1031–9.

**Webb, R. K., van der Walt, J.** and **Runciman, W. B. *et al.*** (1993) Which monitor? The first 2000 AIMS reports, *Anaesth. Int. Care*, 21, pp. 529–42.

**Webster, C., Scheeren T. W. L. and Wan Y. I.** (2022) Patient monitoring, wearable devices and the healthcare information system, *Br. J. Anaesth.*, **128**(5), pp. 756–8.

# Chapter 12 **Blood pressure measurement**

The chapter has links with; Chapters 1, 3, 4, 5, 6, 10, 11 and 13.

## Introduction

Blood pressure measurement occurs either non-invasively or invasively, and usually refers to systemic arterial pressure measurement, but can also refer to systemic venous or pulmonary arterial pressure measurement. In 1733 the Reverend Stephen Hales was the first person to measure the blood pressure *in vivo* in unanaesthetised horses by direct cannulation of the carotid and femoral arteries. In doing so he observed the pulsatile nature of flow in the circulation. In 1828 Poiseuille developed the mercury manometer, and used it to measure blood pressure in a dog. The mercury manometer has, of course, become the standard technique against which other techniques are compared. The earliest numerical information on blood pressure measurement came from direct rather than indirect measurement in 1856 by Faivre, using Poiseuille's device. However, in the last part of the nineteenth century, non-invasive measurement techniques were developed. In 1903, Codman and Cushing introduced the concept of routine intraoperative blood pressure measurement, which at the time was a revolutionary concept. Nowadays it is a fundamental part of minimal monitoring criteria.

## Non-invasive blood pressure measurement

There are several techniques of non-invasive BP (NIBP) measurement, all of which function by occluding the pulse in a limb with a proximal cuff, then detecting its onset again distally, on lowering the cuff pressure. Detection methods include palpation, auscultation, plethysmography and oscillometry. Accuracy of all non-invasive techniques depends on cuff size in relation to the limb concerned, and over which artery the cuff is placed. Such techniques of NIBP measurement are necessarily intermittent. Much discussion has taken place on the accuracy of these devices, and the accuracy of diastolic pressure measurements needs improving, and there are ideas proposed for new non-invasive devices (Tooley and Magee 2009).

### *Palpation*

In the absence of a stethoscope, this technique is simple and reliable. After inflating the cuff on the upper arm to a pressure of above that of systolic, the cuff is then deflated while palpating the brachial artery and the systolic pressure is measured with a mercury column at first detection of the pulse. A study by van Bergen *et al.* (1954) showed that BP can be underestimated by this method by up to 25% at 120 mmHg. Factors that worsen this underestimate include bradycardia and rapid cuff deflation.

### *Auscultation*

Auscultation depends on hearing Korotkoff sounds, first described in 1905. The sounds are described in phases, from I to V, shown in Figure 12.1. The physical origin of Korotkoff sounds is uncertain, but is almost certainly due to resonance set up in tissues from turbulent flow in the artery.

Phase I is the first onset of a *tapping*, high frequency sound, which is synchronous with the pulse, which increases in intensity, which represents the onset of systolic blood pressure, and 5–10 mmHg below which there appears a palpable pulse. In phase II the frequency of the sound is lower, represented by a softening of the sound, and in some patients the sounds in this phase disappear altogether – the auscultatory gap – before the frequency increases again. The presence of an *auscultatory*

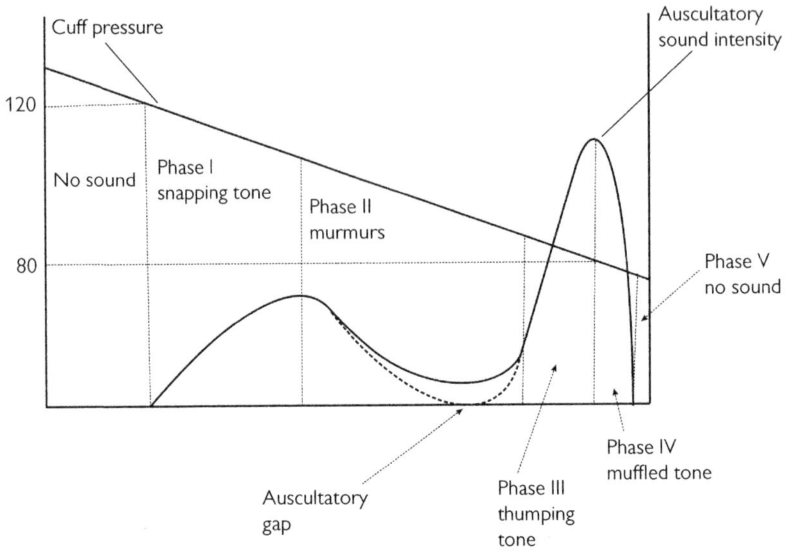


**Fig. 12.1** Graphical representation of cuff deflation and intensity of sounds on auscultation when measuring blood pressure.

*gap* in some hypertensive patients within phase II, indicates the need for a rough estimate of systolic BP by palpation before a more accurate measure by auscultation. The sounds then become sharper in phase III. In phase IV there is an abrupt muffling of the sounds and their complete disappearance in phase V. Diastolic blood pressure corresponds to either phase IV (American Heart Association, children) or phase V (American Heart Association, adults) or both (World Health Organisation). Phase V is closer to real diastolic than phase IV and there is better agreement between observers on phase V onset. However in some hyperdynamic states, phase V may not occur until the cuff is almost completely deflated.

Another error with this method (and with other cuff methods) is using the wrong cuff size (see next). Other causes of inaccuracy include lack of agreement between observers, over-rapid deflation of the cuff, and bradycardia. The studies of Pereira *et al.* (1985) showed that, although there were reasonable positive correlations between direct and auscultatory measurements for systolic ($r$ = 0.93) and diastolic ($r$ = 0.79) pressures, there was a large variation between observers. They showed that auscultation tended to overestimate at lower pressures and underestimate at higher pressures. However, the method is simple and reliable.

## *Oscillometry*

In contrast to historically used oscillotonometry (which uses a double cuff system, one for compressing the limb, the other for sensing pulsations), oscillometry uses a single cuff, both to compress the artery and to detect pulsations. This is the standard contemporary method of NIBP measurement in automated devices using microprocessor technology. If the cuff is automatically inflated to some predetermined level above systolic BP, then deflated continuously or in a stepwise fashion, arterial pulsations are detected on the cuff as systolic BP is reached. As mean arterial pressure is reached, these pulsations reach maximum amplitude, and as diastolic pressure is approached these pulsations diminish and disappear. This process is shown graphically in Figure 12.2. The mechanism inside such a device is shown in Figure 12.3. A single pressure transducer detects the cuff pressure itself continuously as well as the arterial pulsations. Appropriate electronic circuitry digitises and processes the signal, then systolic,

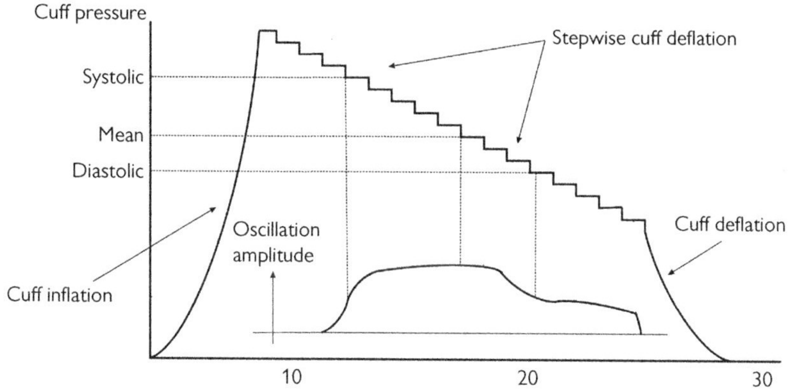


**Fig. 12.2** Graphical representation of the use of an oscillometer, showing decreasing cuff pressure plotted against time in seconds on deflation with increasing transmission of oscillation and the link to measured components of blood pressure.

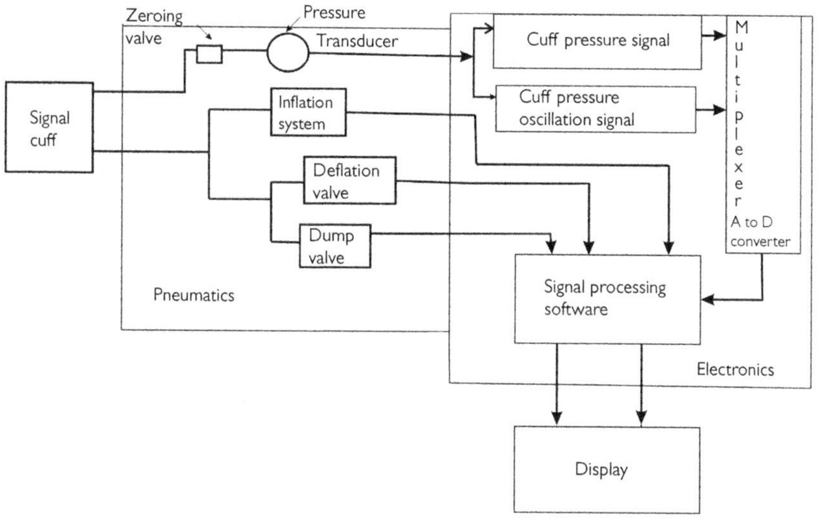


**Fig. 12.3** Hydraulic and electronic components of an oscillometer.

mean and diastolic pressures are displayed. The original Dinamap measured only mean arterial pressure (MAP), where cuff oscillations are at a maximum. It was found to be accurate if the compressible volume within the hydraulic components of the device was kept to a minimum. With the subsequent development of more sophisticated electronic algorithms, systolic BP (SBP), MAP and diastolic BP (DBP) became measurable. SBP is deemed to occur where the rate of increase of the pulsations is at a maximum (rather than the onset of pulsations) and the DBP is measured where the rate of decrease is maximum (rather than the offset). It is generally more difficult to detect diastolic pressure than systolic using this technique. It is also likely that the algorithm checks the measurements with the equation

$$MAP = DBP + \frac{(SBP - DBP)}{3}.$$

This assumes that the pressure waveform is triangular in shape, with DBP at the base, SBP at the apex, with MAP at the triangle's centroid. There are also oscillometric devices that deflate the cuff continuously rather than in discrete steps, and which analyse the overall oscillation envelope.

Excessive cuff movement, rapid BP changes, abnormal pulse rhythms and interchanging cuffs can all exceed the ability of the electronic algorithms to interpret the BP components accurately. Otherwise, these devices have been shown to be convenient and reasonably accurate, although with less accuracy at critically low pressures, particularly diastolic.

## Doppler ultrasound

Blood pressure can also be determined using ultrasound, by detecting blood vessel wall movement or blood flow. In either case the Doppler principle is the applicable physical principle (see Chapter 10). An ultrasonic transmitter and receiver lies against the skin beneath an occluding cuff. As the cuff is deflated and blood flow or vessel movement is detected, there is an audible Doppler frequency shift, whose character changes as the cuff pressure falls through systolic to diastolic. Analysis of frequencies by the device yields SBP and DBP. Doppler techniques have been found to yield higher systolic pressures that an old fashioned sphygmomanometric method (MacDonald *et al.* 2008).

## Cuff size

This is an important factor in determining the accuracy of any NIBP measurement technique. In particular, this factor has implications for NIBP measurement in children and in obese patients. The guidelines of the American Heart Association stipulate that the width of (the inflatable bladder part of) the cuff should be 40% of the mid-circumference of the limb, and that the length of the cuff should be twice this width. A narrow cuff gives a falsely high reading and a wide cuff gives a falsely low one. A cuff reading of blood pressure may indeed not correlate with intra-arterial BP measurement across the whole range of BPs, because there is a non-linear relationship between the pressure in a cuff and its internal diameter around a limb, which is the variable important in compressing the limb concerned.

Morbidity from cuffs includes skin and underlying tissue damage and possible ulnar nerve damage, when used on the arm too close to the elbow.

## Other cuff sites

Sometimes the upper arm is not the most convenient place at which to measure the blood pressure using a cuff. The calf and the ankle are two such alternative sites. It has been found that there is poor agreement between different sites for systolic pressure measurement, but better agreement for diastolic and mean pressures (Moore *et al.* 2008), and that the ankle is the least uncomfortable place for the cuff. If the ankle is used as a cuff site, then the additional presence of an intermittent compression device on the leg must not influence the BP reading, if the measurement is made when the compression device is not in its active phase (Parikh *et al.* 2007).

## Plethysmographic methods

The *Finapres* uses the principle of arterial volume clamp plethysmography, developed by Peñaz and Slurer. Figure 12.4 shows the Finapres. A small, low-volume cuff, which also contains an infrared light source and photo detector, so that the finger is transilluminated, is applied around a finger. The amount of infrared light absorbed depends to some extent on the blood volume in the finger at the time; this is the same technology as the pulse oximeter uses. The finger cuff is relatively non-compliant, and is attached to a small pump and a solenoid valve, which allows rapid small amplitude pressure changes to be applied to the finger. This is linked to a servo-control mechanism with a fast response time. Initially the system determines the MAP during the 'open loop phase', and subsequently the arterial waveform is continuously followed during the 'closed loop phase'.

During the open loop phase, the cuff is deflated from maximum inflation until cuff oscillations are maximum, corresponding to MAP determined by an oscillometric method. The amount of infra-red light absorbed in the finger at this point corresponds to a *set point*. During the closed-loop phase, the

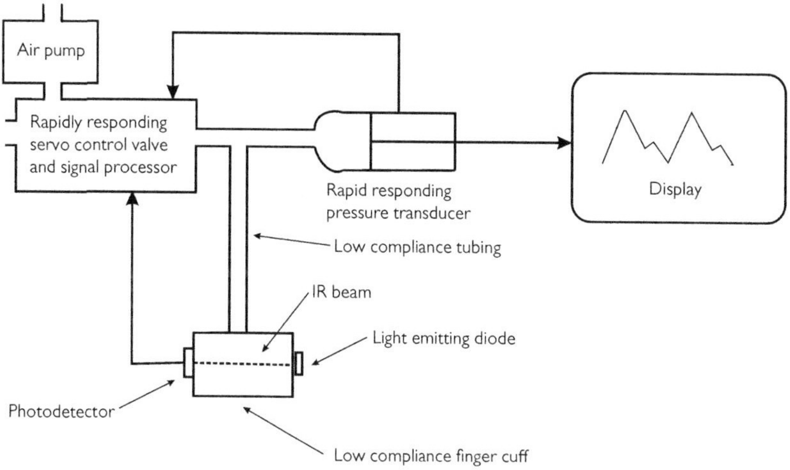


**Fig. 12.4** Peñaz technique for continuous non-invasive technique for blood pressure measurement (Finapres).

cuff pressure is adjusted rapidly to maintain constant IR light absorption in the finger tissues. It does this in the presence of arterial pulsation and vessel distension, as deviations from MAP occur due to intra-arterial pressure rise to systolic BP, and fall to diastolic BP from the set point at MAP. Thus the device tracks arterial pressure and the output is displayed as an arterial waveform.

In order for the accuracy of the device to be maintained, all components of the compressible volume, including the non-distensible cuff, must be kept to a minimum. The whole electro-pneumatic and plethysmographic device, with associated amplifiers, is contained in a box strapped to the patient's arm. Despite variable reports on its accuracy, its small size makes it convenient to use in mobile situations and the fact that it produces a continuous output makes it useful. The use of a modern variant of this device, the 'Nexfin', found that the technique has insufficient accuracy for use in critically ill patients (Hohn *et al.* 2013).

Another device that falls into this category of 'applanation tonometry' and functions in a similar way, but without a cuff, is the 'Tensymeter' (Szmuk *et al.* 2008), a non-invasive device that is used over the radial artery. An actuator applies external pressure to the artery, and a sensor assesses the pulsations at different levels of applied pressure, and uses an algorithm to produce a continuous output of systolic, mean and diastolic pressure.

A device is being developed which uses a combination of photoplethysmography of a peripheral pulse waveform and machine learning to measure blood pressure without using intermittent inflation of a cuff (Chowdhury *et al.* 2020).

## Direct measurement of blood pressure

The direct measurement of arterial blood pressure has some advantages over other blood pressure measurements: the waveform obtained from the data is continuous (as opposed to intermittent), and it can be in real-time and is potentially the most accurate of any blood pressure measurement. Direct measurement is very important in critically ill patients and in those whose cardiovascular system may be compromised. It is important in patients who require physiological or pharmacological manipulation of the blood pressure, e.g. cardiopulmonary bypass, or hypotensive anaesthesia. It also provides a convenient means for taking blood for blood gas analysis. When the waveform is obtained, a number of other indices (Hutton and Cooper 1985; Prys-Roberts 1984) can be obtained, apart from the systolic,

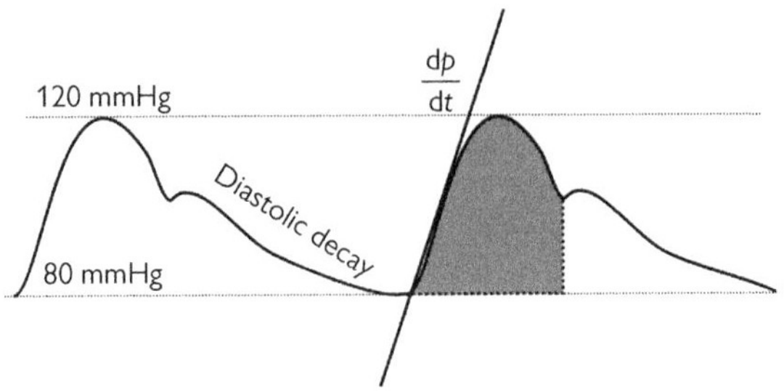


**Fig. 12.5** Arterial waveform showing indices obtained: myocardial contractility (d*p*/d*t*), index of stroke volume (represented by the shaded area), and diastolic decay.

diastolic, mean and heart rate. Myocardial contractility can be assessed from the gradient (d*p*/d*t*) of the arterial upstroke as shown in Figure 12.5.

The area beneath the curve up to the dicrotic notch gives an index of stroke volume, which is also shown in the figure. The characteristics of the diastolic decay give information about the resistance and compliance of the peripheral vascular bed. An abrupt fall in the pressure wave from its peak with no tail can be a sign of reduced peripheral vascular resistance. High peripheral resistance is shown by a shallow diastolic decay, as shown in the diagram. The pulse waveform is used as the basis of pulse contour analysis to estimate cardiac output (see Chapter 13).

# Components of the monitoring system

The components of the direct blood pressure monitoring system include the hydraulic coupling, the transducer, amplification, signal processing, signal display, and power supplies to the various components.

## *Hydraulic coupling*

Ideally, for the greatest accuracy, the pressure transducer should be inserted directly into the site to be measured. Whilst catheter-based transducers do exist, this section deals with transducers that are connected to the measurement site by means of a fluid filled catheter, usually isotonic dextrose or saline. For a correct representation of the waveform, and to control damping and resonance (as discussed at the end of this chapter), the catheter must be reasonably stiff, straight, and the fluid is assumed to be incompressible and must not contain any air bubbles. The catheter terminates at the transducer dome, which is a disposable device containing a flexible membrane, which sits in very close proximity to the diaphragm of the transducer. The pressure change at the measuring site induces a similar change at the membrane, which moves the transducer diaphragm. The amplifier and signal processing have been discussed in Chapter 5. The electrical power to the transducer (for the bridge circuit) is normally obtained, via suitable electrical isolation, from the amplifier.

## *Transducers*

Transducers have already been briefly mentioned in Chapters 3 and 5. This chapter deals with different transducers in more detail specifically used for direct pressure measurement. The most common type of pressure transducer consists of a diaphragm (also called the membrane), one side of which is open to the atmosphere and the other connected to the pressure that is to be measured. Pressure, as mentioned above, causes a displacement of the diaphragm that can be measured in many ways. Strain gauges, resistive, capacitive and inductive, are the main examples, with resistive strain gauges being the most common.

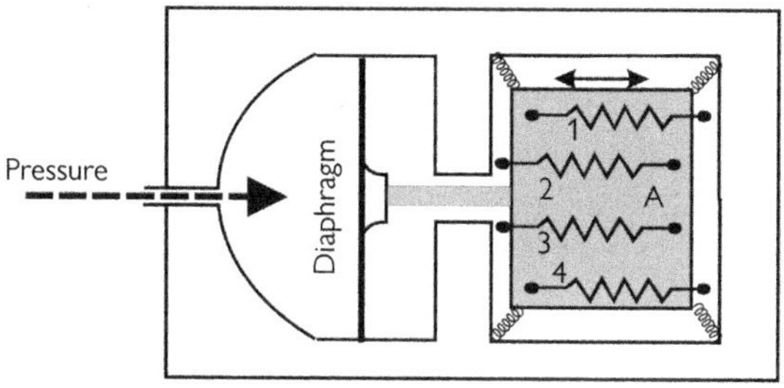


**Fig. 12.6** Diagram of a typical pressure transducer which uses bonded strain gauges. The pressure moves the diaphragm back and forth, which in turn moves the plate A (which is held in place by springs at each corner as shown). With pressure in the direction of the arrow, the movement of plate A causes strain gauges 1 and 4 to be compressed, and 2 and 3 to be expanded.

## *Resistive strain gauges*

The resistance of a wire increases with increasing strain. As the length increases and the diameter decreases, so the electrical resistance can increase; conversely the compression of the wire has the opposite effect. Different materials will have different sensitivities to the stress and strain. In addition different materials will be affected to different extents by temperature in this regard. Strain gauges are constructed to be used in a pressure transducer, as shown in Figure 12.6.

The wire is connected to a flexible base as this is bonded to the structure under measurement. Nickel and platinum wires are often used as they have appropriate sensitivities and temperature coefficients. Silicon wires can be used as they have much higher sensitivity, but are also affected by temperature change to a greater extent, with significant non-linear effects at higher temperatures.

Strain gauges therefore tend to be of two main types: crystals of silicon and metallic. A single crystal of silicon with a small amount of impurity can be used and the variation in performance with temperature can be minimised by connecting four such crystals in a Wheatstone bridge arrangement (see Chapter 4), so that all the bridge resistors are in fact the crystals themselves, all contained within the transducer. Two of the strain gauges are arranged so that their resistance increases with pressure (e.g. resistances 2 and 3 in the diagram) and the other two will decrease with pressure. This bridge arrangement also has the advantage over the bridges already discussed in that the sensitivity to the pressure signal is quadrupled. The temperature will affect all the stain gauge components in the bridge equally and therefore the outputs will not change.

## *Inductance gauges*

The inductance of a coil depends on its geometry, the magnetic permeability of the medium or core on which the coil is wound, the overlap between core and coil, and on the number of turns of the coil (Geddes and Baker 1989). If the core is attached to the transducer membrane, then the dynamic pressure changes will cause the core to be more or less inserted into one coil, as shown in Figure 12.7(a). The inductance will therefore change in proportion to the pressure on the diaphragm. If the inductance is part of a tuned circuit, e.g. resonated at rest at say 5 kHz, and the circuit is also either part of a Wheatstone bridge circuit, or part of an oscillator and frequency-to-voltage-converter circuit, then the blood pressure will produce a voltage proportional to it in both cases.

## *Capacitive based gauges*

If one plate of a capacitor (A in Figure 12.8) is fixed and the other plate is part of the moveable membrane (B in the figure), then the diaphragm movements due to pressure will be translated to a change in capacitance. This movable plate should be as small and stiff as possible, to give maximum high-frequency response. If the capacitor is part of a circuit with a high-frequency wave (typically 8 kHz), and

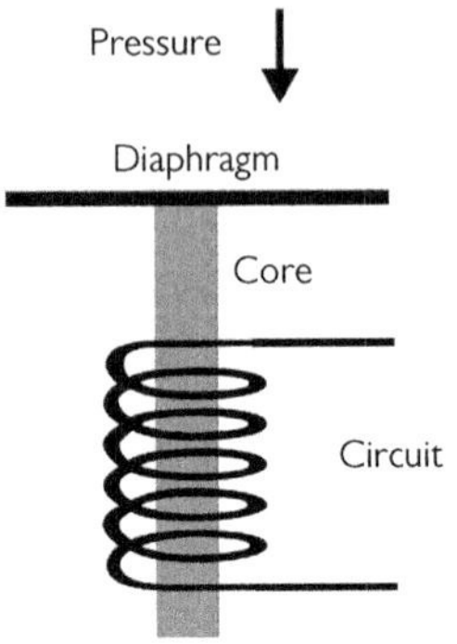


**Fig. 12.7** Diagram showing the principle behind an inductance-based pressure transducer. The pressure moves the diaphragm, which moves the iron core in and out of the coil.

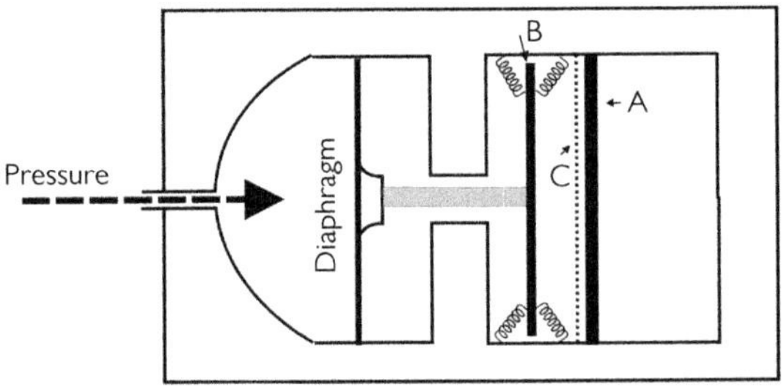


**Fig. 12.8** Capacitive pressure transducer. The pressure pushes the diaphragm in and out, and this alters the position of plate B, which is connected by springs to the body of the transducer. Plate A is fixed, and so the capacitance is proportional to the pressure. C is the dielectric material.

the circuit is connected either to one side of a Wheatstone bridge or to the frequency-to-voltage converter circuit, then a voltage proportional to the pressure will be produced in both cases. The capacitor transducer has high stability to external influences, good temperature stability, and has a good linear pressure range from –30 to 300 mmHg. It can also cope with high voltages from a defibrillator. It does however require more complex driving electronics than the strain gauge example.

## Resonance and damping

In this section, resonance and damping will be discussed, using invasive blood pressure, as a *mechanical* example of resonance, and electrical analogues can also be derived. The mechanical measurement system is shown in Figure 12.9.

A pressure change, due to the blood pressure waveform, will cause fluid to move through the catheter and displace the diaphragm of the transducer. In this example, inertance of the transducer system (mass), resistance of the system (viscous drag or friction) and compliance of the system (elasticity or stiffness) are analogues to electrical inductance, resistance and capacitance, respectively. There is an appropriate electrical circuit to the diagram in Figure 12.9, which is shown in Figure 12.10.

The 'c' subscripts represent the catheter, 't' the transducer, and 'd' the diaphragm and the driving pressure is the blood pressure. In practice, when there is a stiff catheter and a bubble-free fluid, then the compliance of the catheter, and friction and inertia of the transducer are very small. A simplified model is shown in Figure 12.11. The dotted extension is the addition of air bubbles into the system.

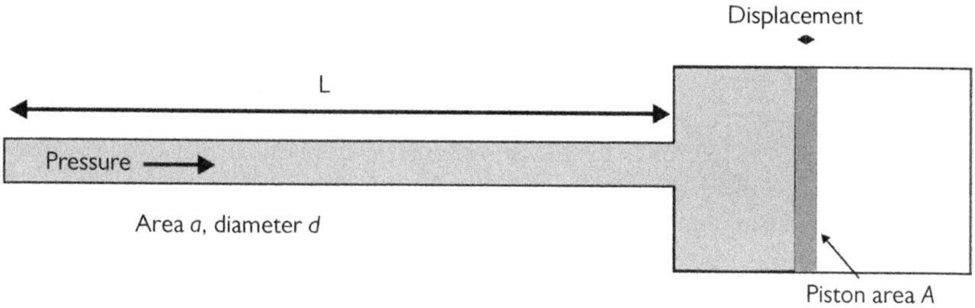


**Fig. 12.9** Diagram of catheter and transducer piston.

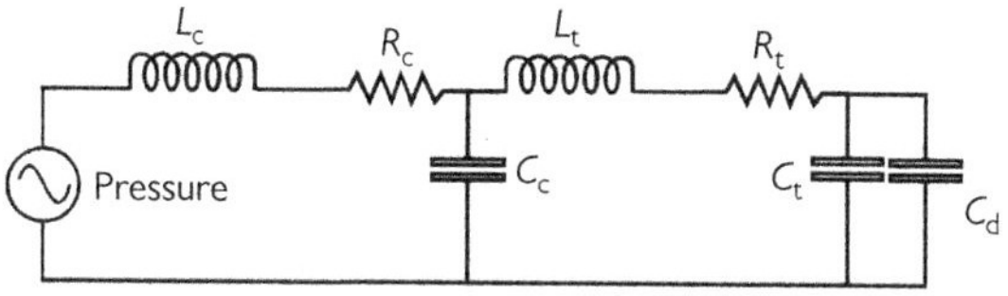


**Fig. 12.10** Electrical analogy circuit of Figure 12.9. See text for explanation.

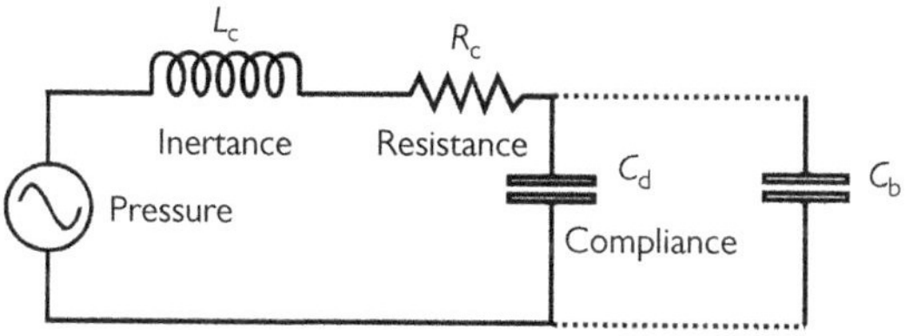


**Fig. 12.11** The dotted extension is the addition of an air bubble into the system (subscript b).

Approximate values can be estimated for the circuit components by using classical mechanical system equations (Brown *et al.* 1999).

$$R_c = \frac{8\eta L}{\pi r^4}, \quad L_c = \frac{\rho L}{\pi r^2}, \quad C_d = \frac{\Delta V}{\Delta P},$$

where $L$ is the catheter length (as in Figure 12.10), $\eta$ and $\rho$ are the viscosity and density of the fluid in the catheter, $r$ is the radius of the catheter ($d/2$ in Figure 12.10), $\Delta V$ is the volume change (related to the displacement in Figure 12.10) and $\Delta P$ is the pressure difference causing that change.

The phenomenon of *resonance* is an issue that needs to be understood in the measurement of blood pressure using arterial lines and transducers. When any physical system has vibration imposed upon it, it will vibrate at a frequency and an amplitude dependent on the relationship between its own physical properties and the externally imposed force. For a measurement system, such a phenomenon produces an unacceptable variation in response to a change in a variable being measured, and the fidelity and accuracy of the measurement is very much impaired. If the external applied force occurs at a frequency which coincides with a harmonic (a multiple) of one of the natural frequencies of the system, then the system will resonate, which means it oscillates at a characteristic *resonant* frequency at an amplitude that may increase dramatically (theoretically to an infinite amplitude) in the absence of any other forces that may prevent that. In practice, all physical systems have such frictional forces that attenuate the amplitude achieved by a system oscillating at its natural frequency. The *damping* in the system is a measure of the frictional force (hydraulic or frictional) acting on the mass and changes the oscillating response to one where the amplitude does not increase as much. If the waveform of the blood pressure is applied to the system, the fluid in the catheter will transmit the pressure to the piston and cause the diaphragm to oscillate in response. If the pressure is removed then the diaphragm will eventually return to the original position. This return can be slow or rapid and the diaphragm may oscillate depending on the relationship between the mass of the system, the elasticity and damping. These factors affect how faithfully the blood pressure signal is transferred to the pressure transducer.

The following mathematical expression describes this (see also Chapter 1):

$$M\frac{d^2x}{dt^2} + k_1\frac{dx}{dt_1} + k_2x = \textit{sum of applied forces},$$

where $M$ is the mass-inertia component, $k_1$ is the damping constant, and $k_2$ is the stiffness of the system.

This can be translated into the electrical equivalent:

$$L\frac{d^2q}{dt^2} + R\frac{dq}{dt_1} + \frac{q}{C} = \textit{applied voltage}.$$

This is equivalent to

$$L\frac{di}{dt} + Ri + \frac{q}{C} = \textit{applied voltage},$$

where $L$ is the inductance, $R$ the resistance (the damping), and $C$ the capacitance. $q$ is the charge and $i$ the current.

The response of the direct blood pressure system can be measured by triggering it with two different inputs. The first is using a *step* function and the second a driven variable frequency sine wave. The step function is a sudden change from no pressure to full pressure, instantaneously, for example by activating a continuous flush device and then suddenly releasing it. The variable frequency is obtained by putting a pressure oscillator into the system that starts at DC (zero frequency) and goes up to 200 Hz. This was discussed in the concept of dynamic calibration in Chapter 3 and shown in Figure 3.6.

If the step is applied, the diaphragm moves to its new position in a time dependent on the damping in the system. The *overshoot* (the displacement beyond the final resting level) will depend on this as well. In solving the second-order differential equation above, the solution can be described as a combination of a sinusoidal waveform inside an envelope of a decaying exponential function, as shown graphically in Figure 12.12. The factor $k_1/M$ describes the amount of damping present in the system, and if it exceeds a certain value the oscillatory component will reduce to zero, which may adversely affect the response of the overdamped system. If it is less than a certain value, the amount of oscillation will become prolonged, and this too reduces the usefulness of a measurement system (underdamped). It is normal to make this factor a non-dimensional *damping ratio, D.* When there is *critical* damping, defined as the damping ratio $D = 1$, the diaphragm will respond as quickly as possible without overshoot. Less damping results in a more rapid response of the diaphragm but there is overshoot. If there were no damping (which is not possible in practice) then the system would permanently oscillate at the natural frequency of the system. A summary of the different types of responses encountered with different damping ratios is shown in Figure 12.12. This demonstrates that the more damping there is, particularly where it is greater than critical damping, the less the overshoot and the more time the system takes to reach the final value. This means that the frequency of the system becomes lower as the damping is increased. When the damping is critical ($D = 1$), shown in curve E, then this is the fastest the diaphragm can reach the final position without overshoot.

$$\text{The resonant frequency of the system: } f_0 = \frac{1}{2\pi}\sqrt{\frac{k_2\,(\textit{stiffness})}{M\,(\textit{mass component})}}$$

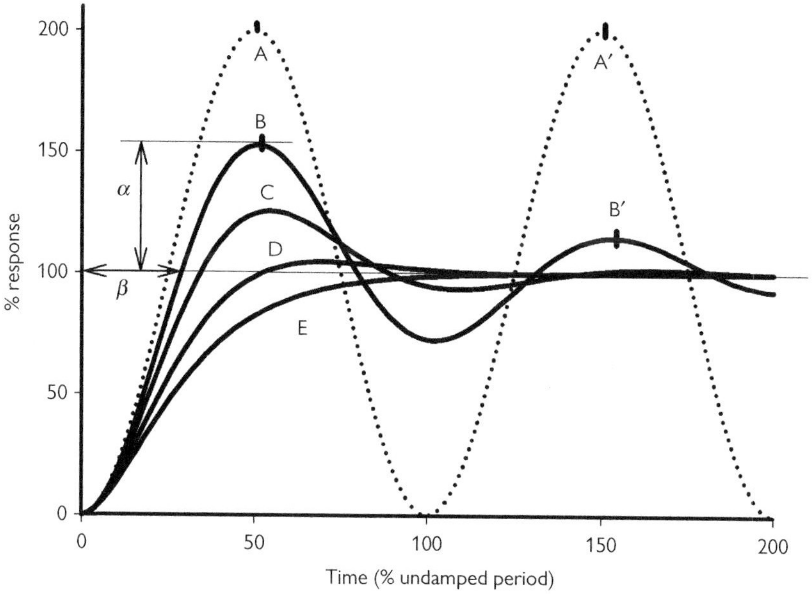


**Fig. 12.12** Diagram showing the system response to a step increase in pressure, with different damping ratios. The dotted response A is with no damping ($D$ = 0). B is with light damping (damping ratio of 0.2). C is with a ratio of 0.4. D is with a ratio of 0.7, E is with damping of 1. The final position is shown by the line that goes through % response = 100. $\alpha$ and $\beta$ are the overshoot and rise-time of response B respectively. The undamped frequency of the system is 1/(A′–A) Hz and the damped frequency with damping ratio of 0.2 is 1/(B′–B) Hz.

The electrical equivalent can be seen to be: $f_0 = \dfrac{1}{2\pi}\sqrt{\dfrac{1/C}{L}}$,

where $C$ is the capacitance, and $L$ the inductance. The damped natural frequency is the reciprocal of time B′–B (from Figure 12.12) and is:

$$f_D = f_0\sqrt{1-(D)^2} \text{ or in the example } f_D = f_0\sqrt{1-(0.2)^2}.$$

Therefore the damped frequency is lower than the natural undamped frequency. The rise time is related to both the resonant frequency of the system and the damping factor. To obtain a more rapid rise response without excessive overshoot, it is necessary to raise the natural frequency of the system (higher frequency = steeper rise time, shorter period). To do this a stiffer diaphragm ($K_2$) is required or a using a lighter mass in the system ($M$), from the equation above.

The second method of looking at the response of the system is to apply a sine wave pressure signal at constant amplitude to the system, but of gradually increasing frequency. The output of the pressure transducer could be similar to Figure 3.6, and the relative amplitude will follow one of the curves in Figure 12.13, depending on the damping of the system.

At low frequencies the output of the system remains at a constant amplitude, independent of frequency, indicating that the system is accurately following the input pressure waveform. However, as the frequency is increased beyond a certain value, the output waveform can increase in amplitude, the peak of the response occurring at the resonant frequency of the catheter–transducer system. At higher frequencies, after this resonant peak, the amplitude of the response declines towards zero.

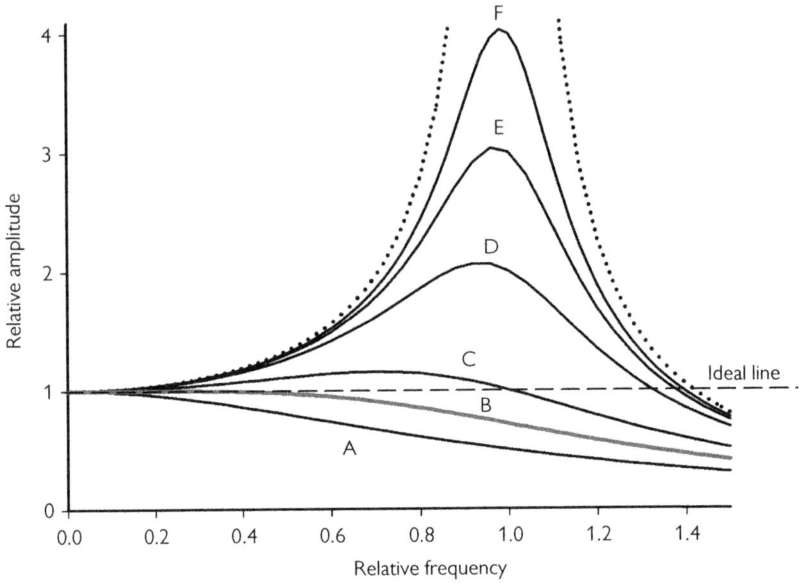


**Fig. 12.13** Frequency response curves of the relative amplitude (ratio of the output wave and the input wave) against the relative frequency (the ratio of the input frequency and the resonant frequency). Curve A is with the damping ratio of 1, B 0.7, C 0.5, D 0.25, E 0.17 and F is with 0.125. The dotted lines represent the system with a damping ratio approaching zero. The dashed line is the ideal frequency response with a relative amplitude equal to 1.

With critical damping $D = 1$ (curve A), the amplitude of the frequency response curve, (as shown in Figure 12.12), falls as the input frequency is increased above 0.1 of the resonant frequency. With less damping (i.e. curves C–F in figure 12.13), the amplitude of motion increases as the resonant frequency is approached, and then decreases. The figure suggests that with $D = 1$, the system can respond faithfully (i.e. no distortion, following the ideal response line) to sine waves of up to about 10% of the natural resonant frequency. If this resonant frequency is much higher than the highest frequency component of the pressure wave of interest, then this is not a problem. When the damping is 0.5 (curve C), then the frequency response is more uniform, but there is more overshoot. A damping factor of 0.7, shown by the response (curve B), is a special case. There is no resonant peak in the response, it follows the ideal response up to about 40% of the resonant frequency. There is a 5% amplitude overshoot (see Figure 12.12 curve D), and also the phase shift is linear up to the resonant frequency. As discussed in Chapter 3, this linear phase shift means that each sine wave frequency component in the pressure signal has a delay in the signal (e.g. due to inertia components) linearly proportional to the driving frequency. This means that all frequency components are delayed by the same amount. These are all important conditions for the faithful reproduction of the pressure signal by the system. With the damping at 0.7, then the shape of the blood pressure is the most faithfully reproduced and the step response is only slightly compromised. However, if the damping is reduced to 0.64 (*optimal* damping), then the response time shortens but the overshoot rises to 7%. This is the best compromise between speed of response and overshoot. Figure 12.14 illustrates this and shows the graph of speed (rise time) against overshoot (see Figure 12.12 as well for a graphical explanation of rise time and overshoot) at different damping values. The frequency response and the phase response are good for the damping of 0.64, but not quite as good as the 0.7.

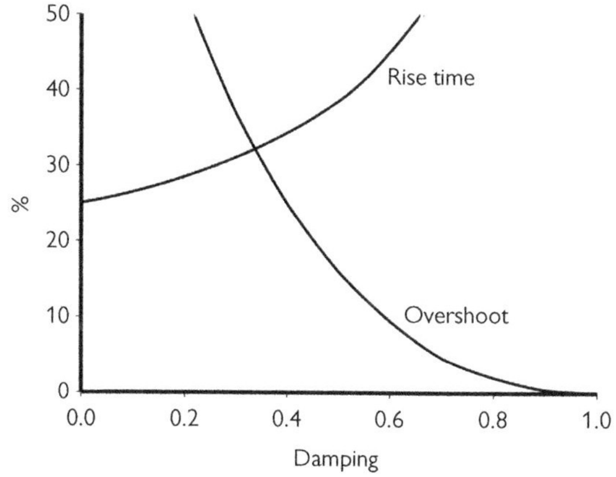


**Fig. 12.14** Damping values verses rise time (% of undamped period) and overshoot (% over final value) in terms of the response to a step function. (Figure 12.12 shows a graphical description of rise-time and overshoot.)

With optimal damping of 0.64, the parameters of the system can be defined as:
Step function input:

- rise time ($\beta$ as defined in Figure 12.12) = 48% of natural frequency.
- overshoot ($\alpha$ in Figure 12.12) = 7% over final amplitude value. Sine wave frequency generator response:
- resonant peak (above ideal response line) = 1.3%
- bandwidth (to 70% of ideal response line) = 0–108% resonant frequency

The damping ratio can be estimated by measuring the overshoot (or rise-time) and using Figure 12.13. Alternatively, if the undamped frequency can be estimated, then the damped frequency can be measured from the $\sqrt{}$step response, and using the equation: $f_d = f_0\sqrt{1-(D)^2}$ where $f_d$, is the damped resonant frequency, $f_o$ is the natural frequency and $D$ is the damping factor.

## Electrical analogue of the damped resonant systems

As well as practically exploring the response of the blood pressure system by mechanical means, the response can be simulated electrically using an analogue as already discussed in Figure 12.11. By choosing values of $C_d$ and $L_c$, and varying $R_c$, the behaviour of underdamped, critically damped and overdamped systems can be explored.

For critical damping ($D$ = 1), the resistance $R_c$ is given by:

$$R_c = 2\sqrt{\frac{L_c}{C_d}}.$$

For any value of $R_c$, the damping is given by:

$$D = \frac{R}{2}\sqrt{\frac{C_d}{L_c}}.$$

The natural resonant frequency $f_o$ is given by:

$$f_0 = \frac{1}{2\pi\sqrt{L_c C_d}}$$ and the damped resonant frequency, $f_d$ is given by :

$$F_d = f_0\sqrt{1-D^2}$$ (which is the same as the mechanical system).

# Other blood pressure measurements

Pressure itself has already been defined in Chapter 3. Blood pressure is normally measured in or around systemic arterial vessels as described in the preceding section. The generator of systemic blood pressure is the left ventricle of the heart. Figure 12.15 shows the variation of BP from heart to capillaries on right and left sides of the circulation. It is possible to measure the left ventricular pressure invasively with an appropriate catheter (see Chapter 13).

Where invasive pressure monitoring is used, the pressure waveform, pulsating between systolic and diastolic values, is transmitted down the arterial tree, normally becoming more spiky towards the periphery of the circulation. This spikiness is because of altered vessel compliance and transmitted waves towards the periphery, and needs to be taken into account when interpreting peripheral arterial traces. Accurate interpretation assumes that electromechanical issues, such as zeroing, calibration, and adjustment of damping have been optimised and that the clinical benefit/risk ratio of using invasive arterial monitoring in the first place has been weighed.

Capillary pressures are low, not usually measurable, and are of the same order of magnitude as oncotic pressures (oncotic pressure is osmotic pressure exerted by large intravascular proteins) in the vessels and surrounding tissues, a fact that governs the transudation of fluid between vessel and tissue. This is countered by the hydrostatic pressure within the capillary, decreasing from the arteriolar end to the venular end of the capillary, driving fluid out of it.

Blood returns from the systemic circulation towards the right atrium via the central veins, whose pressure (CVP) can be measured by a catheter. Normal CVP, when the patient is breathing spontaneously, is ± few mmHg, and therefore accurate zeroing of such a measurement system is important. Venous pressure waveforms have relatively small pulsatile components and a mean value is usually

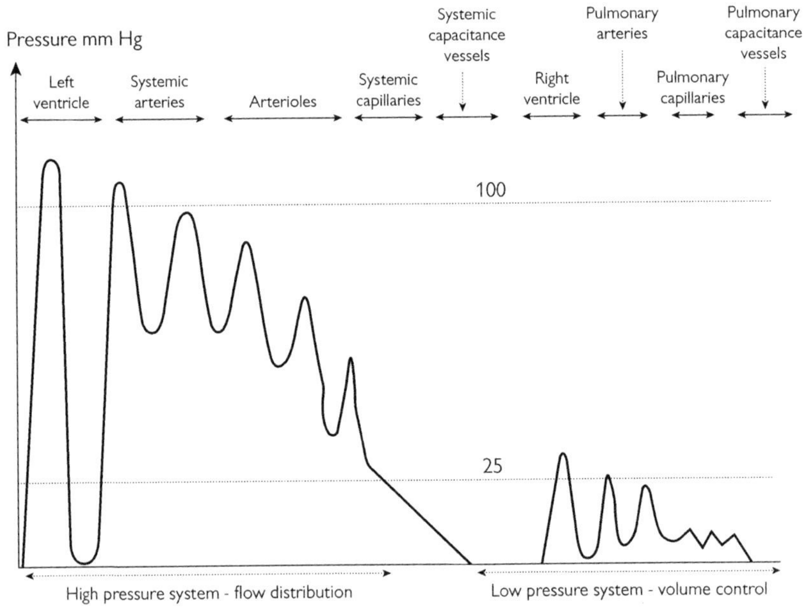


**Fig. 12.15** Pressure distribution across the human circulation.

quoted. This means that, apart from accurate zeroing, a less stringent system of measurement is needed than for an arterial pressure measurement system, and a U-tube manometer often suffices. The CVP represents the filling pressure, not of the left side of the heart, but of the right. Nevertheless, a predictable relationship is assumed to exist between the right atrial filling pressure and the left ventricular end diastolic pressure unless there is heart or lung disease. Under these conditions, left sided filling pressures should be measured, using a pulmonary artery catheter, in order to understand left ventricular function. In general, CVP measurements are interpreted in the light of trends in values rather than the actual values themselves. Pressure measurments may be used to assess volaemic status (Eyre and Breen 2010). Problems with CVP measurement occur when:

- the catheter is too short and not placed in the thoracic cavity;
- the catheter is too long when it is in the right ventricle, measures ventricular pressures and may cause arrhythmias;
- the line is being used simultaneously to deliver fluids;
- compression of intrathoracic veins by positive pressure ventilation, and in particular positive end expiratory pressure is applied;
- microelectrocution risk (see Chapter 6) is now rare.

## *References*


**Brown, B. H., Smallwood, R. H., Barber, D. C., Lawford, P. V.** and **Hose, D. R.** (1999) Chapter 18, pressure measurement, *Medical Physics and Biomedical Engineering*. IOP Publishing, Bristol.

**Eyre, L.** and **Breen, A.** (2010) Optimal volaemic status and prediciting fluid responsiveness, *CEACCP*, **10**(2), pp. 59–62.

**Geddes, L. A. and Baker, L. E.** (1989) Chapter 3, I*nductive Transducers, from Principles of Applied Instrumentation*, Wiley, New York.

**Hohn, A., Defosse, J M., Becker, S., Steffen, C., Wappa, F.**, and **Sakler, S. G.** (2013) Non-invasive continuous arterial pressure monitoringwith Nexfin does not sufficiently replace invasive measurements in critically ill patients. *Br. J. Anaesth.*, **111**(2), pp. 178–84.

**Chowdhury, M. H., Shuzan, M. N. I., Chowdhury, M. E. H. *et al.*** (2020) Estimating blood pressure from the photoplethysmogram signal and demographic features using machine learning techniques. *Sensors*, **20**, pp. 1–24,

**Hutton, P.** and **Cooper, G. M.** (1985) *Guidelines in Clinical Anaesthesia*, Blackwell, Oxford, p. 26.

**MacDonald, E., Froggatt, P., Lawrence, G.** and **Blair, S.** (2008) Are automated blood pressure monitors accurate enough to calculate the ankle brachial pressure index? *J. Clin. Monit. Comput.*, **22**, pp. 381–4.

**Moore, C. *et al.*** (2008) Comparison of blood pressure measured at the arm, ankle and calf, *Anaesthesia*, **63**, pp. 1327–31.

**Parikh, B. R., Simon, A. M., Kouvaras, J. N., Ciolino, R. B., Suthar, T. P.** and **Dorian, R. S.** (2007) Influence of intermittent pneumatic compression devices on noninvasive blood pressure measurement of the ankle, *J. Clin. Monit. Comput.*, **21**, pp. 381–6.

**Pereira, E., Prys-Roberts, C., Dagnino, J., Anger, C., Cooper, G. M.** and **Hutton, P.** (1985) Auscultatory measurement of arterial blood pressure during anaesthesia: a reassessment of the Korotkoff sounds, *Eur. J. Anaes.*, **2**, pp. 11–20.

**Prys-Roberts, C.** (1984) Invasive monitoring of the circulation. In Saidman, L. J. and Smith, N. T. (eds), *Monitoring in Anaesthesia*, 2nd edn, Butterworth, Oxford, pp. 79–115.

**Szmuk, P., Pivalizza, D.** and **Warters, R. D.** (2008) An evaluation of the T-Line Tensymeter continuous non-invasive blood pressure device during induced hypotension, *Anaesthesia*, **63**, pp. 307–12.

**Tooley, M.** and **Magee, P.** (2009) Patent no. WO/2010/061197. Method of measuring blood pressure and apparatus for performing the same.

**Van Bergen, F. H.** ***et al.*** (1954) Comparison of indirect and direct methods of measuring arterial blood pressure, *Circulation*, **10**, pp. 481–90.

## *Further reading*

**Cruickshank, S.** (1998) *Mathematics and Statistics in Anaesthesia*, Oxford University Press, Oxford.

**Geddes, L. A.** and **Baker, L. E.** (1989) Chapter 16, Criteria for the faithful reproduction of an event. From principles of applied instrumentation, Wiley, New York.

# Chapter 13 **Cardiac output measurement**

The chapter links with: Chapters 1, 3 and 12.

## The pulmonary artery catheter

The pulmonary artery catheter was the mainstay of clinical cardiac output measurement for many years, but because of its relatively invasive nature and the lack of improvement in clinical outcome with its use, it is now less often used in a modern clinical environment. Any perceived accuracy of the technique is now considered unnecessary in the face of the risks of its use, and with the introduction of newer non-invasive techniques. Nevertheless, it is worth describing, partly because the technologies involved are still relevant (Coverdale and Patteril 2022; Le Manach *et al.* 2016).

A catheter passed into the right atrium from an easily accessible central vein can be passed through the right ventricle and out into the pulmonary arterial tree while the vascular waveforms are visualised. Figure 13.1 shows the waveforms as they appear to the user. A small balloon at the tip of the catheter allows it to be flow directed and wedged in a pulmonary arterial vessel. At this point the pulsatile waveform is lost and the tip of the catheter is looking ahead, down the pulmonary arterial tree towards the left atrium, a system with a relatively low pressure drop from one end to the other, the flow in that vessel having been brought temporarily to a standstill. Thus, the *pulmonary artery occlusion pressure* (PAOP) or *pulmonary capillary wedge pressure* (PCWP) can be considered a reasonably accurate representation of left atrial pressure or left ventricular filling pressure. This assumes that there is no pulmonary vascular disease, such as pulmonary hypertension, or mitral valve disease, in which case PAOP would not be an accurate representation of left atrial pressure. If the catheter is placed in the apical region of the pulmonary vascular tree, the excess of the alveolar pressure in (positive pressure) inspiration over pulmonary capillary pressure becomes significant, and the latter is a less accurate reflection

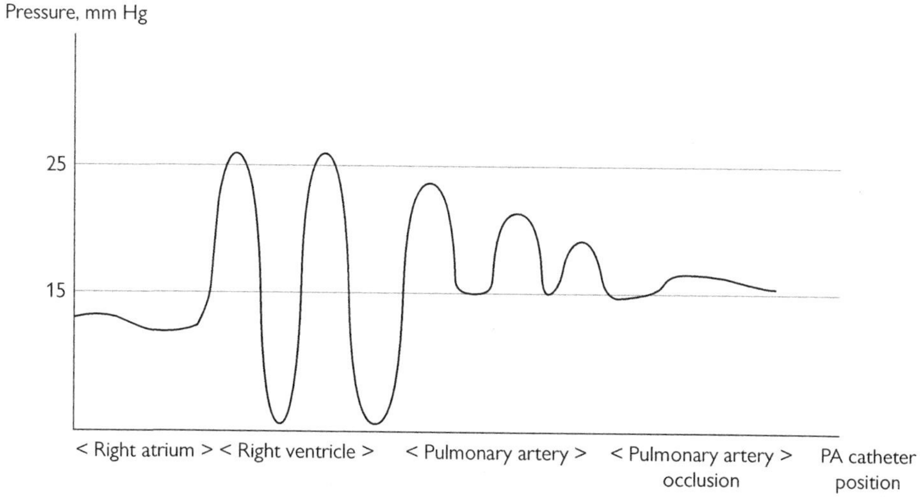


**Fig. 13.1** Pressure waveform trace on insertion of a pulmonary artery catheter.

of left atrial pressure. The balloon should not be over-inflated for fear of rupturing the pulmonary artery, and this is one of its perceived risks that has led to less usage. Once the measurement has been made, the balloon should be deflated so that the pulmonary arterial waveform is once again visible, if necessary withdrawing the catheter a bit to achieve this; failure to do so would result in regional lack of perfusion and may result in pulmonary ischaemia. The same transducer, signal processing and recording requirements are needed as for systemic arterial monitoring. If the patient is undergoing artificial ventilation the PAOP measurement must be made at end expiration, particularly if ventilation with positive end expiratory pressure (PEEP) is being applied. As with a CVP line, it is also possible to cause cardiac arrhythmias with the catheter.

A pulmonary artery catheter can also be used to measure cardiac output using the Fick principle, which states that when a dye is added at rate $m$ to a fluid in flow, and the concentration of the dye changes from $Cv$ before, to $Ca$ after being added to the fluid, the flow rate, $Q$, of the fluid, is given by

$$Q = \frac{m}{(Ca - Cv)}.$$

In Fick's original experiment, $Q$ was the cardiac output itself, the 'dye' was oxygen, so $m$ was oxygen uptake and $Ca$ and $Cv$ were respectively arterial and venous oxygen concentration (content). In measuring cardiac output using a pulmonary artery catheter, the *dye* is typically a bolus of cold dextrose at room temperature or colder, which is therefore used as a thermal dye and the method is the *thermodilution* method. Dextrose is used rather than saline to reduce the chance of creating an electrically conducting pathway that could cause microshock. The bolus of dextrose is introduced into the circulation at a proximal part of the catheter situated in the right atrium, mixes in the circulation, and the change in temperature of the blood is measured at the catheter tip by a thermistor. The curve of temperature T against time may look as in Figure 1.14 (see Chapter 1). The software associated with the catheter deduces cardiac output according to Fick's principle using the formula

$$Q = \frac{V\rho_i c_i (t_b - t_i) \times 60}{\int \rho_b c_b T \, dt},$$

where $Q$ is the cardiac output, $V$ is the volume of injectate, $\rho_i$ and $\rho_b$ are the densities of injectate and blood respectively, while $c_i$ and $c_b$ are the thermal conductivities of injectate and blood respectively; $t_i$ and $t_b$ are the temperatures of injectate and blood. The bottom line represents the area under this curve and the small amount of recirculation of the dye shown at the right-hand end of the curve is ignored in the computation. Note therefore that a large *area-under-curve* represents a small cardiac output and vice versa. Variations in temperature of the pulmonary artery blood will result in some error in computing cardiac output by this method (Moise *et al.* 2002), and overestimation of a low cardiac output has been detected due to the increase in cardiac preload caused by the injectate bolus (Tournadre *et al.* 1997).

The pulmonary artery catheter has become the standard against which other less invasive methods of cardiac output measurement are compared, even though the method itself has fallen out of favour. Several factors have contributed to its demise:

- It is possible to damage the right ventricular wall, pulmonary artery wall or tricuspid or pulmonary valves with the catheter.
- Years of use of the pulmonary artery catheter in life-threatening conditions such as septic shock have failed to alter outcome significantly.
- Non-invasive methods of assessing cardiac output, in particular echocardiography and pulse contour analytical methods, have been developed, which are now much more commonly used with satisfactory results and less morbidity.

It is also possible to sample mixed venous blood from the pre-alveolar pulmonary vasculature, and to measure the mixed venous oxygen saturation ($SvO_2$). When compared with the arterial oxygen saturation ($SaO_2$), this gives useful information about oxygen usage by cells and is characteristically low in sepsis, as is the systemic vascular resistance, which is also measurable with a pulmonary artery catheter.

# Echocardiography

The principles of the use of ultrasound with the Doppler principle have been described in Chapter 10. Doppler ultrasound has many applications, and the qualitative and quantitative assessment of cardiac function is one. The method actually measures the velocity of red blood cells in the aorta, which, when averaged and multiplied by the cross-sectional area of the flow (e.g. of the aorta, either measured by the device itself or calculated from demographic input data gives blood flow as cardiac output.

An appropriate way to visualise the descending aorta near its origin using ultrasound is often via the oesophagus, on the end of a probe, which the patient swallows. The ultrasonic waves on the end of the probe are produced by a piezoelectric crystal in the frequency range 2.5 to 5.0 MHz. The same transducer alternately transmits the wave for 1 $\mu$s and detects the reflected waves for 250 $\mu$s, although other formats of the method use separate transmission and receiving transducers. It is also possible to use a transducer situated on the tip of an endotracheal tube to measure cardiac output with Doppler, thus allowing continuous, intraoperative cardiac output monitoring. Alternatively, the non-invasive transthoracic or suprasternal approach is another route of examination. Whatever route is chosen, correct orientation of the ultrasound probe in relation to the descending aorta is required to ensure an accurate estimate of cardiac output.

The velocity signal from the probe is transformed mathematically and the output is represented as a velocity amplitude waveform plotted against time. This produces a characteristic triangular waveform from which further qualitative information about the circulation may be deduced, as shown in Figure 13.2. Inadequate orientation of the probe with the predominant flow direction within the aorta would give a less well-defined, low amplitude waveform. The *flow time* (FT) is shown in Figure 13.2 as the distance across the base of the triangle on the time base. Since FT is influenced by heart rate, and by ventricular preload and afterload, a *corrected flow time* (FTc) is calculated to index the trace to a heart rate of 60 beats a minute, which might give a typical FTc of about 333 msec. A decreased FTc is seen in hypovolaemia, a decreased preload, and an increased afterload. An increased FTc is seen with a decreased afterload. The *peak velocity* is indicated on the trace by the apex of the triangle. It diminishes with age, increased preload, and increased afterload. Transoesophageal Doppler monitoring can be

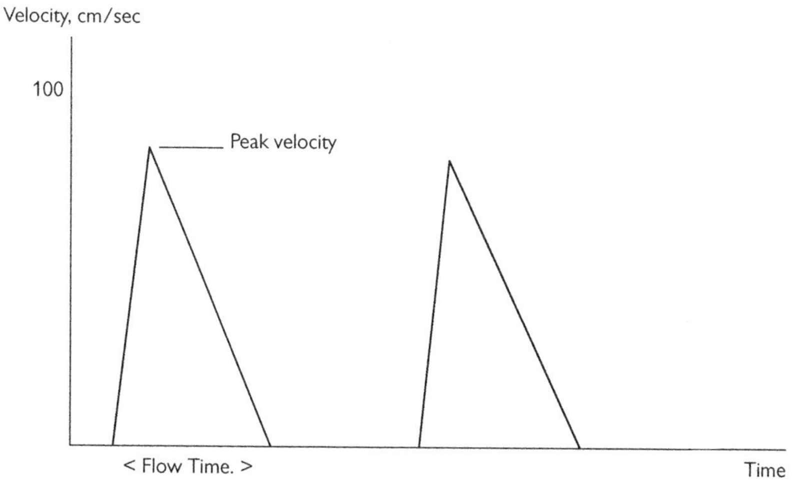


**Fig. 13.2** Velocity vs. time curves obtained to measure cardiac output using echocardiography.

used to assess fluid responsiveness and guide fluid therapy in the operating theatre or in the ICU (Desai and Garry 2018).

As well as measuring blood velocity and deducing cardiac output, an echocardiographic examination of the heart can also look at cardiac structure and function. For example, a cardiologist might be interested in looking at valvular area or dysfunction, abnormal wall movement in ischaemic parts of the heart, end-diastolic and end-systolic volumes, determination of ejection fraction, thrombus detection, detection of air embolus and aortic dissection. It is also possible, by application of Bernoulli's theorem to deduce pressure gradient across, for example, the aortic valve by blood velocity measurement in the aortic root.

Providing the transducer can be appropriately positioned to give results in which the user can feel confident, cardiac output measurements using echocardiography are said to be as accurate as thermodilution methods (Legrant *et al.* 1993) even when used intraoperatively in the presence of cardiac disease (Ryan *et al.* 1992). Clearly, the user must be appropriately trained, and Doppler ultrasound can be used to measure blood flow in vessels other than the aorta from which a degree of atherosclerotic stenosis can be assessed. It has been shown that two-dimensional tranoesophageal echocardiography (TOE) gives results as good as three-dimensional TOE (Cowie *et al.* 2013)

# Pulse contour analysis

A newer non-invasive technique has been developed for cardiac output measurement using mathematical algorithms to analyse the pulse contour obtained from an arterial waveform (as suggested in Chapter 12) (Wiseley and Cook 2001). These are less invasive than a pulmonary artery catheter, but more so than ultrasound, although the method uses invasive monitoring techniques that would already be in place in any case, such as an arterial line and a central venous line. The form of the arterial pressure waveform (the pulse contour) depends not only on stroke volume but also on vascular compliance. The concept of computing stroke volume on the pulse contour was originally described by Otto Frank in 1899 as the *Windkessel model.* To monitor cardiac output by this technique, the device must be regularly calibrated against another technique. The PiCCO and LiDCO devices both use the pulse contour technique, but have different methods of validating the result. It has been noted that the arterial waveform against which a pulse contour method is calibrated must itself have been accurately calibrated, especially in terms of damping and resonance, in order to avoid errors (Foti *et al.* 2022).

## *PiCCO*

The PiCCO (Pulse index Continuous Cardiac Output) device uses an appropriately manufactured specialised arterial cannula with an integrated thermistor to analyse both the arterial pressure waveform and the blood temperature at a peripheral artery such as the radial or femoral artery (Wilde *et al.* 2006). The cardiac output data derived from the pulse contour is calibrated using an intermittent thermodilution technique via a central venous catheter (rather than a pulmonary artery catheter). The cold bolus of fluid is injected into the central vein, and the temperature is measured at the arterial cannula. This is used to update the cardiac output derived from the algorithm used to interpret the pressure waveform contour. The cardiac output is given by:

$$KR\int\left[\frac{P(t)}{SVR}+C(p)\frac{\mathrm{d}p}{\mathrm{d}t}\right]\mathrm{d}t,$$

where $K$ is a calibration constant determined by thermodilution; $R$ is heart rate; $P(t)$ is the mathematical function that describes the pressure waveform with respect to time; $SVR$ is systemic vascular resistance; $C\,(p)$ is the mathematical function describing aortic compliance with respect to the pressure; and $\mathrm{d}p/\mathrm{d}t$ is the rate of change of the pressure waveform curve with respect to time. The terms bracketed under the integral sign are integrated with respect to time. The displayed value is an average of a number of preceding beats.

## *LiDCO*

The LiDCO (Lithium Dilution Cardiac Output) device calibrates the pulse contour derived cardiac output by using a dilution technique with lithium as the 'dye'. A small bolus of dilute lithium chloride is injected into a central or a peripheral vein. Blood is drawn from an ordinary peripheral arterial cannula at a constant rate by a small pump, and it is allowed to flow past a lithium sensitive electrode to a collection system. The lithium electrode system and blood collection system are attached to the arterial line by a T-piece and the whole tubing system is primed with saline. The electrode and its associated software plots a lithium/time concentration curve, from whose area the cardiac output may be calculated in the usual fashion. This is the calibration value that can be used to validate the pulse contour values from the arterial waveform, which uses a different algorithm to deduce the cardiac output from the pressure waveform to the PiCCO device. The lithium delivery system at the venous end is also primed with saline to ensure prompt delivery of the bolus of lithium.

Both pulse contour methods have disadvantages associated with venous and arterial cannulation, such as thrombosis or kinking of the cannulae. The accuracy of both devices depends on the calibration methods described (Johansson and Chew 2007). LiDCO cannot be used with patients on lithium therapy, nor on patients on non-depolarising neuromuscular blockers which interfere with lithium analysis. As with any method that depends on a dilution technique, cardiac shunts will also introduce error into this method of cardiac output measurement. In addition it has been found that pulse contour methods are not satisfactory for monitoring stroke volume changes in response to intraoperative fluid therapy (Nordström *et al.* 2013). There are other devices available that use pulse contour analysis without additional, invasive calibration procedures, such as *Vigileo* and *Heartsmart* but they have been found to be less reliable than the other calibrated pulse contour methods (Sakka *et al.* 2007; Berridge *et al.* 2009). For example, cardiac output measurement and tracking have been found to be affected by the patient's systemic vascular resistance at the time (Suehiro *et al.* 2013).

# Transthoracic electrical impedance

This is included for completeness, but is not a method in common clinical use. The principle depends on the change of electrical impedance in the thorax with a number of activities, such as respiration, but including the change of heart size associated with the cardiac cycle. As the method was developed, a way was found to deduce stroke volume from the change in transthoracic electrical impedance. The method has been found to have a variance of more than 20 to 48% (Tomaske *et al.* 2008), which may explain why it is not in common use, although trials using it have found a reasonable degree of confidence in the method for general surgical patients (Lorne *et al.* 2014), even if the method has been found to be less reliable for critically ill patients (Kupersztych-Hagege *et al.* 2013).

## *References*

**Berridge, J.**, **Warring-Davies, K.**, **Bland, J.** and **Quinn, A.** (2009) A new, minimally invasive technique for measuring cardiac index: clinical comparison of continuous cardiac dynamic monitoring and pulmonary artery catheter methods, *Anaesthesia*, **64**, pp. 961–7.

**Coverdale, G**, and **Patteril, M.** **(**2022**),** Do pulmonary artery catheters have a role in the 21st century ICU? *Br. J. Anaesth.*, **129**(1), pp. 3–7.

**Cowie, B.**, **Kluger, R.** and **Kalpokas, M.** (2013) Left ventricular and ejection fraction assessment with tranoesophageal echocardiography, two dimensional versus 3 dimensional, *Br. J. Anaesth.*, **110**(2), pp. 201–6.

**Desai, N.** and **Garry, D.** (2018) Assessing dynamic fluid responsiveness using transthoracic echocardiography, *B.J.A. Educ.*, **18**(7), pp. 218–22.

**Foti, L., Michard, F., Villa, G., Ricci, Z.,** and **Romagnoli, F.** (2022) The impact of arterial pressure waveform underdamping and resonance filters on cardiac output measurements with pulse wave analysis, *Br. J. Anaesth.*, 129(1), E6–E8.

**Johansson, A.** and **Chew, M.** (2007) Reliability of continuous pulse contour cardiac output measurement during hemodynamic instability, *J. Clin. Monit. Comput.*, 21, pp. 237–42.

**Kupersztych-Hagege, E.**, **Teboul, J.-L.**, **Artigas, A.** ***et al.*** (2013) Bioreactance is not reliable for estimating cardiac output and the effect of passive leg-raising in critically ill patients, *Br. J. Anaesth.*, **111**(6), pp. 961–6.

**Legrant, J. Y.** ***et al.*** (1993) Cardiac output measurement: comparison of esophageal Doppler vs. thermodilution, *Br. J. Anaesth.*, **70**(suppl 1), p. 9.

**Le Manach, Y.** and **Collins, G. S.** (2016) Disagreement between cardiac output measurement devices: which device is the gold standard? *Br. J. Anaesth.*, **116**(4), 451–3.

**Lorne, E., Mahjoub, Y., Diouf, M.** ***et al.*** (2014) Accuracy of impedance cardiography for evaluating trends in cardiac output: a comparison with oesophageal Doppler, *Br. J. Anaesth.*, **113**(4), pp. 596–602.

**Moise, S. F.**, **Sinclair, C. J.** and **Scott D. H. T.** (2002) Pulmonary artery temperature and measurement of cardiac output by thermodilution, *Anaesthesia*, **57**, pp. 562–66.

**Nordström, J.**, **Hällsjö-Sander, C.**, **Shore, R. and Björne, H.** (2013) Stroke volume optimization in elective bowel surgery: a comparison between pulse power wave analysis (Lidco Rapid) and oesophageal Doppler (CardioQ), *Br. J. Anaesth.*, **110**(3), pp. 374–80.

**Ryan, T.** ***et al.*** (1992) Transesophageal pulsed Doppler wave measurement of cardiac output during major vascular surgery: comparison with thermodilution technique, *Br. J. Anaesth.*, **69**, pp. 101–104.

**Sakka, S., Kozieras, J.**, **Thuemer, O.** and **van Hout, N.** (2007) Measurement of cardiac output: a comparison between transpulmonary thermodilution and uncalibrated pulse contour analysis, *Br. J. Anaes.*, **99**, pp. 337–42.

**Suehiro, K.** ***et al.*** (2013) Systemic vascular resistance has an impact on the reliability of the Vigileo-FloTrac system in measuring cardiac output and tracking cardiac output changes, *Br. J. Anaesth.*, **111**(2), pp. 170–7.

**Tomaske, M.**, **Knirsch, W.**, **Kretschmar, O.** ***et al.*** (2008) Cardiac output measurement in children: comparison of Aesculon cardiac output monitor and thermodilution, *Br. J. Anaes.*, **100**, pp. 517–20.

**Tournadre, J. P.**, **Chassard, D.** and **Muchada, R.** (1997) Overestimation of low cardiac output measurement by dilution, *Br. J. Anaesth.*, **79**, pp. 514–16.

**Wilde, R.**, **Breukers R.**, **van den Berg, P. and Jansen, J.** (2006) Monitoring cardiac output using the femoral and radial arterial pressure waveform, *Anaesthesia*, **61**, pp. 743–6.

**Wiseley, N. A.** and **Cook, L. B.** (2001) Arterial flow waveforms from pulse oximetry compared with Doppler flow waveforms, *Anaesthesia*, **56**, pp. 556–61.

# Chapter 14 **Gas pressure, volume and flow measurement**

The chapter links with: Chapters 1, 3, 7, 12 and 22.

## Introduction

Unlike a liquid, a gas is compressible and the relationship between pressure, volume and flow depends on the *resistance* to gas flow (or *impedance* if there is frequency dependence between pressure and flow in alternating flow, see Chapter 4 for the electrical analogy of this) in conduits (bronchi, anaesthetic tubing); it also depends on the compliance of structures being filled and emptied (alveoli, reservoir bags, tubing or bellows). Normal breathing occurs by muscular expansion of the thorax, thus lowering the intrathoracic pressure, allowing air or anaesthetic gas to flow towards the alveoli down a pressure gradient from atmospheric pressure. When positive pressure ventilation occurs, gas is 'pushed' under pressure into the alveoli. Depending on the exact relationship between the ventilator and the lungs, different relationships exist between airway pressure (rather than alveolar pressure, which cannot easily be measured) and gas flow and volume.

## Gas pressure measurement

Gas pressure measurement devices were traditionally in the form of an aneroid barometer, a hollow metal bellows calibrated for pressure and temperature, which contracts when the external pressure on it increases, and expands when it decreases. The movement is linked to a pointer and indicator dial (see Figure 14.1(a)). It is often more convenient to make the device in the shape of part of a circular section, but the principle is the same. This is what the Bourdon gauge, which commonly measures pressure in gas cylinders, looks like (see Figure 14.1(b)).

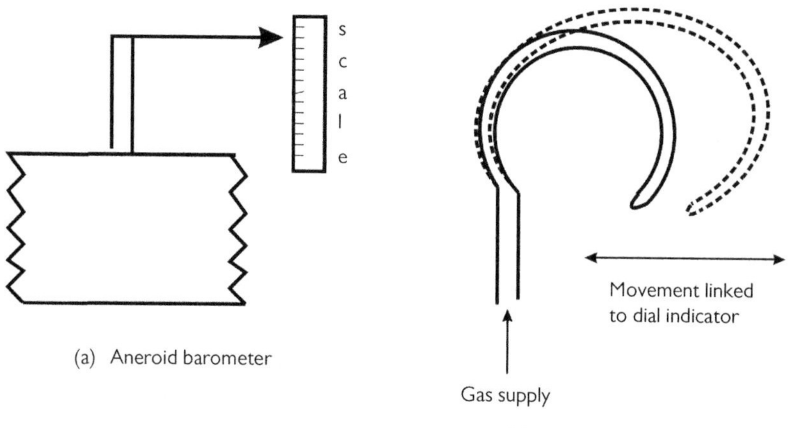


**Fig. 14.1** Two different aneroid barometers for measuring gas pressure.

The detection of movement of the diaphragm of an aneroid barometer can take several forms. The movement can either be linked via a direct mechanical linkage to a pointer, or diaphragm movement can be linked to a capacitative or inductive element in an electrical circuit, such as a Wheatstone bridge. Airway pressure during spontaneous breathing or artificial ventilation is low. The preferred units of measurement are cm $H_2O$ and the range of values is between –20 and +20 cm $H_2O$. The aneroid barometer to measure this will therefore be of light construction, using thin copper for the bellows material. By contrast the pressure in a gas cylinder is of the order of 137 bar (about 141 000 cm$H_2O$, or 1.41 km height of water!) and in an anaesthetic gas pipeline it is of the order of 50 bar (52 000 cm $H_2O$). Therefore, the aneroid barometer will be of much more robust construction.

The strain gauge transducer, one use of which is for invasive blood pressure monitoring (see chapter 12), has evolved into a device that can also measure gas pressure. Modern semiconductor materials exhibit significant piezoresistive properties, whereby their electrical resistance changes with mechanical deformation. A piezoresistive strain gauge, stuck on to a piece of silicon can be used in conjunction with a Wheatstone bridge (see Chapter 4) as a device to measure gas pressure in a ventilator or breathing circuit. There is an hydraulic connection between the patient and the transducer composed of air, the compressibility of which limits the frequency response of the device.

It is also possible to measure gas pressure in a circuit using a static side port in the tubing that leads to a manometer, but the compressibility of gas makes this less suitable than for measuring the static pressure in a liquid.

Where a substance exists in a cylinder as a gas (i.e. above its critical temperature, e.g. oxygen), the pressure gauge effectively becomes the contents gauge for the cylinder, since the pressure and volume changes are inversely related by Boyle's law. Where, however, the substance exists as a combination of a liquid and its associated vapour (i.e. below its critical temperature, e.g. nitrous oxide), the pressure gauge will indicate the saturated vapour pressure, which will remain constant at constant temperature (e.g. 51 bar at room temperature) as long as the vapour pressure can be restored in the cylinder from the liquid reservoir. The pressure gauge in this case is therefore not useful as a contents gauge. If a nitrous oxide cylinder is continuously emptied at a fast rate, the pressure gauge would probably gradually decrease, but this is because the temperature of the contents is falling with continuing vaporisation and with it the saturated vapour pressure.

The measurement of airway pressure in a breathing system or ventilator circuit occasionally may not reflect the alveolar pressure; if there is significant upper airway obstruction, the indicated upstream airway pressure will be high, and the downstream alveolar pressure will be lower than indicated. Under these circumstances adequate lung volume filling on inspiration will not be usefully indicated by the pressure gauge. Since a ventilator consists of components such as bellows and tubing, each of which has its own compliance and flow resistance characteristics, any airway pressure measurement will be altered by these factors and indicated airway pressure may not adequately reflect alveolar pressure. This is particularly true where the frequency of ventilation is high and the volume is small, such as occurs in ventilation of neonates. Under these conditions the frequency response of the measurement system may not be adequate.

A gas pressure gauge can form the basis of a ventilator or breathing system disconnection alarm.

## Gas volume and flow measurement

### *The spirometer*

It is sometimes necessary to do volumetric and other lung function tests on patients preoperatively (Ntima and Lumb 2019a; Ntima and Lumb 2019b). Clinical observation of the patient often gives good qualitative information about gas volume and flow into the patient. For quantitative measurement, the *Bell spirometer*, shown in Figure 14.2, is the simplest device for measuring the various breathing volumes shown in the accompanying graph. The device can measure volumes contained within the trace shown in Figure 14.2, e.g. tidal volume, and inspiratory and expiratory reserve volumes; however,

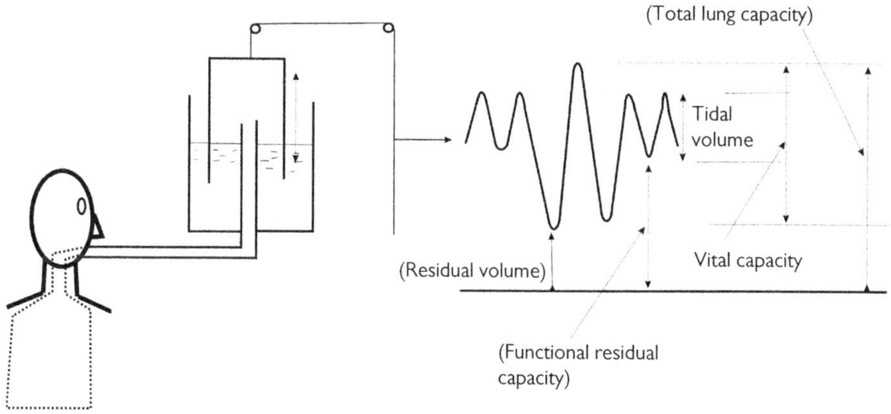


**Fig. 14.2** The Bell's respirometer and the volumes it can measure. (Quantities unmeasurable by the spirometer are in brackets.)

it cannot measure various residual capacities which are contained beyond the trace itself, for example, residual volume, functional residual capacity (FRC), or total lung capacity. Any device that measures flow and mathematically integrates the signal can also be used to calculate tidal volume; *minute volume* is then *tidal volume* × *respiratory rate per minute*.

## *The Vitalograph*

A Vitalograph is often used in a preoperative assessment setting (see Figure 14.3(a)) to measure *forced vital capacity* (*FVC*) and to deduce *forced expiratory volume in one second* ($FEV_1$). It has even more resistance than a Bell spirometer, but is nevertheless a useful clinical tool. On taking a deep breath the patient breathes out hard into the device, breathing out gas at **B**ody **T**emperature and **P**ressure, fully **S**aturated with water vapour (BTPS). As the gas cools to room temperature, the water vapour condenses out, and the filling of the bellows moves a pen pointer, which is linked to a device, which moves a pen chart. Although the measurement is done at **A**tmospheric **T**emperature and **P**ressure with **D**ry air (ATPD), the chart is calibrated to allow final values to be computed at BTPS. The resulting graphs can be used diagnostically as shown in Figure 14.3(b).

## *The Wright's respirometer*

Now a device of mostly historical interest, the Wright's respirometer is a turbine flowmeter, designed to allow the inspired or expired gas flow past some stationary vanes to ensure unidirectional flow, and past some moving vanes linked to a pointer, calibrated so that the amount of gas passing through the device is the expired volume. It is effectively a flow integrator and despite its careful engineering design, the inertia of the moving vane means that it over-reads at high initial flow rates and under-reads at low flow rates; it also under-reads at low flow rates due to friction. Clearly there is also likely to be some inaccuracy where the expired gas contains significant amounts of nitrous oxide, whose density is 50% greater than that of air. However, despite all these potential errors, the device is accurate to within 10% of true values. It is shown diagrammatically in Figure 14.4. A more modern version of this device uses magnetic coupling of the turbine to an electronic measuring scale.

## *The Fleisch pneumotachograph*

The principle of using differential pressure measurement to measure flow, such as the venturi device, and the associated orifice flowmeter, has been discussed in Chapter 5. An evolution of the venturi is the *Fleisch pneumotachograph*, which measures flow and is a device that depends on a linear

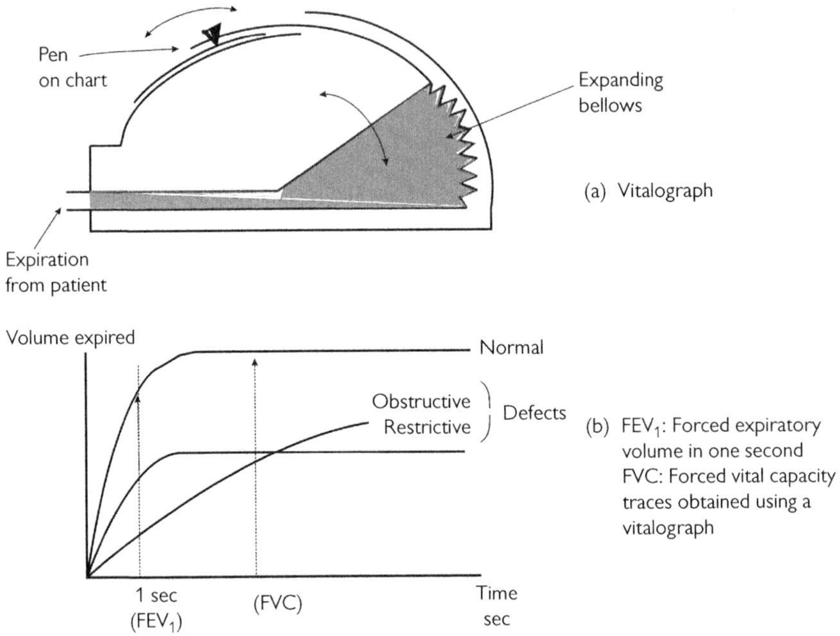


**Fig. 14.3** (a) The Vitalograph; (b) graphical output from the Vitalograph.

relationship between pressure and flow during laminar flow as suggested by Hagen and Poiseuille. It achieves this by dividing the flow through the tube into a large number of parallel, small diameter tubes, thus ensuring laminar flow through each one. The pressure difference between the inlet and outlet is measured and is directly related to flow. This type of device is therefore also known as a *variable pressure drop, fixed orifice flowmeter* and is shown diagrammatically in Figure 14.5. Its accuracy depends on the extent to which laminar flow has been achieved, on the precision of construction and placement of the pressure tappings, the bandwidth of response of the device and the variations in temperature and viscosity of the gas within it. There are variations on the device that, for example, use a mesh rather than a series of parallel tubes, across which the flow may not be laminar, and in which the pressure drop may not be linearly related to flow, but that are still useful flow measurement devices. For all such devices, care must be taken when measuring flows during positive pressure ventilation that there is compliance matching of tubing attachments to the pneumotachograph, and that if a gauze mesh is used, it does not become deformed. In all these flow measurement devices the flow signal is integrated to give volume. This used to be done electronically, but nowadays the flow signal is digitised (see Chapter 4) and integrated mathematically by an algorithm in a microprocessor. Digitisation has reduced the problem of baseline drift and noise to which analogue signals were prone. Further software can use the airway pressure measurement and the volume calculation to draw a pressure/volume loop for each breath, which is a further useful addition to intraoperative airway monitoring (Bardoczky *et al.* 1993).

Another device that uses the principle of differential pressure measurement for flow measurement is the pitot tube, shown in Figure 14.6. One arm of a U-tube comes from the side wall of the flow tube and measures the static pressure, while the other arm faces directly into the flow and measures the dynamic pressure, which is proportional to kinetic energy plus the static pressure; the difference between the two gives a (velocity)$^2$ term, from which flow can be deduced. The pitot tube is better known for its role in measuring aircraft velocity.

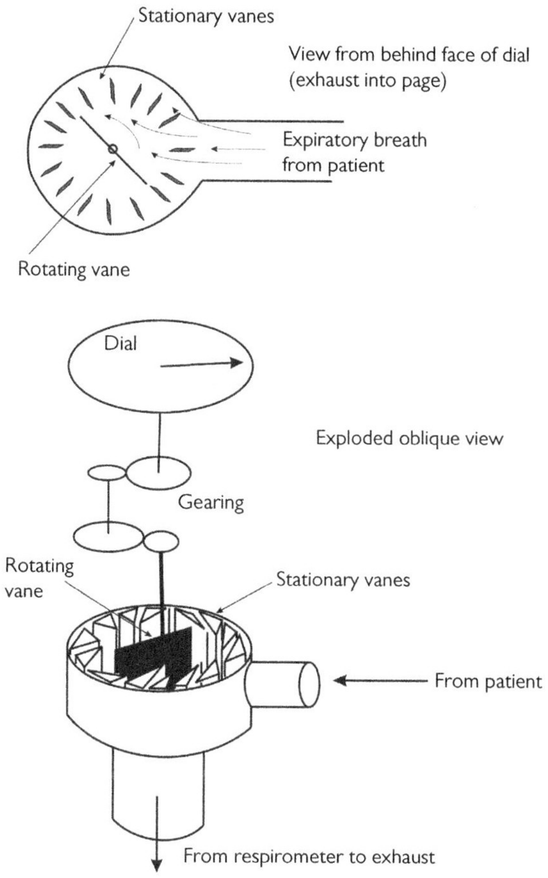


**Fig. 14.4** Diagrammatic sections of the Wright's respirometer.

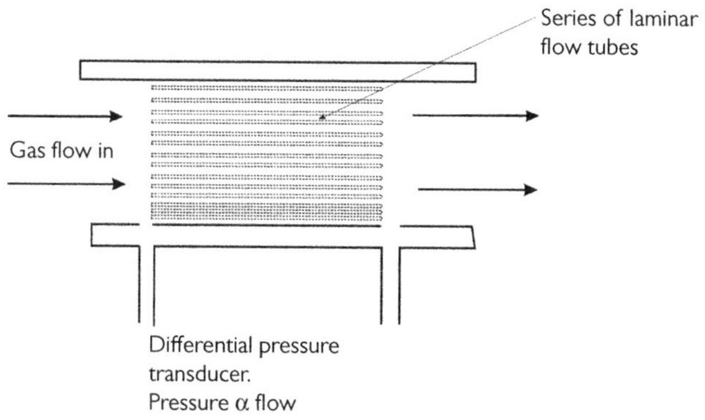


**Fig. 14.5** The Fleisch pneumotachograph.

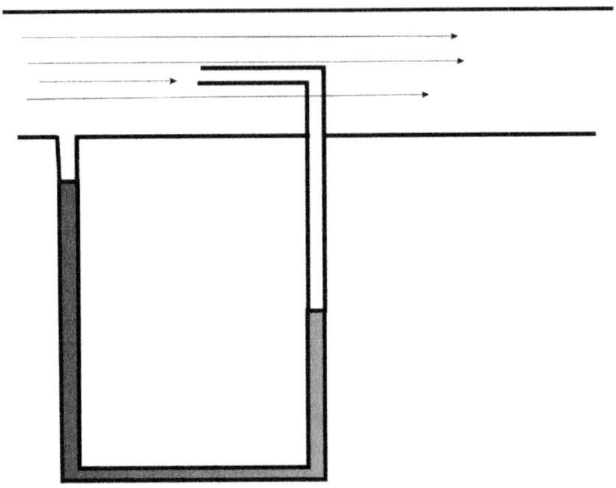

**Fig. 14.6** The pitot tube.

A modern anaesthetic machine is capable of presenting respiratory information graphically in a modified form, using the combined information from pressure, flow and volume measurement; for example, the shape of flow/volume loops is clinically informative, as are pressure/volume loops.

## *Hot wire anemometry*

If a heated wire is placed in a gas stream, the degree of its cooling by the gas flow depends on gas temperature, specific heat and gas velocity (from which flow rate can be calculated). Some ICU ventilators use two anemometer wires, which are maintained at constant temperatures of 800°Cand 1600°C and which form two arms of a Wheatstone bridge (see Chapter 4). Initial calibration of the device measures thermal conductivity of the gas at zero flow and accuracy varies, depending on gas composition.

## *Ultrasonic flow transducer*

The principle of Doppler ultrasound has been described in some detail in Chapter 10 and its use in measuring blood flow has been discussed in an earlier section. Figure 14.7 shows such a device for measuring gas flow. Its principle is based on ultrasonic detection of vortex formation behind a partial obstruction to the flow. It has the advantage that it is not affected by temperature or gas composition, but below a critical flow rate vortices may not be formed to an adequate extent. Another version of an ultrasonic flowmeter has an ultrasonic pulse transmitter and receiver at both ends of a flow measurement tube; pulses are transmitted in both directions and detected at each end; with the gas flow going in one direction down the tube, there is a difference in the time for the pulses to travel in each direction, from which the gas flowrate can be deduced.

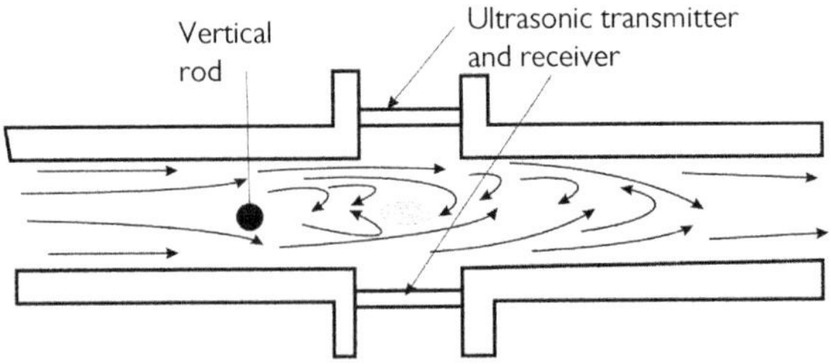


**Fig. 14.7** The ultrasonic flowmeter.

## Measurement of functional residual capacity and dead space

Although not routine in anaesthetic practice, knowledge of these techniques is included for completeness.

## The body plethysmograph

This is shown in Figure 14.8. The patient sits in a sealed box and breathes through a tube attached to a pneumotachograph. He or she then makes respiratory effort against a closed shutter while changes in mouth pressure, $\Delta P$, are recorded. In order to calculate the associated change in the gas volume within the box, which is also a change in lung volume, $\Delta V$, a calibrating syringe is used in the box to link $\Delta P$ and $\Delta V$. Mouth pressure changes can be thought of as intrathoracic pressure changes, since no gas flows under these conditions during panting against a closed shutter. By applying Boyle's law to the thoracic volume, $V$ (the FRC), it can be said:

$$PV = (P + \Delta P)(V - \Delta V),$$

where an increase in pressure $+\Delta P$ leads to a reduction in volume $-\Delta V$ and vice versa. $P$ is $(P_{amb} - P_{H_2O})$, $\Delta P$ and $\Delta V$ are measured or derived; hence $V$ (FRC) can be deduced. The body plethysmograph can also be used to measure airway resistance at different lung volumes.

## Measurement of anatomical and physiological deadspace

One method for measuring anatomical deadspace is based on the *washout method* for measuring FRC, which uses nitrogen as the marker gas (Fowler's method). To measure anatomical deadspace, the method now uses $CO_2$ as the marker gas, which is more readily measurable. The subject takes a deep breath of air and starts to breathe it out. The $CO_2$ is measured at the mouth, and Figure 14.9 shows the familiar square wave of the expired breath, this time plotted not against time, but against total volume expired. Since the last air inhaled has resided in the anatomical deadspace, it is the first to be exhaled with negligible $CO_2$. The boundary between deadspace gas and $CO_2$-containing alveolar gas is not rigid,

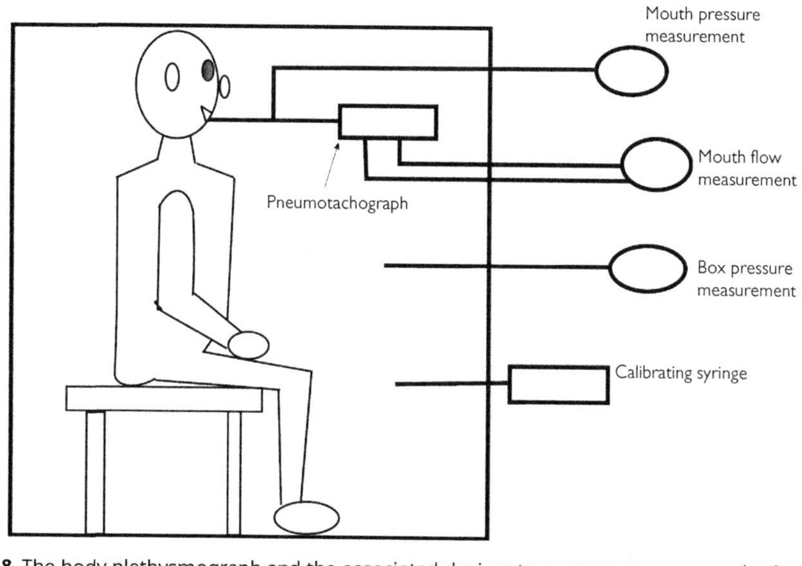


**Fig. 14.8** The body plethysmograph and the associated devices to measure pressure and volume change and allow the deduction of functional residual capacity (FRC).

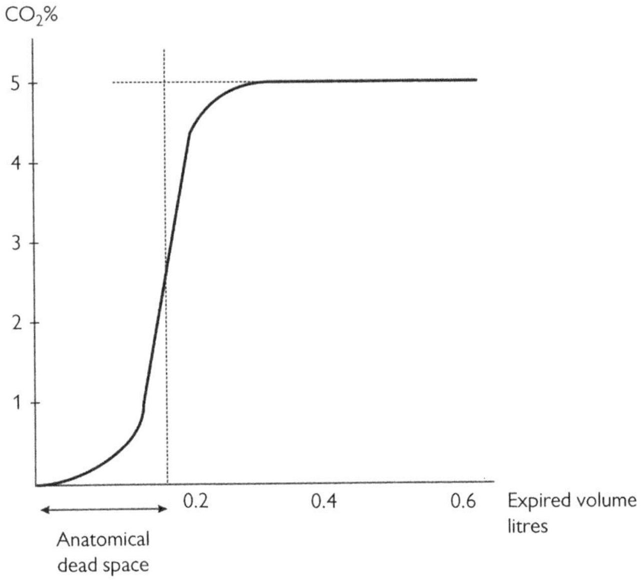


**Fig. 14.9** Fowler's method for measuring anatomical deadspace; clinical trace of exhaled carbon dioxide concentration against time replotted against expired volume.

so the rise in the trace is not quite vertical. Nevertheless, a vertical boundary can be drawn to represent deadspace volume as shown.

*Physiological deadspace* is the functional deadspace where gas exchange does not take place, and includes the anatomical deadspace and also those areas of the lung where gas exchange should occur but does not due to poor or absent perfusion, such as in hypotension or in the presence of a pulmonary embolus. In general, all the $CO_2$ exhaled must come from the alveoli, even if it can only be observed in the mixed expired breath. If $V_A$, $V_D$ and $V_T$ are respectively the alveolar volume, deadspace volume and tidal volume, and $F_{ACO2}$ and $F_{ECO2}$ are the concentrations of $CO_2$ in the alveoli and mixed expired gas, respectively, it can be asserted that:

$$V_T = V_A + V_D$$

and that

$$F_{ACO2} V_A = F_{ECO2} V_T,$$

whence

$$\frac{V_D}{V_T} = \frac{F_{ACO2} - F_{ECO2}}{F_{ACO2}}.$$

If the gas concentrations on the right-hand side are multiplied by ambient pressure and Dalton's law is applied, an expression can be derived in terms of gas partial pressures and this is *Bohr's equation:*

$$\frac{V_D}{V_T} = \frac{P_{ACO2} - P_{ECO2}}{P_{ACO2}}$$

The other method of measuring FRC is the *Helium dilution* technique. Helium gas is highly insoluble in blood and when inhaled, remains largely in the alveoli. A fixed volume of helium, say 10 ml at ATPD, is added to the volume, $V_1$, of a spirometer and the helium concentration, $He_1$, is measured. The spirometer is then connected to the patient at the end of expiration, and breathing continues. The final concentration at equilibrium of helium, $He_2$ is measured. Then

$$He_1 V_1 = He_2(V_1 + FRC).$$

whence FRC is derived.

## *The variable orifice, constant pressure flowmeter*

An example in clinical use here is the peak expiratory flowmeter, in which the peak expiratory flow is measured, and can be as much as 500–800 l $min^{-1}$ in healthy adults. Figure 14.10 shows the device that is commonly used. A flow of gas into the mouthpiece deflects a vane attached to a pointer, which is resisted by a spiral spring. At the same time the expired gas escapes through an annular groove around its circumference.

## *The Rotameter*

This is another example of a variable orifice, constant pressure flowmeter, whose physical principles have been described in Chapter 7 and which is shown diagrammatically in Figure 7.3. Rotameters are standard devices on anaesthetic machines for measuring a steady gas flow being delivered to the common gas outlet, although they have been replaced on modern machines by solenoid flow controllers (Boaden and Hutton 1986), and flow is indicated on an iconic facsimile of a rotameter. Although the Rotameter was patented by Draeger in 1907 for metering carbon dioxide flow in the beer industry, it was not fitted to an anaesthetic machine until 1937. Where the bobbin is conical in shape, the flow is read from the top of the bobbin. Many Draeger bobbins are spherical and the flow is read from the centre of the sphere. By changing the taper on the Rotameter tube it is possible to change the measurement scale; it is therefore important to be aware of the non-linearity on a Rotameter scale. It is also possible to mount two Rotameters in series, one for flows up to 1 l $min^{-1}$, and one for higher flows.

Sources of error in a Rotameter include: failure to mount the tube vertically; the presence of dirt or electrostatic charge on the tube, causing the bobbin to stick; a cracked tube.

When the gas passing through the Rotameter is pressurised, as in positive pressure ventilation or when it is used in a hyperbaric chamber, the position of the bobbin changes without any real change in the flow rate. Under pressure the density of a gas increases from, say $\rho_0$ to $\rho_1$. At a given volume flow rate a larger annular area is needed to maintain the same pressure difference and the bobbin sits high

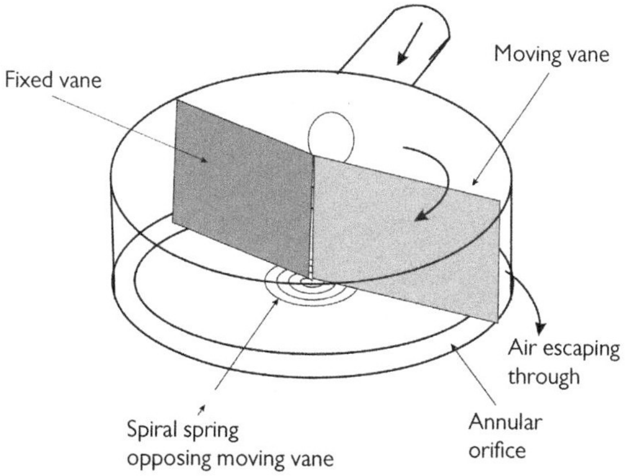


**Fig. 14.10** The peak expiratory flowmeter.

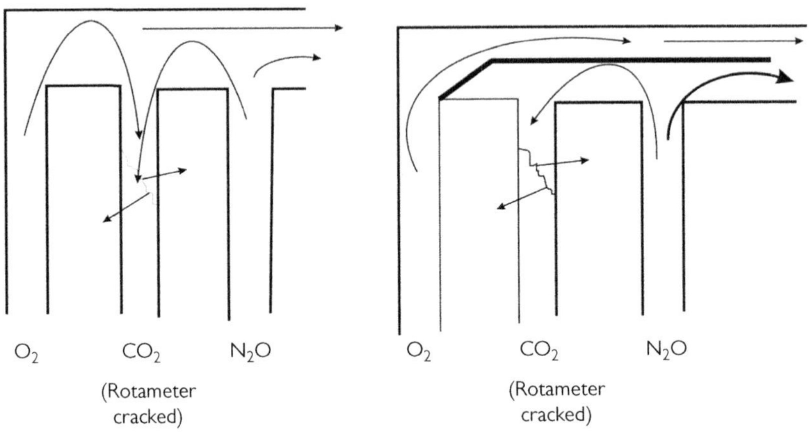


**Fig. 14.11** Rotameter bank in UK ($O_2$ on the left) and the possibility of a hypoxic gas mixture being delivered to the patient in the event of a cracked Rotameter, unless the oxygen outlet is baffled from the other gases.

in the Rotameter tube. It is found that the actual flow rate in the flowmeter, $F_A$, is related to the indicated flow rate, $F_I$, by:

$$F_A = F_I\sqrt{(\rho_0 / \rho_1)}$$
$$= F_I\sqrt{(P_0 / P_1)},$$

i.e. the actual flow rate in the (pressurised) flowmeter is lower than the indicated flow rate, where $P_0$ and $P_1$ are the respective associated pressures. But, when
released to the lungs at atmospheric pressure, the pressure is once again $P_0$ and changes in flows and pressures are related to each other by Boyle's law:

$$F_0P_0 = F_AP_1,$$

where $F_0$ is the actual flow rate to the lung. Hence

$$F_0 = F_A(P_1 / P_0)$$
$$= F_I\sqrt{(P_1 / P_0)},$$

which means that actual flow rate to the lung is higher than indicated.

A safety feature in the design of a bank of Rotameters for different gases includes baffling the oxygen tube so that it is the last gas to be mixed with the other gases. This is shown in Figure 14.11. It is to minimise the chance of delivering a hypoxic mixture to the patient in the event of a cracked Rotameter tube and despite the fact that Rotameter banks in UK are designed historically with the oxygen tube upstream of the others.

## *References*

**Boaden, R. W.** and **Hutton, P.** (1986) The digital control of anaesthetic gas flow, *Anaesthesia*, **41**, pp. 413–18.

**Ntima, N. O**. and **Lumb, A. B**. (2019a) Physiology and conduct of pulmonary function tests, *B.J.A. Educ.*, **19**(6), pp. 198–204.

**Ntima, N. O**. and **Lumb, A. B**. (2019b) Pulmonary function tests in anaesthetic practice, *B.J.A. Educ.*, **19**(7), pp. 206–11.

## *Further reading*

**Clutton-Brock, T. H.** and **Hutton, P.** (1994) Gas pressure, volume and flow measurement. In P. Hutton and C. Prys-Roberts (eds), *Monitoring in Anaesthesia and Intensive Care*, WB Saunders Co. Ltd, Philadelphia, PA, pp. 172–93.

# Chapter 15 **Pulse oximetry**

The chapter links with: Chapters 5, 11 and 16.

## Pulse oximetry

The pulse oximeter is a device for non-invasive, continuous measurement of oxygen saturation. As such it is arguably one of the most important intra-operative monitors at the disposal of anaesthetists, and efforts are being made to make pulse oximeters available at all operating locations throughout the world (Walker *et al.* 2009). Although the device measures oxygen saturation of arterial blood, which is the physiological endpoint of interest, it is not a replacement for monitoring all the events which may lead to hypoxaemia; in other words it does not replace an oxygen analyser at the common gas outlet of the anaesthetic machine. Depending on the site of the probe, usually the ear lobe or finger, there is a variable delay between the onset of a causative hypoxaemic event and detection of hypoxaemia by the pulse oximeter, the delay being longer the more peripherally placed the probe. Appropriate size and design of the probe for accuracy and safety in children is important (Howell *et al.* 1993) and finger probes are more accurate but slower to respond than ear probes (Webb *et al.* 1991). Forehead reflectance probes have been used with good results (Casati *et al.* 2007). It is also true that the human eye is notoriously bad at detecting cyanosis in the range of saturations 81–85%. For additional information on monitoring principles, see Chapter 11. It is clear, however, that in a hierarchy of monitors for anaesthesia, the pulse oximeter is indispensable.

A pulse oximeter uses two separate technologies: one is plethysmography, where reproduction of the pulsatile waveform takes place; the other is spectroscopy, where absorption of light of specific wavelengths by body tissues occurs and is analysed. The spectroscopic aspects depend on the laws of Beer and Lambert, which can be combined to state that the amount of light absorbed by a substance is proportional to the thickness of the substance sample (the path length of the light) and the concentration of the substance. The relationship is a logarithmic one and can be written as:

$$\begin{aligned} \textit{absorption} &= \log_{10}\frac{\text{(intensity incident light)}}{\text{(intensity transmitted light)}} \\ &= \text{constant} \times \text{path length} \times \text{concentration.} \end{aligned}$$

However, there are variations between the Beer–Lambert law and the observations from pulse oximeters in humans (Awad *et al.* 2007).

Figure 15.1 shows the absorption spectra, in the red to infrared range, of various forms of haemoglobin, including oxyhaemoglobin ($HbO_2$) and deoxyhaemoglobin (HHB). Pulse oximeters use light-emitting diodes (LEDs), emitting light of two different wavelengths to measure light transmitted from a probe, usually 660 nm (red) and 940 nm (infrared), in order to compare the spectra of oxyhaemoglobin and deoxyhaemoglobin. The LEDs have a slight temperature dependence on their absorption bands, but this does not significantly affect the accuracy of the pulse oximeter (Reynolds *et al.* 1991).

It can be seen from Figure 15.1 that at 660 nm (red), reduced (deoxygenated) haemoglobin absorbs more light than oxyhaemoglobin, while at 940 nm (infrared), the converse is true. The wavelength at which the curves cross over, 805 nm, is called the *isosbestic point*, and there is a wavelength within this waveband where the curves are farthest apart, 660 nm. A 940 nm LED emits light not far from the isosbestic point and the 660 nm LED emits light close to the point of widest separation of the curves; this gives spectrophotometric information about the total haemoglobin concentration and the difference between oxyhaemoglobin and deoxyhaemoglobin, respectively. Note that the scale is a logarithmic one, so the differences in absorbance are in fact large. The light that is not absorbed is transmitted (*transmitted = input − absorbed*), and the ratio of transmitted light at 660 nm to that at 940 nm

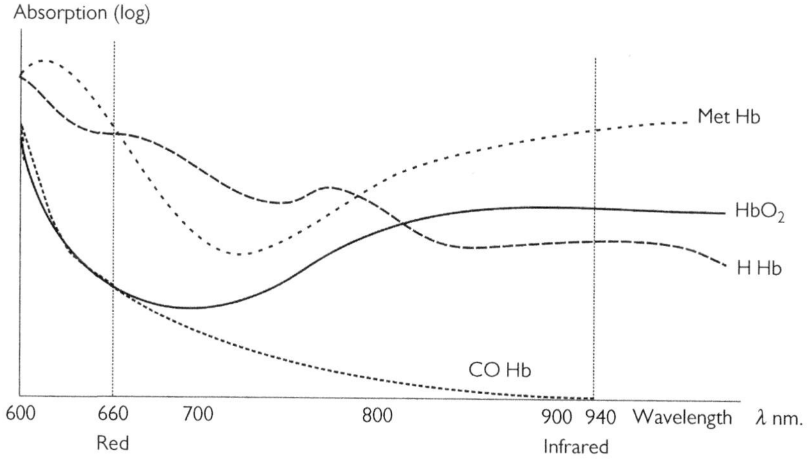


**Fig. 15.1** Light absorption in the red and infra-red bandwidths of various species of haemoglobin.

is calculated. This ratio is used by the oximeter's software to calculate saturation. The two LEDs are switched alternately at a rate of 400 Hz, with the 'LED off' periods in between 'LED on' periods to allow a single photo detector to measure light transmission and to make allowance for the effect of ambient lighting conditions. Absorption of red and infrared light in the tissue of a finger or earlobe is not confined to arterial blood, but also occurs in all other tissues, such as venous blood, muscle, nail, etc., as shown in Figure 15.2. However, only the transmission signal from pulsatile arterial blood is an 'AC'. signal, while all other constant light transmission signals are 'DC'. The amplitude of both AC and DC components from a given blood and tissue sample may well be very different at the two different wavelengths, giving raw signal levels as shown in Figure 15.3(a). Part of the software processing involves scaling the raw signal amplitudes until the DC components are equal, so that the AC components can be reasonably compared and the ratio, $L$, of AC signals at the two measured wavelengths can be calculated. It is then possible for the oximeter's software to look up a value of oxygen saturation, $S_pO_2$, corresponding to different values of $L$. This calibration curve is shown in Figure 15.3(b) and will have been obtained from a multiple wavelength co-oximeter using formal arterial blood samples. Note that when $L = 1.0$, $S_pO_2 = 85\%$. The $S_pO_2$ reading on a pulse oximeter is usually an average of readings over the preceding 10 seconds or so, although this averaging period can be shortened. Errors in the readings can occur with movement and vibration (Langton and Hanning 1990), hypertension, vasoconstriction (Langton *et al.* 1990; Talke and Stapelfeldt 2006), tricuspid valve regurgitation (Stewart and Rowbottom 1991), ambient light, some IV dyes (methaemoglobin causes under-reading), carboxyhaemoglobin (causes over-estimation) and diathermy (Ralston *et al.* 1991). Poor tissue perfusion, hypothermia (Gabrielczyk and Buist 1988), hypotension and hypovolaemia also eventually cause some error (Falconer and Robinson 1990). It has also been shown that the pulse oximeter under-reads $S_{pO2}$ under conditions of low vascular resistance, such as sepsis (Secker and Spiers 1997). Because the plethysmographic signal, which is often displayed alongside the $S_{pO2}$ value, may be subject to internal amplification, its amplitude is no guide to the adequacy of the input signal. However, the width of the plethysmographic trace has been found to be consistently related to changes in systemic vascular resistance (Yang *et al.* 2007). Error can also occur where there has been extrapolation by the device of values of $L$ as in Figure 15.3, outside the calibrated range (Ridley 1988), which has been obtained from arterial blood samples of healthy volunteers breathing hypoxic gas mixtures to give $S_{pO2}$ s in the range 80–100%. Clearly, it would be unethical to try to obtain calibration for saturations lower than this.

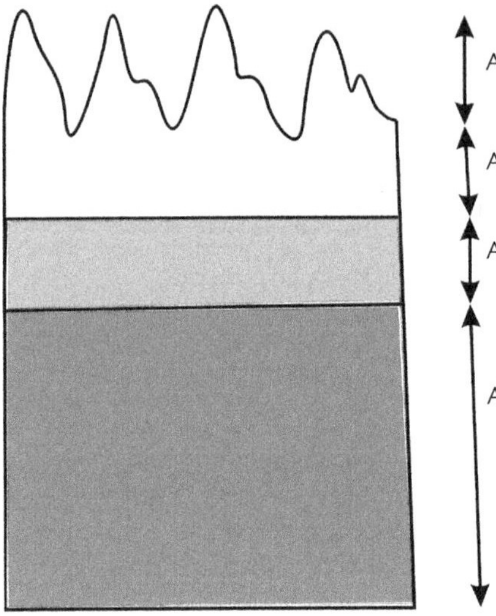


**Fig. 15.2** Absorption in different tissue components by light of a pulse oximeter.

From the preceding paragraphs, it is clear that the pulse oximeter only looks at *functional saturation*, incorporating HHb and $HbO_2$, which is afforded by using two measurement wavelengths. It ignores other Hb components, which are included in a measure of *fractional saturation*, namely methaemoglobin (Met Hb) and carboxyhaemoglobin (HbCO), which can only also be measured using an additional two wavelengths. The absorption spectra of these two groups are included in Figure 15.1. The

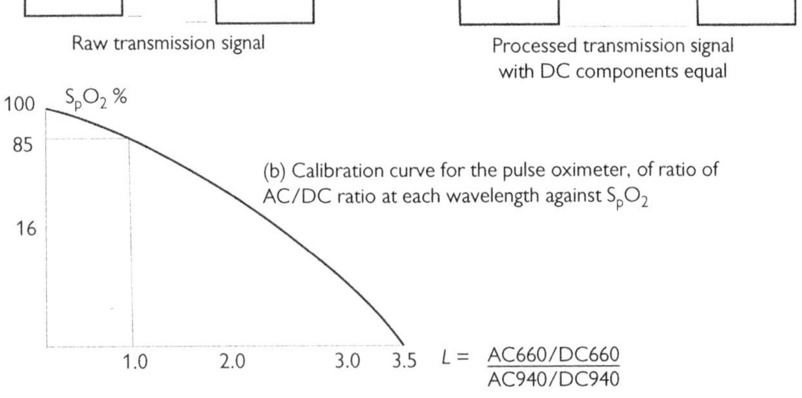


**Fig. 15.3** (a) The processing of 'AC' and 'DC' light transmission signals in a pulse oximeter, normalising the 'DC' component. (b) This gives a ratio that can be plotted to give $S_pO_2$.

carboxyhaemoglobin absorption spectrum resembles that of $HbO_2$ in the red range, and its presence in arterial blood therefore contributes to an overestimate of the $S_pO_2$. Hence, in smokers with significant levels of HbCO up to about 20%, or in victims of carbon monoxide poisoning, the pulse oximeter leads to a false sense of security. Figure 15.1 shows that Met Hb absorbs to similar extents at both wavelengths and if significant methaemoglobinaemia, which can be caused by the local anaesthetic prilocaine, nitrites and nitrates, dominates the clinical picture, the ratio $L$ will be 1.0 and the $S_pO_2$ will tend to be at or near 85% (see Figure 15.3(b)).

Within the range of wavelengths 650 nm to 1000 nm, foetal haemoglobin, HbF, has the same absorption characteristics as adult Hb and therefore the pulse oximeter is accurate in neonates. HbF can, however, affect the accuracy of estimation of $HbO_2$ and HbCO by a four-wavelength co-oximeter. Similarly, although bilirubin does not affect the accuracy of pulse oximeters, it may affect the accuracy of a co-oximeter. Dark nail polish does affect the quality of the signal, and skin colour itself was originally not thought to affect the accuracy of pulse oximeters. However, during the COVID-19 pandemic of 2020, it became apparent that darker skin allowed a falsely high reading of oxygen saturation, and that in order to avoid this bias, pulse oximetric light sources must have a much narrower spectral bandwidth (Cabanas *et al.* 2023; Bierman *et al.* 2024). Improvement of the technology in this respect is particularly important, given the much wider availability of domestic pulse oximeters, and it may be that artificial intelligence will find a role here (Cabanas *et al.* 2025).

## *References*


**Awad, A. A., Haddadin, A. S., Tantawy, H., Badr, T. M., Stout, R. G., Silverman, D. G.** and **Shelley, K. H.** (2007) The relationship between the photoplethysmographic waveform and systemic vascular resistance, *J. Clin. Monit. Comput.*, **21**, pp. 365–72.

**Bierman, A., Benner, K.** and **Rea, M.** (2024) Melanin bias in pulse oximetry explained by light source spectral bandwidth, *Br. J. Anaesth.*, **132**(50), pp. 957–63.

**Cabanas, A. M., Martin-Escudero, P.** and **Shelley, K. H.** (2023) Improving pulse oximetery accuracy in dark-skinned patients: technical aspects and current regulations, *Br. J. Anaesth.*, **131**(4), pp. 640–4.

**Cabanas, A. M., Martin-Escudero, P., Pagan, J.,** and **Mery, D.** (2025) Technical and regulatory challenges in artificial intelligence-based pulse oximetry: a proposed development pipeline. *Br. J. Anaesth.*, **134**(5), 1295–19.

**Casati, A., Squicciarini, G., Baciarello, M., Putzu, M., Salvadori, A.** and **Fanelli, G.** (2007) Forehead reflectance oximetry: A clinical comparison with conventional digit sensors during laparotomic and laparoscopic abdominal surgery, *J. Clin. Monit. Comput.*, **21**, pp. 271–6.

**Falconer, R. J.** and **Robinson, B. J.** (1990) Comparison of pulse oximeters: accuracy at low arterial pressures in volunteers, *Br. J. Anaesth.*, **65**, pp. 552–7.

**Gabrielczyk, M. R.** and **Buist, R. J.** (1988) Pulse oximetry and postoperative hypothermia. An evaluation of the Nellcor –100 in a cardiac surgical ICU, *Anaesthesia*, **43**, pp. 402–4.

**Howell, S. J., Blogg, C. E.** and **Ashby, M. W.** (1993) Howell modified sensor for pulse oximetry in children, *Anaesthesia*, **48**, pp. 1083–95.

**Langton, J. A.** and **Hanning, C. D.** (1990) Effect of motion artefact on pulse oximeters: evaluation of four instruments and finger probes, *Br. J. Anaesth.*, **65**, pp. 564–70.

**Langton, J. A., Lassey, D.** and **Hanning C. D.** (1990) Comparison of four pulse oximeters: effects of venous occlusion and cold induced vasoconstriction, *Br. J. Anaesth.*, **65**, pp. 245–7.

**Ralston, A. C., Webb, R. K.** and **Runciman, W. B.** (1991) Potential errors in pulse oximetry III. The effects of interference, dyes, dyshaemoglobins and other pigments, *Anaesthesia*, **46**, pp. 291–5.

**Reynolds, K. J. *et al.*** (1991) Temperature dependence of the light emitting diode and its theoretical effect on the pulse oximeter, *Br. J. Anaesth.*, **67**, pp. 638–43.

**Ridley, S. A.** (1988) A comparison of two pulse oximeters. Assessment of accuracy at low arterial saturations in paediatric surgical patients, *Anaesthesia*, **43**, pp. 136–40.

**Secker**, **C**. and **Spiers**, **R**. (1997) Accuracy of the pulse oximeter in patients with low systemic vascular resistance, *Anaesthesia*, **52**, pp. 127–30.

**Stewart**, **K. G.** and **Rowbottom**, **S. J.** (1991) Inaccuracy of pulse oximeters in patients with severe tricuspid regurgitation, *Anaesthesia*, **46**, pp. 668–70.

**Talke**, **P.** and **Stapelfeldt**, **C.** (2006) Effect of peripheral vasoconstriction on pulse oximetry, *J. Clin. Monit. Comput.*, **20**, pp. 305–9.

**Walker**, **I. A.**, **Merry**, **A. F.**, **Wilson**, **I. H.** ***et al.*** (2009) Global oximetry: an international anaesthesia quality improvement project, *Anaesthesia*, **64**, pp. 1051–60.

**Webb**, **R. K.**, **Ralston**, **A. C.** and **Runciman**, **W. B.** (1991) Potential errors in pulse oximetry II. The effects of changes in saturation and signal quality, *Anaesthesia*, **46**, pp. 207–12.

**Yang**, **S.**, **Batchelder**, **P. B.** and **Raley**, **D. M.** (2007) Effects of tissue outside of arterial blood vessels in pulse oximetry: a model of two-dimensional pulsation, *J. Clin. Monit. Comput.*, **21**, pp. 373–9.

# Chapter 16 **Respiratory gas analysers**

The chapter links with: Chapters 5, 11, and 17.

## Introduction

The purpose of respiratory gas analysis during anaesthesia is to identify and measure the concentrations, on a breath-by-breath basis, of the individual gases and vapours in use. It may also be useful as a guide to respiratory or cardiac function, or to identify trace contaminant gases. Different techniques use different physico-chemical properties of the gas or vapour. An understanding of the physical principle underlying each method is necessary in order to recognise the value and limitations of each.

In terms of the device's ability to respond on a breath-by-breath basis, there are two important components: the time taken for the gas to be sampled from the anaesthetic machine or breathing system, the *delay time*; then there is the time taken for the device to measure the gas concentration, the *response time*. This is depicted in Figure 16.1. Most of the delay occurs in the delay time or *transit time* and can be reduced either by analysing the gas sample close to the airway, or by using as short and thin a sampling tube and as high a sampling flow rate to the analyser as possible (Chan *et al.* 2003); the sampling flow rate is usually of the order of 100 to 200 ml $min^{-1}$. If minimal fresh gas flow rates are being used in a circle anaesthetic breathing system and the sampled gas is not returned to the breathing system, then a high gas sampling rate could represent a significant gas leak. Figure 16.1 shows a sigmoid curve of recorded gas concentration change in response to a square wave input change. The response of a gas analyser is often expressed as the time taken to produce a 90–95% response to a step or square wave input change. A square wave change in gas concentration can be produced by moving a gas sampling tube rapidly into and out of a gas stream, by bursting a small balloon within a sampling volume containing a gas sample, or by switching a shutter to a gas sample volume using a solenoid valve.

An important part of the use of gas analysers is zeroing and calibration since they are all prone to drift in both zero and gain. These days zeroing is often done automatically on switching on the analyser and at predetermined intervals. However, the calibration – that is to say the linearity and gain of the output signal for a known input – has periodically to be checked with calibration gases. Some devices can only measure the concentration of one gas, others can estimate several gases.

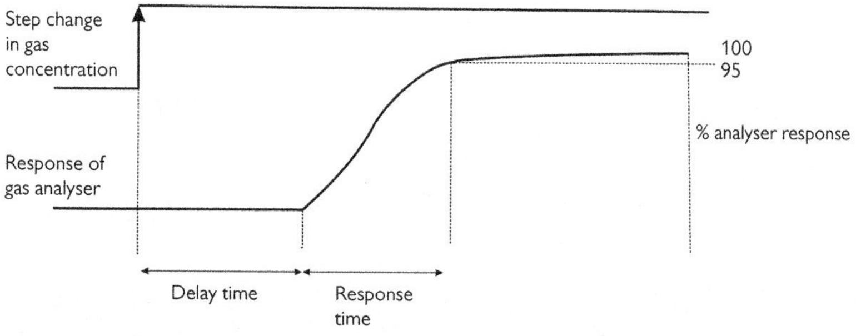


**Fig. 16.1** Response of a gas analyser to a step change in gas concentration.

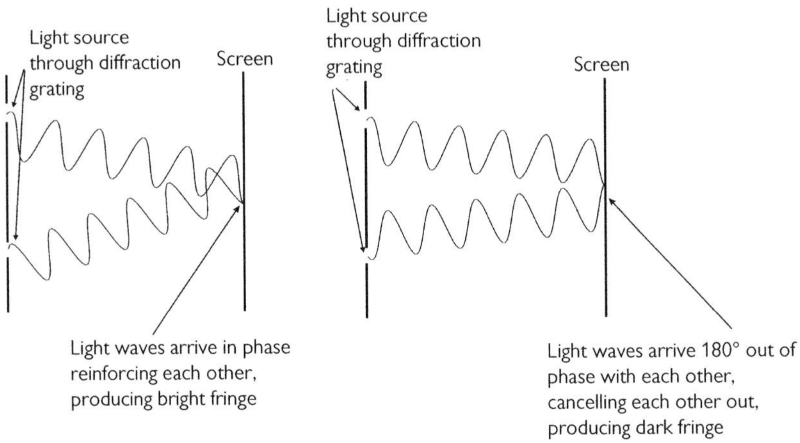


**Fig. 16.2** Light refractometry. Interference fringes caused by light waves arriving in phase and 180° out of phase.

## Refractometry

This method uses different refractive indices of gases to identify and calibrate gases. It is included here, not because it is routinely used in anaesthesia, but because it is still a laboratory standard against which other methods are compared. The refractive index of a transparent medium is given by:

$$\mu = \frac{\textit{velocity of light in a vacuum}}{\textit{velocity of light in the medium}}.$$

$\mu > 1.0$ because the velocity of light in a vacuum, $3.0 \times 10^8$ m s$^{-1}$, is always greater than in any other medium. The delay in the passage of light through a gas depends on the number of gas molecules present; therefore, the refractive index depends on its pressure and temperature. Refractometry depends on the principle that interference bands are formed when light waves from a source, which pass through two slits, are focused on to a screen. Figure 16.2 shows that when the transverse waveforms of light from the two slits arrive in phase with each other, they reinforce each other, producing a bright band of light; when they arrive 180° out of phase, they cancel each other and a dark band is produced; hence *interference fringes* are produced and the clearest fringes are produced when a monochromatic (single wavelength) light source is used.

### *The Rayleigh refractometer*

This is shown in Figure 16.3. Light from a tungsten source passes through a pair of vertical slits and a convex lens, the upper part of the pair of light beams emerging parallel from the lens; these beams are then passed through two tubes, A and B, one of which contains the gas to be analysed, the other a gas of known refractive index. The lower portion of light from the slits does not pass through the tubes containing the gases. After passing through another lens to the eyepiece, an upper and lower set of interference fringes are visible, each set being formed by virtue of the interference of light beams from the slits. When tubes A and B are initially filled with the same gas, the upper fringe pattern assumes a position that can be lined up with the lower reference fringe pattern. If the gas in, say tube A, is changed to a gas to be analysed, the upper fringe pattern shifts because of the differential path lengths of the light in A and B. If one of the two glass plates, X and Y, say Y, is rotated to increase the path length through B, to match that through A, then the upper fringe pattern comes back into line with the lower one. The amount of rotation of Y, on a carefully calibrated scale, can be made to be proportional to the gas concentration in A.

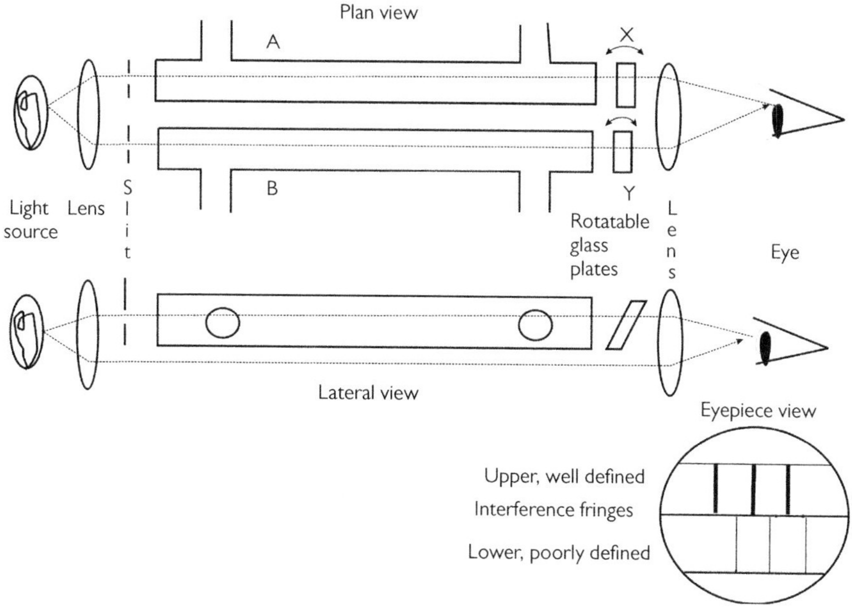


**Fig. 16.3** The Rayleigh refractometer.

Figure 16.4 shows a portable refractometer, in which the light beam from a common source is split into two beams by a prismatic glass plate, thus allowing a reference light path and one that passes through the sample. The returning light paths form an interference fringe pattern, which is viewed through an eyepiece.

Since all gases possess the physical property of refractive index, all gases can be analysed by this method. Although highly accurate, it does not lend itself to breath-by-breath analysis because of its large size and the lack of ability to analyse changing gas concentrations. Nevertheless, it is used as the standard method against which others are calibrated.

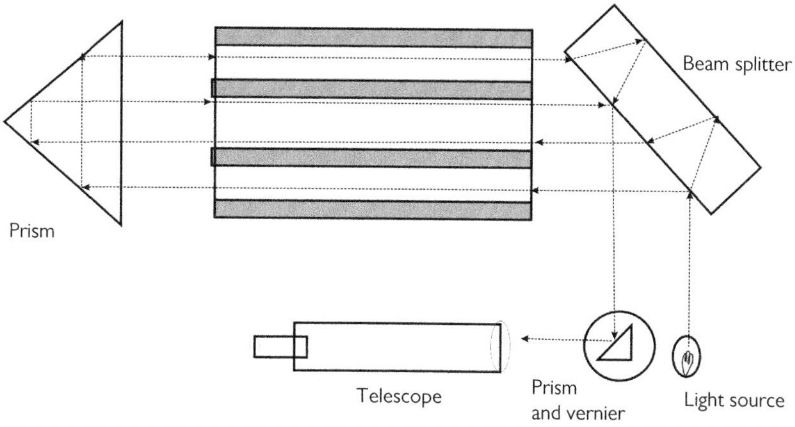


**Fig. 16.4** Portable refractometer. See text for details.

# Infrared spectroscopy

Molecules that contain two or more different atom species (polyatomic) (i.e. $CO_2$, $N_2O$, $H_2O$, but not $O_2$ or $N_2$) absorb infrared radiation because of the nature of the bond between the dissimilar atoms. This property can be used to analyse gases such as carbon dioxide, nitrous oxide and all anaesthetic vapours, but not oxygen or nitrogen. The absorption $A$ of the IR light is related to the intensities of incident light $I_i$, the transmitted light $I_t$, the extinction coefficient $\varepsilon$, the path length $L$ and the concentration $C$ of the absorbing medium by the *Beer–Lambert* law:

$$A = \log_{10} \frac{I_i}{I_t} = \varepsilon LC.$$

The principle of an infrared gas analyser (*Luft* or non-dispersive type) is shown in Figure 16.5. Because $CO_2$ analysis is arguably as important as pulse oximetry for patient safety during anaesthesia, these devices are now commonly available in the anaesthesia workplace. Figure 16.5 shows an infrared (IR) light source emitting radiation in the range 1–15 µm wavelength. The light passes through a 'chopper' wheel rotating at 25–100 Hz, which ensures that the infrared light is only intermittently passed further down the device; this also prevents overheating of the gas sample. The light is then passed simultaneously through a pair of tubes, one of which contains a reference gas, the other of which contains the gas for analysis. Because of the differential IR absorption in the two chambers, differential amounts of IR light are transmitted to a pair of detector cells filled with air, separated by a diaphragm. The pressure in the two halves is therefore different from separate amounts of IR heating and, because the chopper wheei ensures that the IR input is oscillating, the diaphragm oscillates as well. It is usually part of an electrical capacitance and this signal is amplified and displayed as a gas concentration proportional to the number of molecules of gas present.

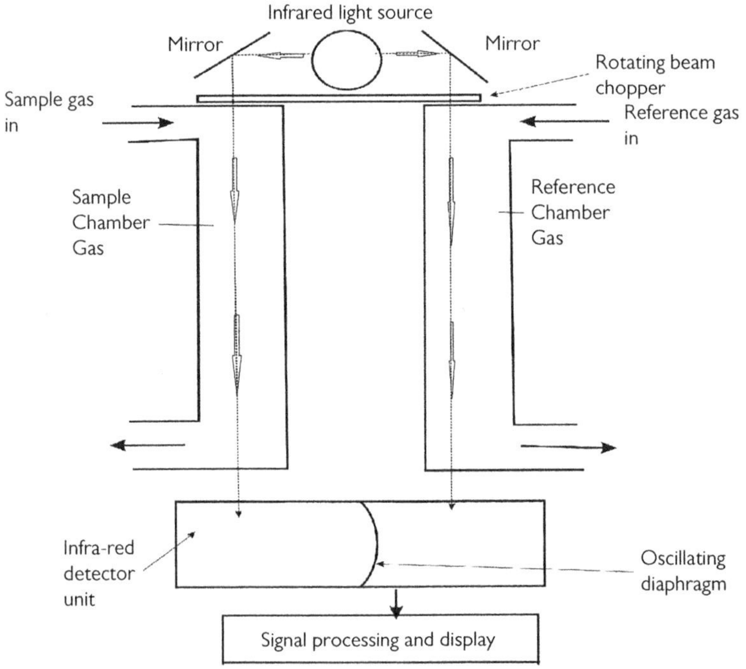


**Fig. 16.5** Infrared gas analyser (Luft head).

There are a number of sources of error in infrared spectroscopy. Major bands of absorption of IR for $CO_2$, $N_2O$ and CO occur in the 4.3, 4.5 and 4.7 μm wavebands, respectively, and there is considerable overlap in the 3–5 μm range. Therefore, there is significant interference between the spectra of these three gases, particularly between $CO_2$ and $N_2O$ in the 4.3 μm range. Another source of error is due to the phenomenon of *collision broadening*, where the absorption spectrum of one gas is actually broadened by the presence of another. This is due to transfer of interatomic bond energy between colliding $N_2O$ and $CO_2$ molecules. There are electronic correction factors incorporated into the analysers to allow for different mixtures of $N_2O$ and $CO_2$. It has also been found that an infrared spectrometer under-reads the $CO_2$ values in a gas mixture containing 79% helium in oxygen (Ball and Grounds 2003). It has been reported that a gas mixture containing desflurane produces some error in an infrared gas analyser (Scheeren *et al.* 1998), as does cyclopropane (Mason and Lloyd-Thomas 1991) and alcohol (Foley *et al.* 1990).

A further source of error with this device is related to the fact that its output signal is proportional to the number of molecules present, which is really the partial pressure of the gas. Therefore, the pressure in the sample and reference cells and the ambient pressure are all important variables against which the device must be calibrated. This includes pressure changes due to sampling through a narrow bore tube from the breathing system, as well as changes in back pressure from positive pressure ventilation. If the pressure of the measured gas mixture increases without any real change in the fractional concentration, then the partial pressure of the gas under investigation also increases. If the software of the device converts partial pressure to fractional concentration, there will be an erroneous increase in the indicated fractional concentration. Likewise, if the analyser is calibrated at sea level and then used at altitude, such that there is an altered relationship between the gas partial pressure and ambient pressure, then error will result. Therefore, calibration should be done under the intended working conditions and repeated relatively frequently. Another solution is to have the device calibrated for partial pressure rather than concentration, in which case error due to atmospheric pressure changes remains small. Most devices remain stable but, as well as two or three point calibration, response time should also be routinely checked. Despite long sampling lines and low sampling rates (100–200 ml $min^{-1}$), the 90–95% step response time should remain under 150 ms. In this respect, the water vapour sampled with the gas sample sometimes blocks the sampling tube, but most devices have either a water trap or a sampling line made of a material that absorbs water vapour. In this case, an electronic correction is made to the result to allow for the presence of the water vapour in the expired breath sample. Alternatively, water itself is a powerful absorber of IR light, and its partial pressure can be measured, usually at a different wavelength from the other constituents being analysed.

Modern IR analysers may use photocells rather than differential pressure chambers to detect IR transmission and may use narrow bandwidth filters for the different gases being sampled. For example, in the Datex-Engstrom device, $N_2O$ is measured at 3.9 m, $CO_2$ at 4.3 m and volatile agents at 3.3 m. It cannot distinguish volatile agents from each other unless it is 'informed' or different agents are analysed at different wavebands. Regular automatic calibration takes place using compressed vapour canisters. Note that exhaled ethyl alcohol or acetone will interfere with the readings. Any residual error due to interference between $CO_2$ and $N_2O$ is taken care of electronically. The accuracy of the IR analyser is about 0.1% in a range of $CO_2$ of 0–10%.

## Mass spectrometry

A mass spectrometer is capable of analysing a gas mixture on the physical principle of separating the components in a magnetic field according to their molecular mass and charge. Providing the constituents of the gas mixture are known, provision of appropriate detectors can be made and any gas can be analysed. Error occurs where an unknown constituent is introduced into the mixture, such as the propellant in bronchodilators, or acetone in the breath of a diabetic. Error can also occur where the molecules have the same molecular mass (see below). Although a mass spectrometer was developed for clinical use in 1958 (Fowler 1958), it is still used more often in the laboratory than in the operating room. It has been used in remote sampling, multisite and timesharing modalities.

## *Basic principles*

The mass spectrometer has three stages, shown in Figure 16.6. In the first stage the sampled gas is drawn into a low-pressure sample chamber. Only a small fraction of this gas is drawn into the second stage and through a *molecular leak*, which is in the main part of the analyser. The third stage is the electronic amplification and display of the signal.

The second stage of the analyser is virtually under a vacuum. In the ionisation chamber the gas molecules are bombarded by a transverse beam of electrons, as shown in Figure 16.6, and thereby become ionised by losing an electron. They then pass towards a plate to which a negative voltage has been applied, termed the *acceleration plate*, and through a slit in this plate, the molecular leak. From this point the path of the ions is influenced by a magnetic field. The field thus deflects and separates the ions according to their *mass:charge* ratio. Since most molecules have been ionised to carry a single positive charge, separation is mainly on the basis of mass, lightest ions being deflected the most, heaviest ions the least. The ions reach photo-voltaic detectors, where electronic registration, amplification and display of the signal occurs, proportional to the rate of arrival of ions and therefore to partial pressure of the gas.

The way in which the magnetic field is produced and ions are detected on the plates has two variants, resulting in two types of instrument. The earlier form was the *magnetic sector* type, where the magnetic field lies at right angles to the path of ions and is produced by a combination of electric and fixed magnetic fields. By varying the voltage on the acceleration plate, the velocity of the ions entering the magnetic field can be changed. This can allow the deflected ion beam to be directed across the detector plate and different components to be detected in turn. It is therefore possible to separate components of the gas sample according to mass:charge ratio.

More commonly seen these days, is the *quadrupole mass spectrometer*. This device is more compact and allows better discrimination between components. The magnetic field is produced by a combination of D.C. electric and A.C. radio frequency fields. As shown in Figure 16.6, the quadrupoles consist of four rods with opposite pairs electrically connected. By careful tuning of the radiofrequency component

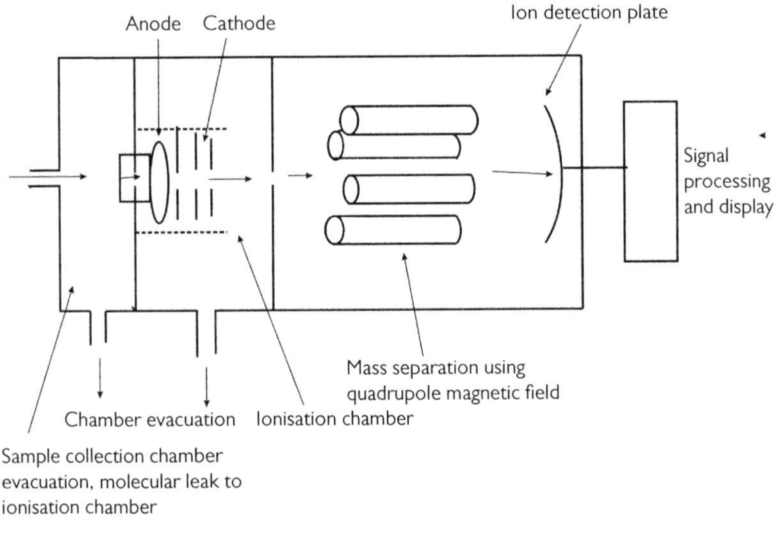


**Fig. 16.6** The mass spectrometer.

of the magnetic field, only ions of a given mass:charge ratio proceed through the quadrupole to the detector, all other ions oscillating and colliding with the walls of the device. By a combination of changing the voltage on the acceleration plate (the cathode) and of judiciously tuning the magnetic field, a spectrum of mass:charge components can be detected and quantified. By scanning at 50 Hz it is possible to produce a continuous record of gas concentrations.

The respiratory mass spectrometer is accurate, giving good gas identification and quantification. It requires only about 20 ml $min^{-1}$ gas sampling rate, with a 100 ms response time. However, it does have some disadvantages. The second stage of the device operates under almost vacuum conditions; this requires a high quality, continuously running pump. If the device itself is at some distance from the sampling site, significant delay time may be added to the response time. Water condensation can be avoided by heating the sampling tube, but the response time for water vapour may still be longer than for other components.

Some molecule types may lose two electrons rather than one on ionisation, and appear to the magnetic field with a double charge. They then behave like an ion with half the mass, which leads to confusion in interpretation. Furthermore, the ionisation process can lead to fragmentation of a molecule, so that a mass spectrum appears at the output rather than a peak. However, this anomaly is useful to distinguish the gas components with the same molecular mass, such as $N_2O$ and $CO_2$ (44 Da), or $N_2$ and CO (28 Da). $N_2O$ is fragmented into NO, $O_2$, $N_2$, N and O, while $CO_2$ is fragmented into $O_2$, $C_2$, C and O. Rather than trying to detect and distinguish both gases at 44 Da, $N_2O$ can be detected at a subordinate peak of 30 Da and $CO_2$ at 12 Da. Because the fragmentation is predictable, the amplitude of the subsidiary peak can be used as a measure of the parent peak and therefore of gas concentration. Using appropriate low-pass and high-pass filters, obfuscating peaks in the spectra can be removed.

## Raman spectroscopy

When light falls on an object, it is reflected and scattered by the object. Most of this scattering occurs without any loss of energy or change of wavelength and is known as *Rayleigh scattering*, which allows us to see the object with scattered waves in the visible spectrum. A small fraction of the incident light, about $10^{-6}$, is scattered with a loss of energy and a change of wavelength characteristic of the molecule off which the light is being reflected; this is *Raman scattering*, first observed in 1928 by the Indian physicist, after whom the technique is named. Raman spectroscopy has been used in industry for years as a means of identifying solids, liquids and gases, but has had to await the advent of powerful laser light sources and sensitive photocell detectors to be useful in a clinical setting for breath-by-breath analysis.

Figure 16.7 shows the schematic layout of a Raman spectroscope, incorporating an Argon laser source of wavelength 485 nm, high reflectance mirrors to concentrate the laser beam, a gas sampling chamber, appropriate optics, a detection system, and signal processor and display system. Table 16.1 shows characteristic wavelength or frequency changes that identify different gases. If plotted graphically, the amplitudes of the frequency-shifted peaks are proportional to the gas concentrations. In Raman spectroscopy each gas is independently analysed, including $CO_2$, $N_2O$, volatile agents, $O_2$, $N_2$ and water vapour. The response time is around 100 ms and the device is therefore capable of breath-by-breath analysis. The sample is not altered by the process and can therefore be returned to the breathing system, which is a significant advantage in low flow anaesthesia (Lockwood *et al.* 1994), although there is some overlap between gas species (Lawson *et al.* 1993). However the devices require a great deal of electrical power and are noisy.

## Piezoelectric gas analysis

A pair of piezoelectric crystals, connected to an electrically active circuit, is made to resonate with a characteristic frequency difference. One of the crystals is coated in silicone oil, which absorbs a volatile anaesthetic agent to which it is exposed. This changes the natural frequency of the crystal, and the frequency difference between the crystals changes by an amount dependent on the amount of volatile

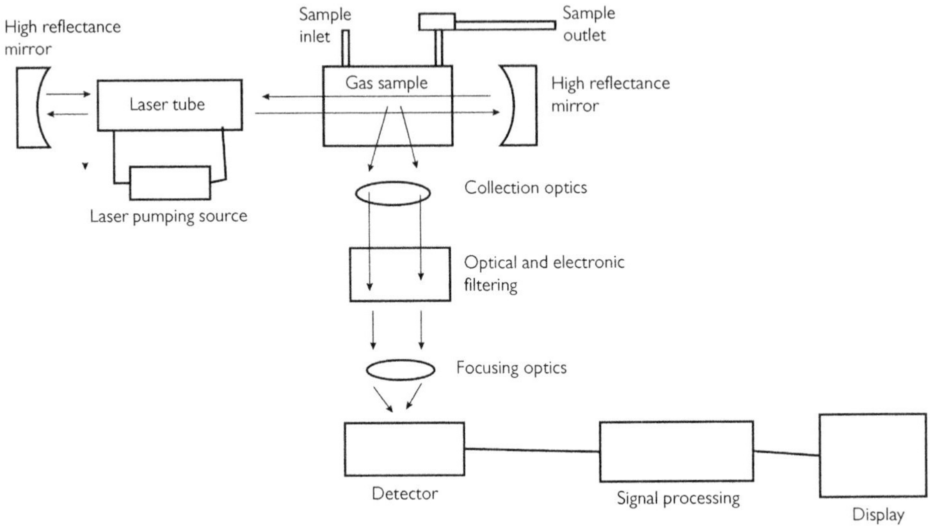


**Fig. 16.7** The Raman spectroscope.

**Table 16.1** Characteristic frequency shifts of substances with Raman spectroscopy

| Gas | Frequency shift $cm^{-1}$ |
|---|---|
| Isoflurane | 995 |
| Halothane | 717 |
| Enflurane | 817 |
| $N_2O$ | 1285, 2224 |
| $CO_2$ | 1285,1388 |
| Oxygen | 1555 |
| Nitrogen | 2331 |
| Water | 3650 |

agent absorbed. Manual identification of the agent is required, but the device is remarkably accurate and stable (Humphrey *et al.* 1991).

## Paramagnetic oxygen analyser

Gas molecules are influenced by a magnetic field in two different ways because of their structure. Most are repelled by the field and are called *diamagnetic* molecules. Two gases, oxygen and nitric oxide, are attracted into the field and are called *paramagnetic*. This property enables oxygen concentrations to be analysed and is the result of the presence of unpaired electrons in the outer shell of an oxygen molecule (see Chapter 3), which is able to generate force in a magnetic field. A paramagnetic oxygen

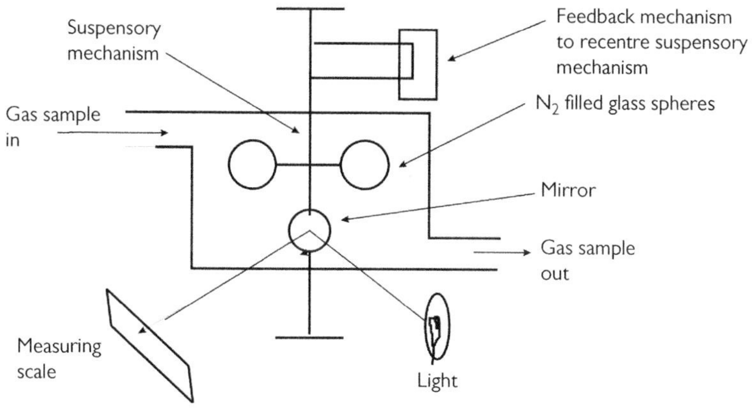


**Fig. 16.8** The paramagnetic oxygen analyser.

analyser is shown in Figure 16.8 of the sort originally developed by Pauling in 1946. In this device, the two suspended glass spheres are filled with nitrogen, a weakly diamagnetic gas. The glass spheres are arranged in a dumbbell shape, suspended between the poles of a magnet by a thread, tensioned to keep the dumbbell in the plane of the magnetic field. Zeroing should be carried out in the carrier gas destined to have oxygen added to it at a later stage. When an oxygen-containing gas mixture is drawn through the analyser, oxygen is attracted into the magnetic field, displacing the nitrogen-filled spheres from it. The detection system can either be a deflection measurement or a *null deflection* type, which measures the current required in the circuitry to restore the pointer to its null point. These devices are accurate to within 0.1% $O_2$, but are adversely affected by pressurisation, vibration, water vapour and high flow rates; there is also a slow response time of up to 1 minute.

To overcome these disadvantages, a development of the device in which there is an electromagnet that produces an alternating magnetic field at a frequency of 110 Hz is shown in Figure 16.9. A reference gas, usually air, enters one arm of the tube, and the sample gas enters the opposite arm at the same rate. As the alternating magnetic field amplitude rises, oxygen molecules from both tubes are attracted towards it in proportion to their concentrations, and as the amplitude falls, the opposite happens. This causes an opposite and proportional alternating in pressure change upstream in the tubes, which is detected by a pressure transducer, placed in such a way as to measure the difference in pressure changes between the tubes, and which detects the 20–50 μbar pressure oscillations thus created. The detected

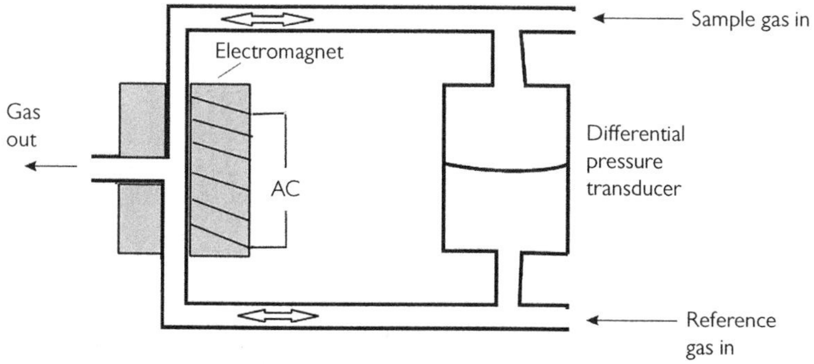


**Fig. 16.9** Modern paramagnetic oxygen analyser.

pressure oscillations are transduced into a sound signal, whose amplitude is directly proportional to the $O_2$ concentration of the sample gas, the device having been calibrated against the reference gas. It has been reported that a gas mixture containing desflurane interferes with the accuracy of a paramagnetic oxygen analyser (Scheeren 1998).

## Polarography and fuel cells

These two techniques are combined in one section because they use the same electrochemical principle in slightly different ways.

The Clarke polarographic electrode is shown in Figure 16.10(a). It consists of a cellophane-covered platinum cathode and Ag/AgCl anode in a phosphate and KCl electrolyte, between which a potential difference of −0.6 V is applied by the battery as shown.

At the anode, the following reactions take place:

$$4Ag \Rightarrow 4Ag^+ + 4e^-$$
$$4Ag^+ + 4Cl^- \Rightarrow 4AgCl.$$

Electrons are provided by the ionisation of the silver anode, and are consumed by the $O_2$ in the gas or blood sample. At the cathode, the following reaction takes place:

$$O_2 + 2H_2O + 4e^- \Rightarrow 4OH^-.$$

The current generated by the reaction represents the consumption of electrons at the cathode and is proportional to the $pO_2$ of the gas sample. Figure 16.10(b) shows that a plateau of current is reached for a given voltage, which represents the rate limitation of the diffusion of $O_2$ from the electrolyte solution. The height of the plateau is proportional to $pO_2$.

The problem with the polarographic electrode is the dependence on a battery and the reduction of $N_2O$ at the cathode when it is contaminated by $Ag^+$ ions. A fuel cell is a similar device that consists of a gold cathode and a lead anode. The same reaction occurs at the cathode as in the polarographic electrode. Note that no polarising voltage is required in this circuit. Their response time is slow, making them acceptable but less suitable for breath-by-breath analysis than other methods (Roe *et al.* 1987).

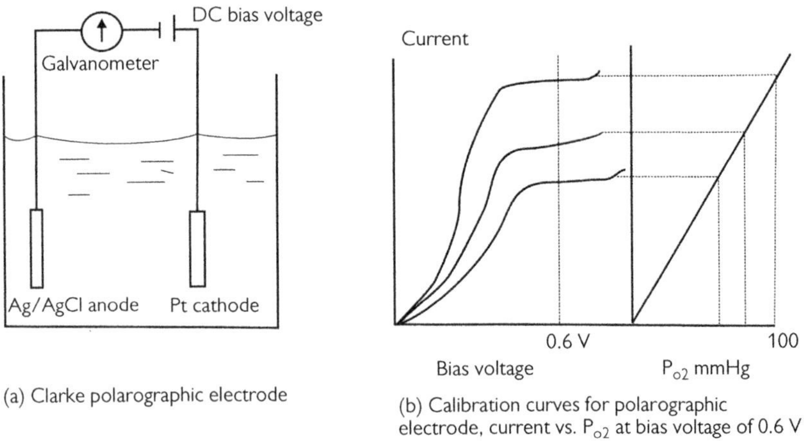


**Fig. 16.10** (a) The Clarke polarographic electrode. (b) Calibration curves for the polarographic electrode.

## Nitric oxide (NO) measurement

NO is a pulmonary vasodilator used in ICU, with toxic side effects such as methaemoglobinaemia and has a toxic by-product of $NO_2$, which must therefore also be detected. There is a chemoluminescent method of NO analysis, in which NO reacts with ozone to produce photoluminescent $NO_2$ molecules, whose light intensity can be detected. Another means of detecting the resulting $NO_2$ is to measure the electrical potential difference in an electrolyte, generated by the reaction between NO and the electrolyte (Etches *et al.* 1995). In both detection techniques, parallel detection cells are used to detect any $NO_2$ in a mixed-gas sample containing NO.

## Preoperative exercise testing

This section has been put in this chapter because the process involves the use of the gas analysers described above. It has become more common, both in the general community and in preoperative assessment of patients, to apply some physiological science to the process in order to classify surgical risk for a particular patient, and its value has become increasingly recognised (Moran *et al.* 2016). This involves monitoring the patient's oxygen consumption and carbon dioxide output with exercise and plotting $CO_2$ output against $O_2$ consumption in ml $kg^{-1}$ $min^{-1}$. These physiological variables may be calculated from *gas concentration difference* (*input –output*)×*tidal volume* × *respiratory rate*. Figure 16.11 shows such a plot, which generally consists of a line with two distinct slopes. At low exercise rates the slope is slightly under 1, corresponding to aerobic metabolism. As the rate of physical work increases, there is an abrupt increase of slope corresponding to a change of metabolism to aerobic plus anaerobic, and this point is termed the anaerobic threshold. Clearly the more work a patient is able to do before anaerobic metabolism starts, the greater is his or her physical capacity. A patient with an anaerobic

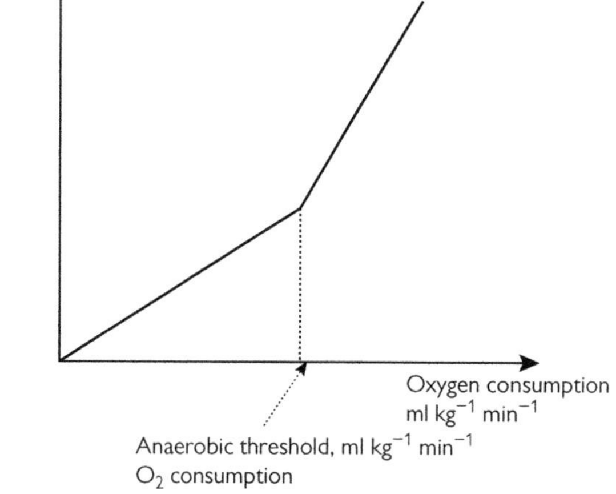


**Fig. 16.11** Plot of carbon dioxide production against oxygen consumption to produce anaerobic threshold in exercise testing.

threshold of as low as 11 ml $O_2$ $kg^{-1}$ $min^{-1}$ is deemed to be at significant additional cardiovascular risk for major surgery (Older and Hall 2007). Although there is some variance in the curves produced by such testing, it is found that inter-observer variance in determining the anaerobic threshold is clinically acceptable when classifying patients' surgical risk preoperatively (Sinclair *et al.* 2009).

## References

**Ball, J. A. S.** and **Grounds R. M.** (2003) Calibration of three capnographs for use with helium and oxygen mixtures, *Anaesthesia*, **58**, pp. 156–60.

**Chan, K. L., Chan, M. T. V.** and **Gin, T.** (2003) Mainstream vs. sidestream capnometry for prediction of PaCO2 during supine craniotomy, *Anaesthesia*, **58**, pp. 149–55.

**Etches, P. C., Harris, M. L., McLinley, R.**, and **Finer, N. M.** (1995) Clinical monitoring of inhaled nitric oxide: comparison of chemoluminescent and electrochemical sensors, *Biomed. Instrum. Technol.* **29**, 131–40.

**Foley, M. A. *et al.*** (1990) The effect of exhaled alcohol on the performance of the Datex Capnomac, *Anaesthesia*, **45**, pp. 232–4.

**Fowler, K. T.** (1958) *A mass spectrometer for the rapid and continuous analysis of gas mixtures in respiratory research*, PhD thesis, University of London.

**Humphrey, S. J. E., Luff, N. P.** and **White, D. C.** (1991) Evaluation of the Lamtec anaesthetic agent monitor, *Anaesthesia*, **46**, pp. 478–81.

**Lawson, D., Samanta, S., Magee, P. T.** and **Gregonis, D. E.** (1993) Gas monitoring in the OR: stability and long term durability of Raman spectroscopy, *J. Clin. Monit.*, **9**, pp. 241–51.

**Lockwood, G. G., London, M. J., Chakrabarti, M. K.** and **Whitwam, J. G.** (1994) The Ohmeda Rascal II. A new gas analyser for anaesthetic use, *Anaesthesia*, **49**, pp. 44–53.

**Mason, D. G.** and **Lloyd-Thomas, A. R.** (1991) Cyclopropane and the Datex Capnomac, *Anaesthesia*, **46**, pp. 398–9.

**Moran, J., Wilson, F., Guinan, E. *et al.*** (2016) Role of cardiopulmonary exercise testing as a risk assessment method in patients undergoing intra-abdominal surgery: a systematic review, *Br. J. Anaesth.*, **116**(2), pp. 177–91.

**Older, P.** and **Hall, A.** (2007) The role of cardiopulmonary exercise testing in the preoperative evaluation of surgical patients. In Cashman, J. and Grounds M. (eds) *Recent Advances in Anaesthesia and Intensive Care*, vol 24, Cambridge University Press, Cambridge, pp. 1–20.

**Roe, P. G., Tyler, C. K. G., Tennant, R.** and **Barnes, P. K.** (1987) Oxygen analysers. Evaluation of five models, *Anaesthesia*, **42**, 175–81.

**Scheeren, T. W. C. *et al.*** (1998) Error in measurement of oxygen and carbon dioxide concentrations by the Deltatec II metabolic monitor in the presence of desflurane, *Br. J. Anaesth.*, **80**, pp. 521–4.

**Sinclair, R. C. F., Danjoux, G. R., Goodridge, V.** and **Batterham, A. M.** (2009) Determination of the anaerobic threshold in the preoperative assessment clinic: inter-observer measurement error, *Anaesthesia*, **64**, pp. 1192–5.

## Further reading

**Magee, P. T.** (2011) Physiological monitoring: gases. Chapter 15 in Davey, A. and Diba, A. (eds) *Ward's Anaesthetic Equipment*, 6th edn, WB Saunders Co. Ltd, Philadelphia, PA, pp. 337–50.

# Chapter 17 **Blood gas analysis**

The chapter links with: Chapters 1 and 16.

## Introduction

Acid-base balance is finely balanced in normal physiology (Shaw and Gregory 2022), and is frequently disturbed in complex ways in critical illness, or by the treatment the patient is receiving, including artificial ventilation (Park and Sidebotham 2023). A blood gas machine has electrodes to measure pH, $pCO_2$ and $pO_2$ and often measures Hb and some biochemistry as well (King and Campbell 2000; Shaw and Magee 2022). Derived values from such a device include $O_2$ saturation, $O_2$ content, bicarbonate, base excess and total $CO_2$.

## The $pO_2$ electrode

This is the Clarke electrode, which was described in the previous chapter on gas analysers and is suitable for both respiratory and blood $O_2$ analysis.

## The pH electrode

A *pH unit* has been defined in Chapter 1 as

$$pH = \log_{10} \frac{1}{[H^+]}$$

In words, this can be described as 'the negative logarithm, to base ten, of the hydrogen ion concentration'.

The physical principle on which the pH electrode is based depends on the fact that when a membrane separates two solutions of different $[H^+]$, a potential difference exists across the membrane. In a pH electrode, such a membrane is usually made of glass and the development of a potential difference between the two solutions is thought to be due to the migration of $H^+$ into the glass matrix. If one solution consists of a standard $[H^+]$, the pH of the other solution can be estimated by measurement of the potential difference between them. The glass membrane used is selectively permeable to $H^+$. No current flows in this device, which does not wear out, in contrast to the Clark electrode, in which current does flow and that does need periodic replacement.

The pH measurement system is shown diagrammatically in Figure 17.1. It consists of two half cells. In one half it has an Ag/AgCl electrode and in the other a $Hg/HgCl_2$ (calomel) electrode. Each electrode maintains a fixed electrical potential. The Ag/AgCl electrode is surrounded by a buffer solution of known pH, surrounded by the pH sensitive glass. Outside the glass membrane is the test solution, usually blood, whose pH is to be measured. It is the potential difference across the glass, between these two solutions, which is variable. The blood or other solution is separated from the calomel electrode by a porous plug and a potassium chloride *salt bridge* to minimise KCl diffusion. The potential difference across the system is about 60 mV per unit of pH change at 37°C. The internal electrical resistance is high and, in order to maximise the device's accuracy, a voltmeter (or other measuring device) of very high internal resistance must be used to minimise current drawn from the system.

The pH electrode actually responds to $H^+$ activity rather than $[H^+]$. These two variables coincide at infinite dilution of solution, but might otherwise differ, because of molecular interaction between ionic species. The electrode is therefore calibrated against standard buffer solutions of pH 6.841 and 7.383.

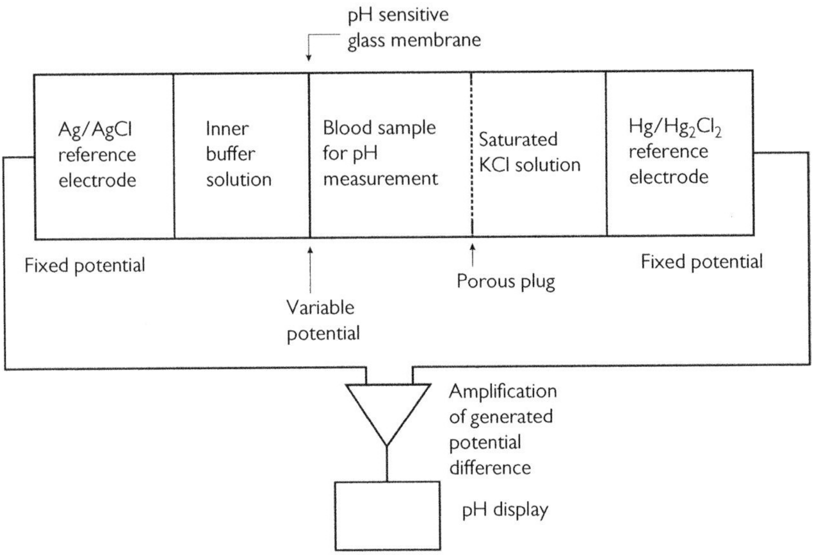


**Fig. 17.1** pH electrode.

# The $pCO_2$ electrode

There is a dynamic equilibrium between $H^+$ and $CO_2$ by virtue of the following reactions:

$$CO_2 + H_2O \Leftrightarrow H_2CO_3 \Leftrightarrow H^+ + HCO_3^-.$$

In other words, there is a relationship between pH and $pCO_2$. The *Henderson–Hasselbalch* equation describes this relationship:

$$pH = pK_a + \log_{10}\frac{[HCO_3^-]}{[H_2CO_3]}$$

$$= pK_a + \frac{\log_{10}[HCO_3^-]}{\alpha pCO_2},$$

Where $\alpha$ is the Ostwald solubility coefficient, 0.003 mmol $l^{-1}$ $mmHg^{-1}$ at 37°C. $pK_a$, the association constant of the chemical reaction concerned is 6.1 and is the pH at which $H_2CO_3$ is 50% associated. Both $\alpha$ and $pK_a$ vary with pH and thus lend the calculation some inaccuracy. It was Astrup, the Danish physiologist, who noticed that there was a linear relationship between pH and $pCO_2$.

The $pCO_2$ electrode is essentially a pH electrode with a difference. The sensitive glass membrane is covered with another membrane that is selectively permeable to $CO_2$. In the original design a layer of water was trapped between the two membranes, allowing the reaction described above to occur. A later modification had salt and bicarbonate solution in this space. A $pCO_2$ electrode therefore allows a $pCO_2$ change to generate a pH change, which is measured by the electrode.

# Derived variables from a blood gas machine

*Buffer base* is the sum of all bases in the blood capable of buffering pH changes. These include $HCO_3^-$, Hb, $PO_4^{3-}$ and the anionic parts of protein. A respiratory driven change in status, marked by, for example, the addition of $CO_2$, results in the formation of carbonic acid. Thus:

$$CO_2 \Leftrightarrow H_2CO_3 \Leftrightarrow H^+ + HCO_3^-$$

and $H^+$ is buffered by the

$$\text{total buffer base} = HCO_3^- + Hb^- + PO_4^{3-} + \text{protein}^-.$$

The buffer base can be considered to be a limitless source of buffering capacity unless the haemoglobin component is significantly reduced. The *base excess*, an indication of metabolic rather than respiratory acid-base disturbance, is defined as the amount of titratable acid required to correct a blood sample to a pH of 7.40 at a $pCO_2$ of 5.3 kPa and at 37°C.

*Standard bicarbonate* is the bicarbonate in a fully oxygenated blood sample at a $pCO_2$ of 5.3 kPa and at 37°C.

## Errors in blood gas measurement

These include (for all electrodes):

- air bubbles in the sample;
- excess heparin;
- gas storage in container with plastic walls;
- failure to store samples at low temperature;

and for the $O_2$ electrode only:

- metabolism in the sample;
- $O_2$ consumption in a Clarke electrode;
- material used in the electrode membrane;
- polarising voltage;
- protein deposition on the pH electrode;
- signal processing errors.

## Temperature and blood gas analysis

Blood gas analysers measure blood gas variables at 37°C. A fall in body temperature means that $CO_2$ is more soluble in blood and that $CO_2$ production slows, leading to a fall in $pCO_2$. This shifts the $O_2$ dissociation curve to the left, increasing the $O_2$ content. However $O_2$ solubility also rises, decreasing $pO_2$ and $O_2$ content. pH increases with a fall in temperature.

Hypothermia itself does not alter the blood gas values at 37°C and arterial blood taken at lower temperatures should be corrected to 37°C before clinical decisions are made on the results (Rupp and Severinghaus 1986).

## Transcutaneous blood gas analysers

$pO_2$ can be measured transcutaneously by applying a Clarke polarographic electrode to the skin. If the skin is 'arterialised' by heating it, a reasonable value for $pO_2$ can be obtained. A modified $pCO_2$ electrode is used to measure transcutaneous $pCO_2$. A common $O_2/CO_2$ permeable membrane and electrolyte solution is used, ensuring a common pH for both measurements. Actual measured values do not correlate well with arterial values, but trends are clinically useful and the device is still used in neonatology.

## Intravascular blood gas analysers

These are microminiaturised versions of the pH, $pCO_2$ and $pO_2$ electrodes described above.

## *References*

**King, R.** and **Campbell, A.** (2000) Performance of the Radiometer OSM 3 and ABL 505 blood gas analysers for the determination of Na, K, and Hb concentrations, *Anaesthesia*, **55**, pp. 65–9.

**Park, M.** and **Sidebotham, D.** (2023) Metabolic alkalosis and mixed acid base disturbance in anaesthesia and critical care, *B.J.A. Educ.*, **23**(4), pp. 128–35.

**Rupp, S. M.** and **Severinghaus, J.** (1986) Hypothermia. Chapter 57 in Miller, R. (ed.), *Anesthesia*, 2nd edn, Churchill Livingstone, p. 2000.

**Shaw, I.** and **Gregory, K.** (2022a) Acid-base: a review of normal physiology, *B.J.A. Educ.*, **22**(10), pp. 396–401.

**Shaw, I.** and **Magee, P.** (2022b) Acid-base quantification: a review of developing technology, *B.J.A. Educ.*, **22**(11), 440–7.

## *Further reading*

**Al-Shaikh, B.** and **Stacey, S.** (2002) *Essentials of Anaesthetic Equipment*, 2nd edn, Churchill-Livingstone, London, pp. 164–6.

**Clutton-Brock, T. H.** and **Venkatash, B.** (1994) *Blood gas monitoring. Chapter 16 in Monitoring in Anaesthesia and Intensive Care*, Hutton, P. and Prys-Roberts, C. (eds) WB Saunders Co. Ltd, pp. 242–55.

# Chapter 18 **Electrophysiology and stimulation**

This chapter contains: the electrocardiogram, artefacts and interference; the electroencephalogram, data collection and analysis; evoked response, auditory evoked responses; monitoring neuromuscular blockade and the electromyogram, nerve stimulators, electrodes, responses.

The chapter links with: Chapters 3, 4 and 19.

## Introduction

This chapter covers the processing and application of electrical signals from the body, in particularly the *electroencephalogram* (EEG), the *electrocardiogram* (ECG), and the *electromyogram* (EMG). The EEG and ECG will be considered in their monitoring capacity. The EMG will be discussed along with simulation and neuromuscular blockade and monitoring.

## The electrocardiogram

The electrocardiogram (ECG) is a surface reflection of the propagation of electrical depolarisation and repolarisation over the various contractile chambers of the heart. Depolarisation is the trigger for releasing the stored contractile energy in the cardiac muscle. Each chamber also produces electrical action and polarising recovery potentials associated with the mechanical contribution of the recovery. The ECG can be divided into two major components: one associated with the propagation of excitation and recovery of the atria; the other with these events occurring in the ventricles. Excitation of the atria gives rise to the P wave, after which the atrial contractions propel blood into the ventricles. An atrial recovery wave exists, but it is rarely seen, as it is obscured by ventricular excitation, which is signalled by the QRS wave. During the later part of the QRS wave, ventricular contraction commences. Recovery of the ventricles is preceded by the T wave. The ECG labels, i.e. PQRST, are shown in Figure 18.1.

To localise the direction of excitation and recovery of the heart chambers (and also to estimate the extent of cardiac injury), a variety of electrode arrangements can be used. The electrodes (which are normally disposable silver–silver chloride as described in Chapter 5) are positioned on easily located anatomical landmarks such as the right arm (RA), the left arm (LA), and the left leg (LL), with the right leg usually providing the reference or common. The standard (1, II, III), augmented (aVR, aVL, aVF) and

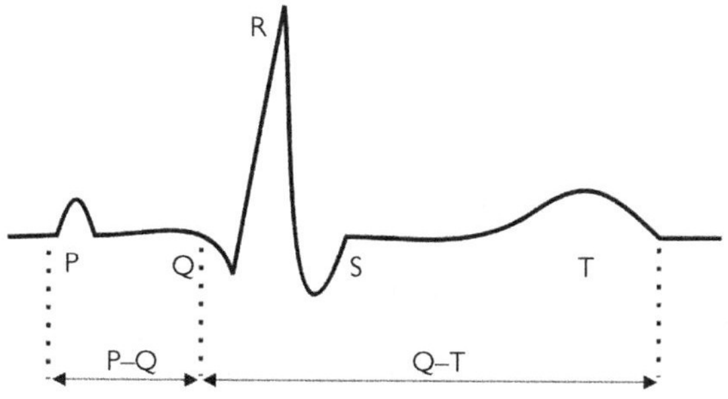


**Fig. 18.1** Diagram of an ECG showing the standard labels of various parts of the waveform.

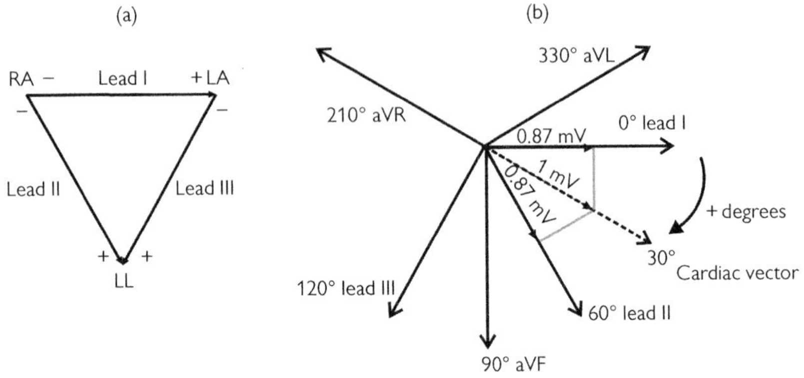


**Fig. 18.2** Calculation of cardiac vectors.

precordial (V) leads are routinely recorded by electrocardiographers. It is possible to locate the direction of excitation and recovery by considering that the direction of the event (excitation or recovery) is at right angles to the isoelectric lead (i.e. the lead with equal forces in the positive and negative). This can be demonstrated by forming an equilateral triangle (Einthoven's triangle), such as in Figure 18.2(a). This gives the direction of the leads, for example, lead I is RA to LA. The amplitude of lead I (0.87 mVin Figure 18.2(b)) is drawn and a right angle (perpendicular) is dropped down from this as shown in the figure. Similarly the lead II voltage of 0.87 mV is drawn along the lead II axis and the perpendicular drawn. This will interact with the lead I perpendicular and this dotted line will be the cardiac direction or *vector*. The vector will be 1 mV, 30 degrees, and lead III will have zero amplitude, indicating that the vector is at right angles to this lead.

## *Indices obtained from the ECG*

The bandwidth required for full 12-lead ECG analysis is from 0.05 to 100 Hz. Real-time monitoring in anaesthesia or intensive care generally requires three leads, both arms and left leg. Lead II (RA, LL) lies close to the normal cardiac electrical axis, permitting the best (maximum amplitude) P and R waves, and can be very useful for diagnosing certain arrhythmias. The ECG can be recorded graphically, usually on a time scale of 0.04 s $mm^{-1}$ (25 mm $s^{-1}$) but also the ECG can be digitised, using a sampling rate of typically 1 kHz, and *algorithms* (computer programs) are used to calculate the position of various parts of the waveform (e.g. R wave).

Many algorithms can be developed to calculate R–R intervals (i.e. reciprocal of heart rate), but a simple and effective one is to first *differentiate* the ECG waveform (Coleman and Bolton 1979) by taking the digitised waveform and creating an approximation of the differential in another part of the memory. This is demonstrated in Figure 18.3. Sample A in the raw signal is subtracted from B, and this forms the first sample in the (approximation) differentiated signal as shown. The next sample will be C – B, and so on.

If the whole raw waveform is treated in this manner, then the (approximated) differentiated wave will result, as indicated in Figure 18.4. As shown in the diagram, this method has the advantage of removing baseline wander due to respiration, removing the T wave (the large wave at the end of the raw signal) and enhancing the R wave. Once the position of the R wave has been detected, then the number of samples till the next R wave will be related to the R–R time interval. For example if there are 1000 samples between detected R waves, and the sampling rate is 1 kHz, then the R–R time interval will be 1 s and the heart rate will be 60 beats per min (BPM). A digital *refractory* period can be built into the algorithm so that the next R wave will not be searched for until a certain time has passed, e.g. 0.5 s. This enables artefacts not to be counted as a genuine R wave.

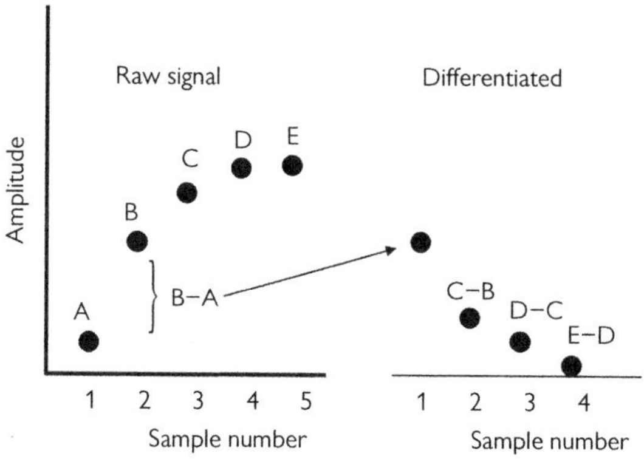


**Fig. 18.3** Diagram showing principle of digital differentiation of a small signal. The raw signal consists of five samples at amplitudes A–E. The approximation of the differentiated signal is created by taking the differences of the raw samples, i.e B–A, C–B, D–C, and E–D.

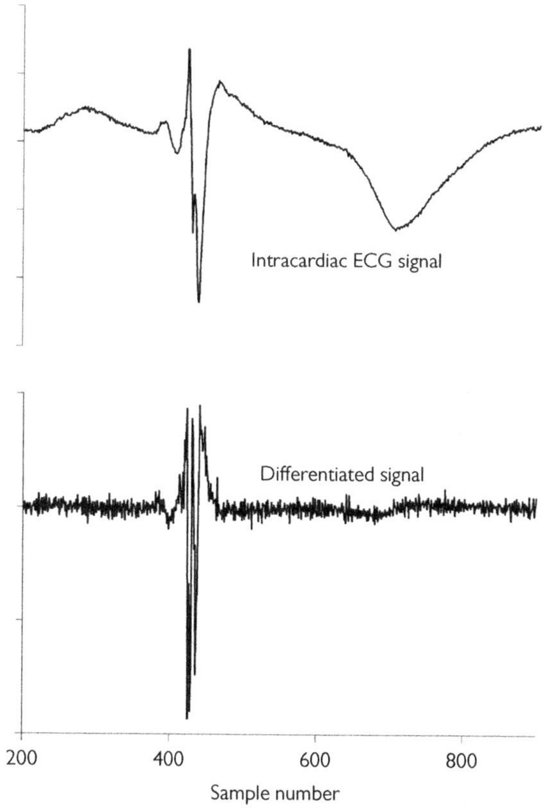


**Fig. 18.4** An intracardiac ECG signal sampled at 1 kHz and the approximation to the differentiated signal.

Other indices can be derived from the ECG such as S–T segments and this can provide prompt detection of myocardial ischaemia. Normally the detection is if the ST line is greater than 0.1 mV below the isoelectric line. As in the detection of R waves, a suitable algorithm used on the digitised waveform can produce this measurement automatically.

### *Artefacts and interference*

Although the amplitude of the ECG is larger than that of the EEG, it is still a small potential (0.1–6 mV) and artefacts and interference can cause problems in interpretation. Mains interference can be minimised by ensuring good electrode contact and a high common mode rejection ratio in the differential amplifier, as discussed in Chapter 5. Filters can be used with success to produce a cleaner signal, although the filter parameters must be chosen with care. Mains filters can only be used in the monitoring mode (rate detection). In the diagnostic mode of ECG analysis, the bandwidth must be 0.05–100 Hz, and the mains filter would remove some of the frequency components of the ECG signal, so should not be used. Low-pass filters set to 100 Hz can be used to remove the higher frequency components of the EMG signals.

## The electroencephalogram

The waves that can be recorded from the surface of the head are the summated result of postsynaptic potentials, which are the responses generated by the pyramidal cells to rhythmic discharges from the thalamic nuclei. The frequencies and amplitude of the thalamic discharges, and of the EEG itself, are determined by the excitatory and inhibitory connections between the thalamic cells. During activation, inputs to the reticular formations abolish the rhythmic discharges in the thalamic nuclei and cause the EEG to become desynchronised, i.e. not one frequency alone but a mixture of low-amplitude frequencies. During de-activation single high frequencies appear. The EEG is made up of a range of frequencies between DC and around 40 Hz. In the frequency domain, the EEG is often divided into frequency bands, which are described as delta (< 4 Hz), theta (4–7 Hz), alpha (8–13 Hz) and beta (13–40 Hz). Normally alpha activity can be recorded from the surface of the brain only during relaxation with the eyes closed and this is the de-activation state. If the subject carries out mental activities or eye opening, the waveform becomes *desynchronised* and at a higher frequency but lower amplitude. The amplitude of the normal EEG is between 10 and 50 $\mu$V, but the range can be between 1 and 100 $\mu$V. The EEG is affected by sleep and anaesthesia. Anaesthetic drugs, whether intravenous or volatile affect the EEG. Low drug doses cause an increase in amplitude of the signal and an increase in frequency, so that the dominant frequency is in the beta range. Higher doses cause the EEG frequency to decrease in a dose dependent manner, with the amplitude remaining high. Very high doses cause very low frequency, low amplitude signals, mixed with bursts of high amplitude and higher frequency. There are also bursts of no activity as well, and this is called *burst suppression*.

Other drugs such as opioids also change the EEG and there are other factors affecting it such as oxygenation levels, $pCO_2$, temperature and noxious stimulation. Reduced cerebral oxygenation causes slowing of the EEG, as does hypocapnia, and hypothermia. Noxious stimulation, unless the patient is heavily analgesed causes an increase in EEG frequency. Because all these things affect the EEG, if processed properly, it can be a useful monitor in theatre, especially for monitoring the depth of anaesthesia and as an awareness monitor.

### *EEG data collection*

The EEG is normally collected by using small silver–silver chloride electrodes (see Chapter 5). These need careful application using a suitable preparation paste to minimise the electrical impedance of the electrode skin interface. This will reduce interference and maximise the signal transfer to the amplifier (see Chapter 5). For secure fixing, the electrodes are fixed in an electrolyte gel and secured typically by collodion. For monitoring purposes, 2–6 sites plus a *ground* or reference are used, compared with 21

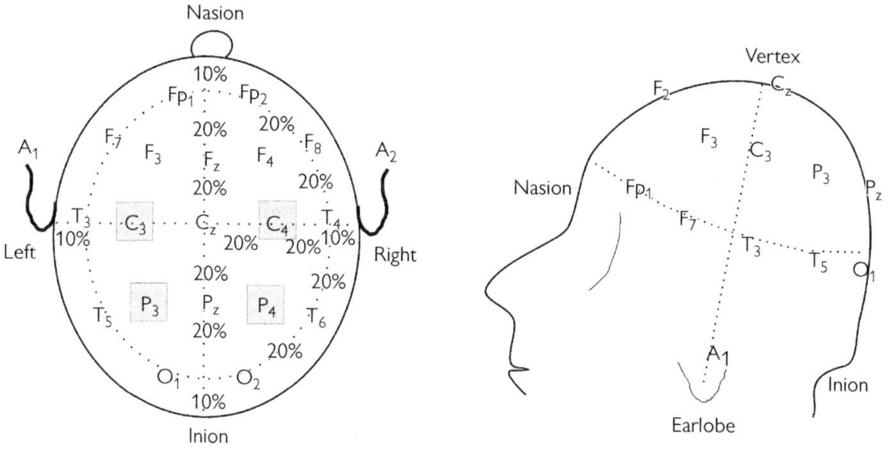


**Fig. 18.5** The 10–20 system for electrode placement. Fp is frontal pole, F is frontal, C is central, P is parietal, O is occipital, T is temporal. Even numbered electrodes are on the right and odd on the left. The midline joining the nasion and inion is defined as subscript Z. The measurements are related to distances on the line drawn from the nasion to the inion. 10% along this line, there is a circumference drawn around which the first ten electrodes are located. 30% along this mid-line is the frontal electrode, then the central electrode after another 20%. The rest of the electrodes follow a similar pattern – most of the inner electrodes are spaced 20% apart. The boxed electrodes are typical monitoring locations referred to in the text.

sites or more for routine diagnostic EEGs in the clinical neurophysiological laboratory. There is a standardised electrode location method used in clinical neurophysiology called the 10–20 system (Jasper 1958), in which the 21 electrodes are fixed at reproducible locations. The system is shown in Figure 18.5, and it employs skull landmarks as reference points to locate the electrodes. There are 19 scalp electrodes and 2 earlobe ones. The optimal sites for monitoring used are those least likely to pick up unwanted potentials of biological or external origin. Bilateral centroparietal placements such as $C_3$–$P_3$ and $C_4$–$P_4$ (Maynard 1984; Prior 1987) (see Figure 18.5) are preferable to those including frontal or temporal electrode placements, because of the risk of picking up slow wave activity due to eye movements or sweating and faster components from scalp or facial EMG. The electrodes are connected to an isolated differential amplifier, which minimises 50 Hz and other external electrical interference being amplified. After amplification, the signal is band-pass filtered, normally to between 0.1 and 32 Hz. Depending on the signal processing methods used to quantify the EEG signal, the filtered signal can be processed by analogue electronics or converted by an ADC (as described in Chapter 5) and processed digitally.

## *Electroencephalogram analysis*

The EEG, an example of which is shown in Figure 18.6, is a complex (comprising many different frequencies) time domain waveform and, for monitoring purposes, it needs to be data reduced and is usually quantified to a single number. Most analysis techniques examine *epochs* (short time periods) of EEG, usually in the range 2–16 s (there are mathematical reasons why this range is chosen). Analysis can be in time (time domain) or frequency (frequency domain).

## *Time domain analysis*

This analysis, which is discussed in Chapter 3, is where the amplitude or power of a signal is considered against time. These analyses include maximum amplitude or zero crossing frequency (number of times the EEG crosses the zero voltage line) per epoch, as demonstrated in Figure 18.7.

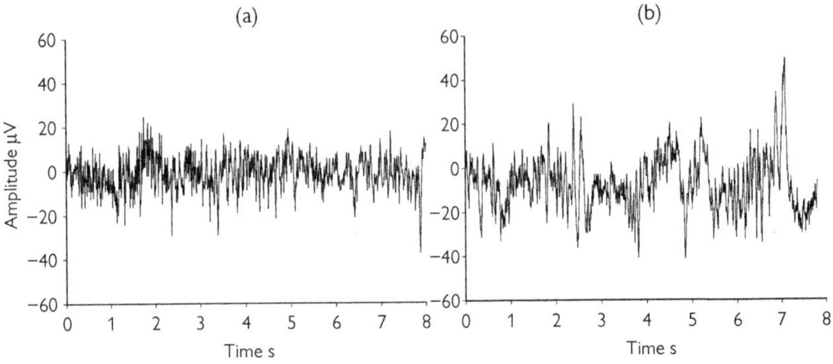


**Fig. 18.6** Example of two 8 s EEG epochs. The signal is collected from $C_3$–$P_3$, and (a) is from an awake patient, receiving a very low dose of propofol, and (b) is from an unresponsive patient receiving a high infusion of propofol (Forrest *et al.* 1994).

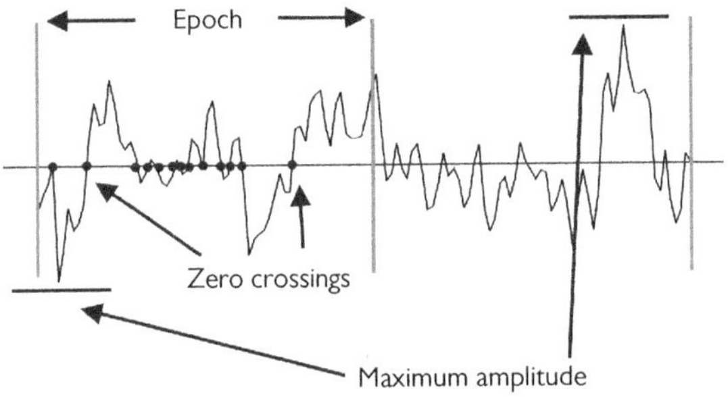


**Fig. 18.7** Diagram illustrating simple time domain analysis of the EEG waveform. In this example, the zero crossings frequency in the first epoch is 12. The maximum amplitude is the maximum amplitude value (positive or negative) in each epoch. The number of turns (i.e. change of direction of the signal) in each epoch could be another measure, as could the integrated voltage per epoch.

## *Frequency domain analysis*

The EEG can also be examined in the frequency domain, and this can reveal hidden information or clearer patterns than can be seen in the time domain. The EEG, as in time domain analysis, is broken down into epochs. It is then converted (by Fourier analysis) into many different sine waves, all at individual amplitudes and starting points (phase) as already demonstrated in Chapter 3, Figures 3.3 and 3.4. The frequency resolution of the frequency analysis is determined by the length of the epoch where $\text{epoch}^{-1}$ is the frequency resolution. For example, if the epoch length was 4 s, then the resolution of the spectrum would be 0.25 Hz, i.e.1/4 Hz.

Quantification of the frequency spectrum in anaesthesia has been well studied using indices such as the *median power frequency* (MPF) and the *spectral edge frequency* (SEF). A spectrum is produced of each from the EEG. From this spectrum are obtained single indices such as the MPF and SEF. The MPF is the frequency value at which 50% of the power is below and 50% above that value and the SEF is at which 95% of the power is below that frequency. This is demonstrated in Figure 18.8.

The MPF and SEF have been studied during single-drug anaesthesia and correlate well with drug levels and clinical effect (Schwilden *et al.* 1989; Forrest *et al.* 1994). The problem with these indices is that they tend to have different values with different drugs and also have the problem of the *biphasic*

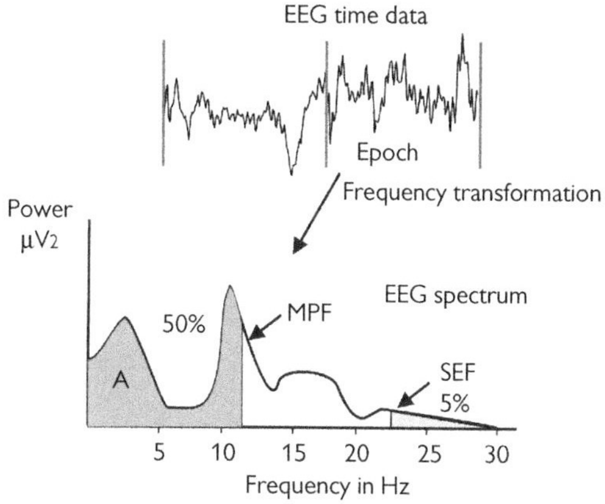


**Fig. 18.8** The MPF and the SEF. The diagram shows an epoch of EEG that is transformed to a spectrum. The MPF and SEF are obtained from this. The MPF is the frequency value where 50% of the power of the spectrum is below it (shown as the shaded part A). The SEF is the frequency value where 5% of the power of the spectrum is above it, or 95% below.

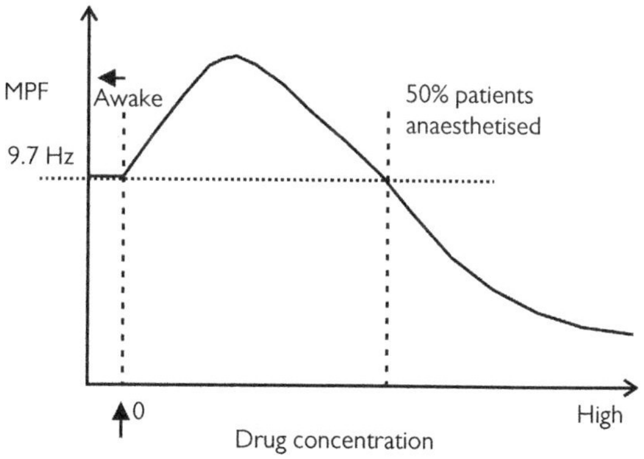


**Fig. 18.9** The biphasic response of the MPF. The diagram shows the MPF at different concentrations of an anaesthetic drug (propofol). Awake patients with no anaesthetic have an MPF of 9.7 Hz but this value is also when 50% of them will be unconscious at a later stage in the research procedure.

*effect*. This is where many anaesthetic agents initially increase the EEG frequencies and therefore the MPF. As the dose of the anaesthetic is increased, the EEG frequency (and therefore the MPF) will decrease. There is therefore an MPF value for awake and the same MPF value will be for some level of anaesthesia as well. This is shown in Figure 18.9 where the value of 9.7 Hz is both the MPF for all awake, drug-free patients and the value at which, by coincidence, 50% of the patients will be anaesthetised (Forrest *et al*. 1994).

## Evoked responses

The cortical responses and potentials so far described (EEG) are *spontaneous*, but another group of cortical potentials can be considered as *evoked*. This is where a short external stimulus is given and the response to that is measured. The stimulus can be auditory, visual or somatosensory (electric shock or

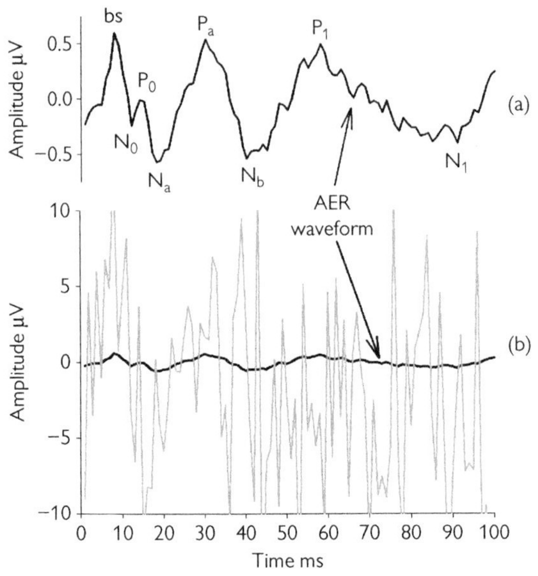


**Fig. 18.10** An auditory evoked response waveform (a), which is a magnified version of the waveform in (b), which shows it submerged in the spontaneous EEG background signal. bs = brainstem wave voltage. $P_n$ are positive waves with subscripts 0, a, b, 1, etc. $N_n$ are negative waves with subscripts 0, a, b, 1, etc.

mechanical). The response is normally lower amplitude than the background EEG, and therefore submerged in the EEG. This is demonstrated in Figure 18.10(b), which shows an *auditory evoked response* (AER), sometimes called an auditory potential, submerged in the EEG. This AER consists of a number of labelled waves as shown in Figure 18.10(a) but each modality (i.e. visual, auditory, etc.), although having a similar wave, has different labels. It is the *latency* and amplitude of each wave that is of interest. The latency is the time delay of the wave from the stimulus (at time zero).

As the AER is submerged, it cannot be visualised directly. Usually *coherent* averaging is used to reduce the *random* background EEG to an average voltage lower than the evoked response; this allows the evoked potential to be obtained and visualised. In a steady state clinical or physiological condition, the stimulus will normally elicit a repeatable response from the cortical electrodes. The EEG will also be present, and will overwhelm the response. The averaging technique is demonstrated in Figure 18.11. The stimulus is given at time 0 and the EEG following it for 100 ms (sweep 1) is stored in computer memory. This sweep contains both the EEG and the AER. After enough time has elapsed for the response to fade away (i.e. greater than 100 ms in this example) another stimulus is given and the EEG (sweep 2) is stored in another memory. The two submerged evoked responses will be very similar, but the background EEG will dominate and appear as a random signal, i.e. the EEGs will be very different from each other. If, for example, 500 stimuli are given sequentially, and all of the *sweeps* (or time periods) of the EEG are added together (in time), the amplitude of the evoked response will be multiplied by 500 times (because it is in the same time frame each time), but the EEG will have largely cancelled out, due to its random nature. In the example, a time point at 15 ms after each stimulus is shown. The EEG values at this time will be part random EEG and part AER. The AER component at 15 ms can be considered in this example to be -0.1 μV. The amplitude values will be (*the EEG value – the AER value*): 20–0.1, –20–0.1, –15–0.1, 12–0.1, 3–0.1μVfor sweeps 1, 2, 3, 4 and 5, respectively. The average of this simple example will be the summation of these divided by the number of sweeps. This is (0 – 0.5)/5, which is 0.1, or the value of the AER

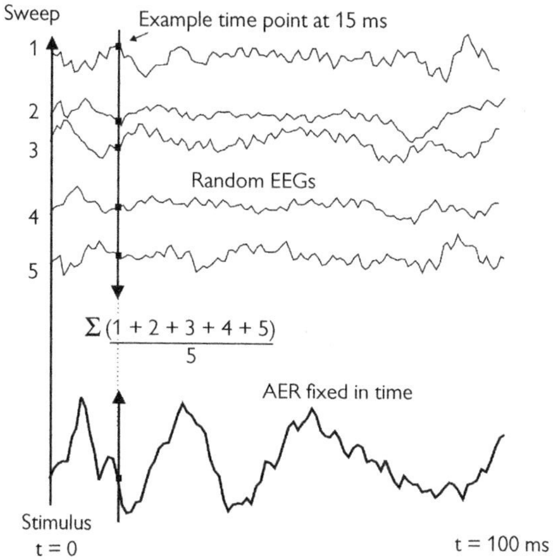


**Fig. 18.11** The principle of averaging to obtain the AER. Many sweeps of the random EEG are averaged (5 in this example) to obtain the AER (lower trace). Amplitude values at a time of 15 ms are added together and averaged. The EEG background will tend to zero, but the AER will be reinforced.

only. The EEG values have been *averaged* out. If all time points are considered in a similar manner, the EEG will tend to zero and the complete AER will appear.

Different waves in the evoked response come from different parts of the brain. For example, the first 10 ms of the auditory response come from the brainstem and the 10–50 ms come from the auditory cortex. All three modalities auditory (Thornton and Sharpe 1998), visual (Uhl *et al.* 1980) and somatosensory (Clark and Rosner 1973) are affected by anaesthesia; the visual responses are the largest responses, but they have not been studied extensively because of the problem of the patient seeing the chequerboard stimulus (a chequerboard in which the black and white squares reverse at a certain frequency) during the operation. Somatosensory responses tend to be affected by both anaesthetic drugs and muscle relaxants. The auditory responses seem to be the best modality for anaesthesia monitoring – the brainstem part of the response is robust to anaesthesia, but the 10–80 ms seem to change in a dose-related manner. Electrodes are normally connected as in EEG monitoring, but in

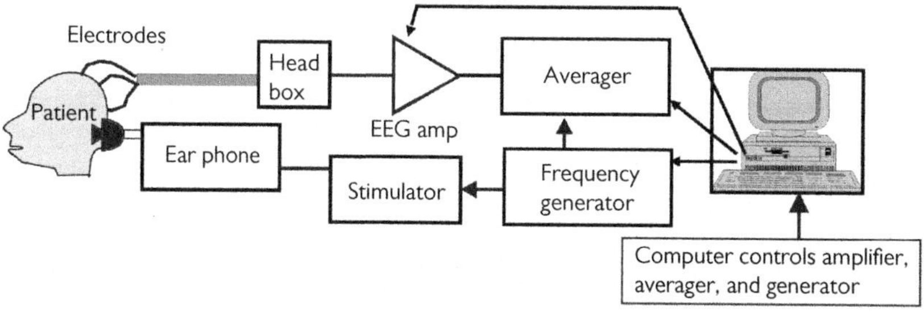


**Fig. 18.12** Diagram of an averaging for the auditory evoked response. The frequency generator outputs a pulse every, e.g. 100 ms, and this synchronises the averager and presents a click or tone to the patient.

specific locations, usually the vertex-mastoid gives the optimum response for auditory responses, but vertex–inion placement prevents interference from myogenic responses such as the post auricular response, which can overwhelm the AER (Tooley *et al.* 2004).

### *Obtaining the evoked responses*

To obtain the AER, the EEG signal is fed, via a suitable head box, to a patient isolated differential amplifier and then to a signal averaging device. The principle of operation is shown in Figure 18.12. In this example, a frequency generator is running at 10 Hz. This means that a stimulus pulse is generated every 100 ms. This pulse is supplied to an auditory stimulus generator that supplies a click or tone to a patient earphone. The pulse also synchronises the averager so that each new sweep is added to the previous sweep in the computer memory.

## Monitoring neuromuscular blockade and the electromyogram

In clinical nerve stimulation, three different types of nerve stimulation are used: single twitch, tetanic and the train of four. In stimulation, a supramaximal stimulus is used. This is where the stimulation amplitude (or intensity), usually provided by electrical current stimulation, is measured 25% above that for a maximal response.

### *Stimulations*

Single supramaximal current impulses can be applied at frequencies of between 0.1 and 1 Hz, the lower frequency of 0.1 Hz allows greater biochemical recovery in the *off* time so the mechanical responses do not *fade*, which means tests take longer with the lower frequency. The frequency used to induce a tetanic (total) contraction is 50 Hz for 5 s. There is no fade during this stimulation if a depolarising neuromuscular blocker is used. If a non-depolarising neromusclar blocker is used, this can cause fade during this response. After the tetanic stimulus is switched off, there is an enhancement of the response to lower frequency stimulations, such as the supramaximal single twitch stimulus or the *train-of-four*, called *post-tetanic facilitation* (PTF). In *train-of- four* (TOF) stimulation, supramaximal stimuli are applied at intervals of 0.5 s (2 Hz) and this can be repeated every 12 s. The ratio of the amplitude of the fourth to the first pulse is called the TOF ratio and this is inversely proportional to the degree of neuromuscular blockade (provided by a non-depolarising relaxant). The PTF can be a useful response to determine the degree of blockade when it is total. When no response is obtained to a single stimulus, the number of responses in a train of four detectable after the tetanic response can be a useful measure (Viby Mogensen *et al.* 1981).

### *The nerve stimulator*

The electrical stimulator used must be a constant current device, which means that the current delivered is independent of the electrode impedance, even though the electrode impedance may change with time, or between patients. Special circuits comprising operational amplifiers and capacitors need to be used to ensure that. Ideally, the constant current should be the same value whether the electrode impedance is zero or near infinity, but in practice the range of impedance across which the current is constant is from near zero to around 20 kΩ. The current should be in the range 10 to 50 mA and a square wave of pulse width 0.2–0.3 ms at a frequency between 0.1 and 1 Hz. The timing circuits should be able to give TOF, single twitch, double burst (two 50 Hz periods of 40 ms, separated by 750 ms off period) and tetanic stimulations. Nerve stimulators are also used to carry out local anaesthetic nerve blocks. An insulated needle is used as the active electrode, with the inactive electrode applied to the skin. The current will be much less electricity applied to the skin surface, a value of 0.5–1 mA, which allows the needle to approach the nerve without damaging the nerve prior to injection. It is important that a lower threshold is detected with the stimulator to confirm that the nerve itself has not been entered by the needle.

## Skin electrodes

The electrodes used are normally, silver–silver chloride, mentioned previously, and tend to be pre-gelled. They can be EEG-type electrodes or specialised ones. The site should be cleaned and prepared. The median and ulnar nerves are the two most often used for stimulation, although the facial and common peroneal nerves are also used. Two electrodes must be used to complete the circuit.

## Measuring the response

Although any motor nerve may be suitable, it has to be accessible and suitable for use with surface electrodes so that the response can be measured. Therefore only a limited number of nerves have been used as discussed previously. Most often the ulnar nerve is stimulated and the evoked response is evaluated visually, mechanically, electrically or clinically.

## Mechanical responses

In this case, the thumb acts on a force–displacement transducer. The transducer and the rest of the hand and arm are fixed. Movement of the thumb pulls or pushes the transducer, shown in Figure 18.13, where the force applied is converted to an electrical signal. This can be amplified and supplied to a computer or a chart recorder. The arm must be rigidly fixed and the transducer should be placed correctly in relation to the muscle. Other mechanical methods include the measurement of acceleration by using a piezoelectric transducer fastened to, for example, the thumb (Jensen *et al.* 1988).

## Electrical responses

Electrical responses to the stimulators include the EMG. This signal can be measured via surface or needle electrodes and is a summation of the many motor unit potentials. The EMG recorded is the result of the stimulation and is therefore *evoked*. Three electrodes (positive, negative and reference) supplied to a differential amplifier (as discussed in Chapter 5) will be needed to sense the signal. The EMG

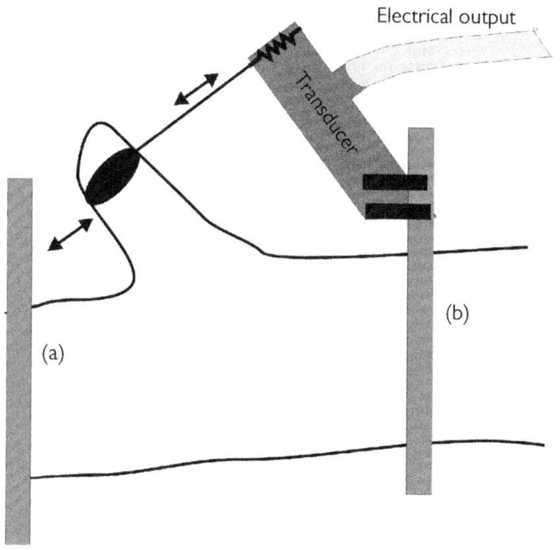


**Fig. 18.13** An example of the measurement of the mechanical evoked muscle response. A and B are clamps to keep the hand and transducer fixed. The thumb is connected to a strain-gauge transducer. The movement of the thumb compresses or extends this and via the transducer electronics produces an electrical output.

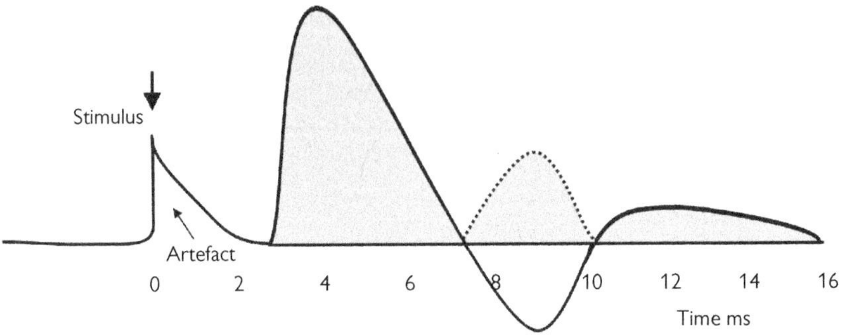


**Fig. 18.14** The evoked EMG. The stimulus is at time zero, and the stimulus artefact lasts for about 3 ms This is excluded from the quantification of the wave. The wave from 3 ms till 16 ms is first rectified, and this is shown by the shaded areas (the dotted curve replaces the negative part of the waveform. The rectified waveform is then integrated by measuring the total shaded area.

is recorded in a similar manner to the EEG, but it is of much larger amplitude and the bandwidth of the signal is much higher (typically 0–4 kHz). The EMG can be processed and filtered and an algorithm can be used to provide quantification output from a computer. A simple measure could be the integrated evoked EMG (Carter *et al.* 1986). This is where the EMG activity is rectified (i.e. the negative values are multiplied by -1) and then the area summated. This is shown in Figure 18.14. The signal is normally integrated from after the stimulus artefact until about 13 ms after the stimulus.

The electrical signals can be simple to set up, mechanical transducers are eliminated, and the electrode site (for example, the arm) can be out of sight. The EMG is able to detect changes that persist into the recovery period that the mechanical responses can not (Harper *et al.* 1986).

## *References*

**Coleman, J. D.** and **Bolton, M. P.** (1979) Microprocessor detection of electrocardiogram R-waves, *J. Med. Eng. Technol.*, **3**(5), pp. 235–41.

**Carter, J .A., Arnold, R., Yate, P. M.** and **Flynn, P. J.** (1986) Assessment of the Datex Relaxagraph during anaesthesia and atracurium-induced neuromuscular blockade, *Br. J. Anaesth.*, **58**(12), pp. 1447–52.

**Clark, D. L. and Rosner, B. S.** (1973) Neurophysiological effects of general anaesthetics, *Anaesthesiology*, **38**, pp. 564–82.

**Forrest, F. C., Tooley, M. A., Saunders, P. R.** and **Prys-Roberts, C.** (1994) Propofol infusion and the suppression of consciousness – the electroencephalogram and dose requirements, *Br. J. Anaesth*, **72**, pp. 35–41.

**Harper, N. J. N., Bradshaw, E. G.** and **Healy, T. E. J.** (1986) Evoked electromyographic and mechanical responses of the adductor pollicis compared with the onset of neuromuscular blockade by atracurium or alcuronium during antagonism by neostigmine, *Br. J. Anaesth.*, **58**, pp. 1278–84.

**Jasper, H. H.** (1958) The ten twenty electrode system of the international federation, *Electroencep. Clin. Neurophysiol.*, **10**, pp. 371–5.

**Jensen, E., Viby-Mogensen, J.** and **Bang, U.** (1988) The accelerograph: a new neuromuscular transmission monitor, *Acta Anaesthesiol. Scand.*, **32**, pp. 45–8.

**Maynard, D. E., and Jenkinson, J. L.** (1984) The cerebral function analysing monitor, *Anaesthesia*, **39**, pp. 678–90.

**Prior, P. F.** (1987) The EEG and detection of responsiveness during anaesthesia and coma. In Rosen, M. and Lunn, J. N. (eds) *Consciousness, Anaesthesia and Pain in General Anaesthesia*, Butterworths, London, p. 37.

**Thornton, C.** and **Sharpe, R. A.** (1998) Evoked responses in anaesthesia, *Br. J. Anaesth.*, **80**, pp. 771–8.

**Tooley, M. A.**, **Stapleton, C. L. Greenslade G. L.** and **Prys-Roberts, C.** (2004) The auditory evoked response during propofol and alfentanil anaesthesia, *Br. J. Anaesth.*, **92**, pp. 25–32.

**Uhl, R. R.**, **Squires, K. C.**, **Bruce, D. L.** and **Starr, A.** (1980) Effect of halothane anaesthesia on the human cortical visual evoked response, *Anesthesiology*, **53**, pp. 273–6.

**Viby Mogenson, J.**, **Howardy-Hansen, P.**, **Chraemer-Jorgensen, B.**, **Ording, H.**, **Engbaek, J.** and **Neilson, A.** (1981) Post-tetanic count (PTC): a new method of evaluating an intense nondepolarising neuromuscular blockade, *Anesthesiology*, **55**, pp. 458–61.

## *Further reading*

**Casey, C. P.** *et al.* (2022) Distinct EEG signatures differentiate unconsciousness and disconnection during anaesthesia and sleep, *Br. J. Anaesth.*, **128**(6), p. 1006e1018.

**Morley, A.** and **Strandvik, G.** (2012). Depth of anesthesia and neurophysiological monitoring. In Davy, A. J. and Dibi, A. (eds) *Ward's Anaesthetic Equipment*, 6th Edition, Saunders Elsevier, London, pp. 369–83.

**Sewell, L.**, **Abbas, A.** and **Kane, N.** (2019). Introduction to interpretation of the EEG in Intensive care. *B.J.A. Educ.*, **19**(3), pp. 74–82.

**Schwilden, H.** (1989) Use of median EEG frequency and pharmacokinetics in determining the depth of anaesthesia. In Jones, J. G. (ed.) *Clinical Anaesthesiology. Depth of Anaesthesia*, Bailliere Tindall, **3**(3), pp. 603–22.

**Sykes, M. K.**, **Vickers, M. D.** and **Hull, C. J.** (1991) Monitoring the nervous system. In *Principles of Measurement and Monitoring in Anaesthesia and Intensive Care*, Blackwell Scientific Publications, Oxford.

# Chapter 19 **Monitoring depth of anaesthesia**

This chapter contains: cerebral function monitors; the compressed spectral array monitor; bispectral index monitors; entropy monitors; Narcotrend monitors; patient state index monitor; auditory evoked response-based monitors; respiratory sinus arrhythmia-based monitors; emerging trends and artificial intelligence.

The chapter links with: Chapters 5 and 18.

## Introduction

There are, and have been, many monitors designed to monitor depth of anaesthesia and to give an indication of awareness during surgery, which use electrical signals obtained from the human body. Some have been designed as research devices, some have been available commercially, but have been withdrawn, and some are still available. Most, but not all, are based on the spontaneous electroencephalogram (EEG) and the auditory evoked response (AER). Some have been designed to use properties of the electrocardiogram (ECG), such as heart rae variability. Although useful, all of the discussed monitors have shortcomings, and they are not 100% sensitive and specific to discriminate between consciousness and unconsciousness, and none correlate exactly with clinical states and levels of anaesthesia. The UK National Institute for Health and Care Excellence (NICE) published guidelines in 2012 for depth of anaesthesia monitoring in high-risk patients and patients using Total Intravenous Anaesthesia (TIVA) under neuromuscular blockade. It recommended using Bispectral Index, Entropy and Narcotrend monitors, and these are all covered in this chapter.

## Depth of anaesthesia monitors using the EEG

### *Cerebral function monitor*

The design of the commercial monitor, the *Cerebral Function Monitor* (CFM) was based on simple time domain measures already discussed (Maynard *et al.* 1969). The CFM took the EEG from a single pair of parietal electrodes. The signal was amplified and passed through a band-pass filter and differentiator, which had the effect of accentuating the gain of the higher end of the 2–15 Hz pass band. The output of this specialised filter was integrated to produce a voltage output, which varied with time. It was plotted on a logarithmic scale. The trace gave an indication of the power of the EEG and the width of the line gave an indication of the signal's variability. A schematic of an example of a CFM trace is shown in Figure 19.1(a). The machine was further developed into the *Cerebral Function Analysing Monitor* (CFAM) (Maynard and Jenkinson 1984). This machine produced two outputs, as shown in Figure 19.1. There was a similar CFM trace, and also a display of frequency domain data consisting of the EEG displayed as traditional EEG frequency bands. The CFM and CFAM were further developed into digital versions with many different names, such as CFAM4 and Olympic Brainz and Brainz (BRM3), and the dominant market for all these devices is the paediatric and neonatal one (Azzopardi, 2015).

### *Compressed spectral array monitor*

The first use of a monitor that used frequency analysis for anaesthesia was using the *Compressed Spectral Array* (CSA) (Bickford *et al.* 1972), and a simplified example is shown in Figure 19.2.

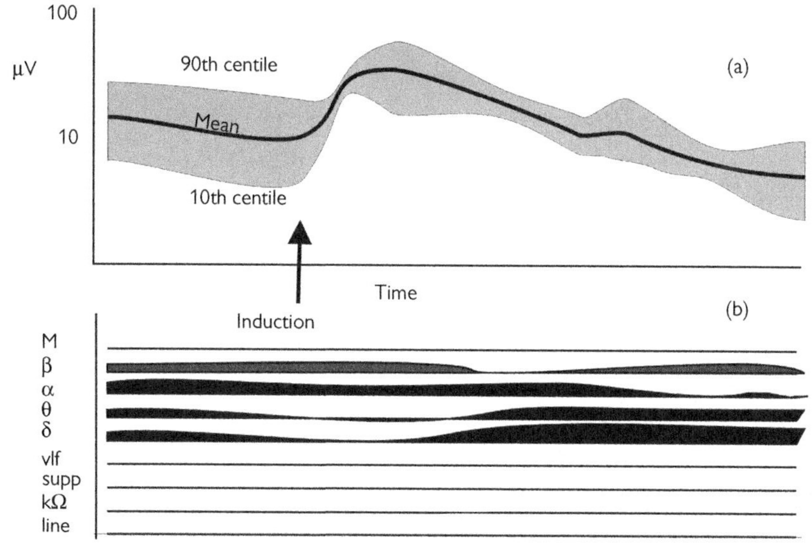


**Fig. 19.1** Schematic of the CFM trace (a) and the CFAM traces (a) + (b). In trace (b), M = muscle, $\beta$, $\alpha$, $\theta$, and $\delta$ are the traditional EEG bands, vlf = very low frequency, supp = burst suppression, k$\Omega$ = electrode impedance, line = mains interference. The figure shows a simulated example of the expected traces during induction of anaesthesia (Maynard and Jenkinson 1984).

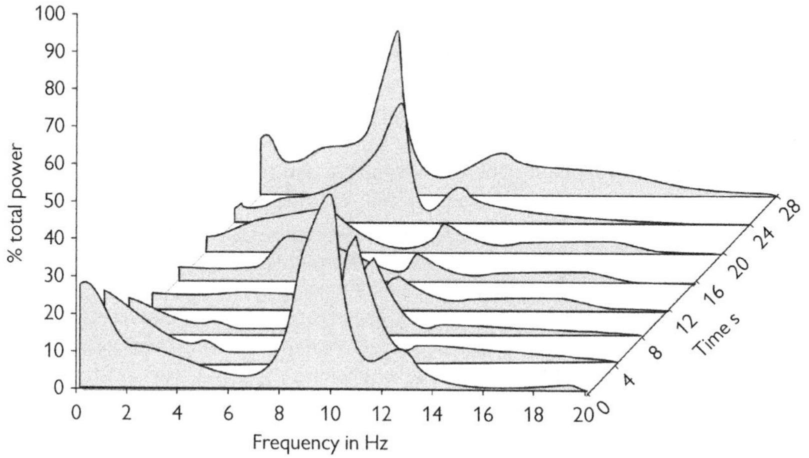


**Fig. 19.2** A simplified version of the compressed spectral array. This shows the EEG power spectrum obtained from 4 s epochs obtained at different time points. Historical spectra are shown at time 4 s, 8 s, etc. This display gives the impression of a subject being anaesthetised (24 and 28 s) and awake (4 and 0 s).

Although this technique displays information in real time with the added advantage of historical information as well, the display was often difficult for the untrained eye to interpret. Frequently, the goal of quantifying the data was not achieved. Alternative forms of the CSA were the *Density Spectral Array* (DSA), where the amplitude information was conveyed by the brightness of the trace, frequency on the ordinate and time on the abscissa (Fleming and Smith 1979). Although these techniques have gone out of fashion, they are now being used to complement newer monitors with the trend to use raw EEG and spectral-based displays (Hight *et al*. 2023; Mogianos and Persson 2025).

## *Bispectral index monitors*

The BIS monitor is the most extensively studied monitor in the anaesthetic literature, and so it will be described in some detail. The monitor uses an index called the *Bispectral Index* (BIS), which attempts to eliminate the biphasic effect mentioned previously and get around the fact that different anaesthetic agents affect the EEG in different ways. This commercial monitor (the BIS monitor, developed initially by Aspect Medical Inc, currently marketed by Medronic-Covidien, Dublin, Ireland) uses a complex algorithm that produces an index between 0 (deeply unconscious) and 100 (awake), with 40–60 as the recommended values for general anaesthesia. The BIS number is designed to be drug independent, i.e. sedation should give the same number irrespective of what drug is producing that effect (Johansen and Sebel 2000). The analysis involved in the algorithm is based on the frequency and time domain measures already described (frequency analysis =beta ratio, time domain analysis= burst suppression indices) but it is dominated by bispectral analysis (Rampil 1998). Bispectral analysis is a *higher-order* (more complex than simple Fourier transformation) spectral analysis based on the phase relationships of individual frequency components to each other. Information *hidden* in the frequency spectrum may be uncovered if the bi-spectrum is included in the analysis algorithm. This can be explained by considering, in a thought experiment, two situations that have different brain states, such as awake and anaesthetised, but the simple frequency spectra are identical. This example demonstrates that the EEG spectra alone cannot discriminate between the two clinical states (see Figure 19.3, which shows the spectrum of two EEG processes, EEG 1 and EEG 2). The spectrum of EEG 1, which represents clinical state 1, can be considered to be produced by the summation of four dominant frequencies, all having independent phases (i.e. they are not coupled together). The spectrum of EEG 2 or clinical state 2 can be considered to be produced by the multiplication of two different frequency generators. The effect of multiplication will be to produce a spectrum consisting of the frequency sum of the two generators, the frequency difference, and double each generator. The phases of these frequencies will be coupled together. It is plausible that the two different clinical states will give these different mathematical situations. For example, awake EEG is non-synchronised EEG that could be produced by independent generators as above and the anaesthetised EEG is often more synchronised. Therefore the two spectra, EEG 1 and 2 will have been produced by different brain processes (e.g. awake and anaesthetised), but have identical simple spectra morphologies. If the bi-spectra of EEG 1 and 2 were calculated, they would be very different because of the very different phase relationships, and may be useful as the dominant component in an algorithm to discriminate between clinical states. The BIS monitor actually uses the relationship between frequency values known as the *bicoherence*; this measure approaches zero when there is no relationship between components (as in the awake state) and approaches one where there is a fixed relationship (as in the deeply anaesthetised state mentioned).

Although the BIS machine is very useful in clinical practice and seems to predict awareness (Myles *et al.* 2004), there are a number of situations where it is not so useful, such as using nitrous oxide-related anaesthesia, opioid dominant anaesthesia, and when interference from other devices is present (Coste *et al.* 2000; Dahaba 2005). Many studies have detected awareness without recall (using the isolated forearm technique), Russell (2013), when BIS indicates non-awareness, and there are other issues with using BIS (Hajat *et al.* 2017).

The BIS monitors use a clever electrode array attached easily to the forehead, with good signal quality. However, this may not be the optimal site for monitoring, and there can be issues with the frontal electromyogram (EMG) confusing the BIS algorithm (Hight et al. 2023).

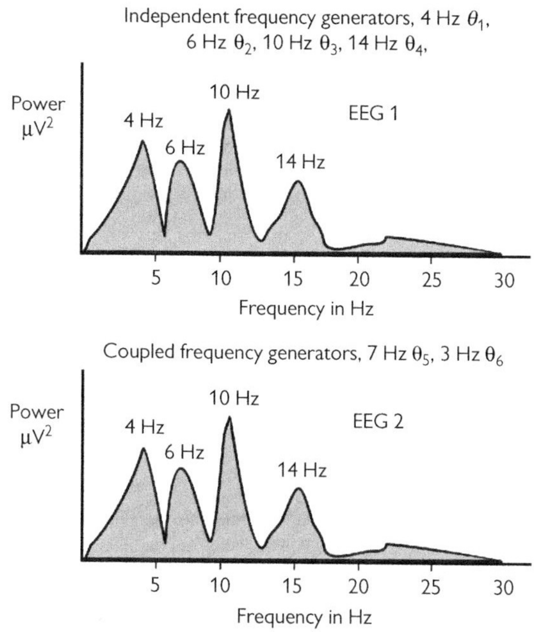


**Fig. 19.3** Two identical EEG spectra, EEG 1 and EEG 2, which are produced by different brain processes, such as awake and anaesthesia. The frequency generators sum together and produce the surface EEG. The generators in EEG 1 are not synchronised or coupled together, but the generators in EEG 2 are coupled. EEG 1 is produced by four separate generators, 4, 6, 10, and 14 Hz. These produce a spectrum dominated by these frequencies, as shown. EEG 2 is produced by the multiplication of two generators 7 and 3 Hz. This might be the process that occurs under anaesthesia. The multiplication of 7 and 3 Hz will produce the sum (10 Hz), the difference (4 Hz), double 7 Hz (14 Hz) and double 3 Hz (6 Hz). In this case all the frequencies are coupled together, because of their common origin, and so the phase relationships will be very different from those of EEG 1.

## *Entropy*

The concept of *entropy* for physiological signals is derived from the concept of thermodynamic entropy for physical systems. In the context of signals, the entropy is about the irregularity, complexity or unpredictability of the EEG signal. In a simple example, shown in Figure 19.4, a signal that has one state, i.e. a pure sine wave, shown in Figure 19.4(a) has an entropy of zero, whereas white

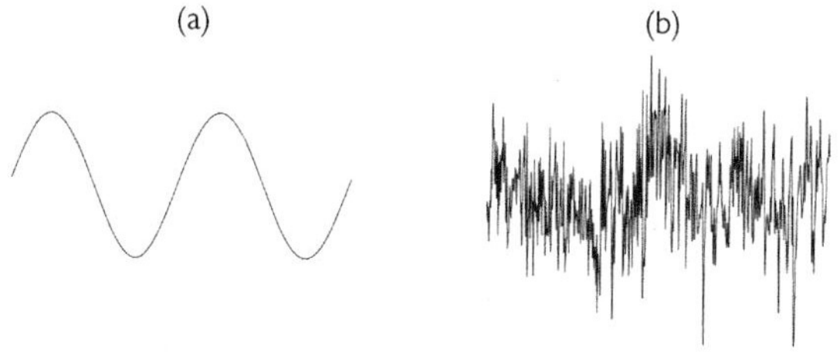


**Fig. 19.4** Diagram showing two states of a signal: (a) represents a simple signal that has an entropy of zero, and (b) is a complex, white noise-like signal that has an entropy approaching one.

noise, i.e. a random, unpredictable signal such as described in Figure 19.4(b), has an entropy approaching one. An awake EEG is much more complex and unpredictable than an anaesthetised EEG, which is much more sine wave like. This means that the entropy value of the EEG should change with clinical state. The commercially available entropy module (GE Healthcare, Madison, WI, USA) calculates entropy over time windows of variable duration and produces two entropy values, State Entropy (SE) and Response Entropy (RE) (Viertio-Oja *et al.* 2004). SE is an index between 0 and 91 using the frequency range 0.8 to 32 Hz and RE is an index between 0 and 100 using the frequency range 0.8 to 47 Hz. The higher index number represents awake values. RE includes higher frequencies than SE, and therefore frontal EMG is included more. The theory is that patients waking up or actually responding to noxious stimuli will have more frontal EMG and therefore RE will be different from SE in these situations. The two indices are displayed and their similarities and differences are supposed to facilitate the monitoring process. Studies have reported promising results and similarities to the BIS monitor (Bonhomme *et al.* 2006) but others also indicate caution (Takamatsu *et al.* 2006).

### *Narcotrend*

The Narcotrend (MonitorTechnik, Bad Bramstedt, Germany) is a monitor that uses an algorithm based on pattern recognition of the EEG. Standard ECG electrodes are used for this device. The EEG signal is amplified and analysed by multivariate statistical analysis to classify the signal into fifteen different stages, A–F, where A is awake, $C_0$ is light anaesthesia, $D_0$ is general anaesthesia and $F_1$ (general anaesthesia with increasing burst suppression), depending on the clinical state of the patient. These letters were initially based on the classical Kruger anaesthetic clinical states and visual analysis of the EEG. The fifteen stages are then converted into an index of 1–100 where, for example, A is 95–100, $C_0$ is 75–79, $D_0$ is 57–64 and $F_1$ is 1–4 (Kreuer *et al.* 2004).

### *Patient state index*

The patient state index (PSI) uses a scale of 0–100, with 100 being awake. The PSI algorithm uses four channels of qualitative frequency analysis of the EEG and uses this information to estimate depth of anaesthesia, together with the changes that occur between the hemispheres and anterior and posterior regions of the cortex. A recent commercial device using this index is the Sedline device (Massimo, Irvine, CA, USA).

## Depth of anaesthesia monitors using the AER

### *Auditory evoked response monitors*

There have been several versions of commercial AER (also called auditory evoked potentials, AEP) monitors produced, which have been based on the early cortical responses of the AER between 10–80 ms, which are also termed the mid-latency auditory evoked response. There have been two different streams of these monitors. One stream was marketed and produced by Danmeter (A/S Odense, Denmark) and includes the A-line monitor, the A-line ARX and the AEP/2 monitor, which have all been validated in various clinical trials (Bruhn *et al.* 2006, Litvan *et al.* 2002). The other stream was the system produced by Glasgow University in the UK called the aepEX system, and was marketed by MDM (Essex, UK) (Nishiyama 2009). All of these commercial devices are no longer available, although they are still used in clinical practice. All of the monitors use similar principles, but have variations on the sophistication of the processing used. The A-line and the aepEX are produced using coherent averaging, already described in chapter 18, but differ in their method of producing an index from the evoked response waveform. The more recent versions of the Danmeter monitors used autoregressive modelling to produce a faster average, and the AEP/2 monitor used a combination of spontaneous EEG and AER to produce an index.

## Depth of anaesthesia monitors using the ECG

### *Respiratory sinus arrhythmia-based monitors*

Monitors have been developed to measure depth of anaesthesia that do not use the EEG, but are based on the ECG. They were based on the concept of *heart rate variability* (HRV) (Pomfrett 1999). HRV is where the heart rate, as measured by the reciprocal of the R–R ECG interval, is measured. This rate is normally plotted against uneven time points and then extrapolated into a continuous waveform with equal time points. The waveform is converted to the frequency domain and it was found that the spectrum of this correlates with the depth of anaesthesia (Jeanne *et al.* 2009). Two commercial devices were developed (the Fathom and the Anemon-1) but are no longer available. Although the method seems to have gone out of favour, there are some recent references that suggest it could be still a useful method with further development (Zhan *et al.* 2021; Gentile and Introna 2025).

### *Emerging devices*

There are many newer and emerging devices available. The cerebral state function monitor (previously marketed by Danmeter, now by Danmeter-Goalwick) uses *fuzzy logic* analysis using a single-channel EEG. Med-Storm Innovation AS have produced the pain-nociceptive sensor, which produces an awakening index. This uses changes in both spontaneous and evoked skin conductance as its measure. A new device that seems to be in current practice is the Quantium consciousness index (q-CON), marketed by Quantium Medical, Barcelona, Spain. This is a device using a single-channel frontal EEG. It uses an algorithm based on using the power in the various frequency bands of the EEG, compared to the full frequency EEG band between 1–44 Hz. Burst suppression and EMG are part of the algorithm. The algorithm uses a novel adaptive neurofuzzy inference system in its analysis. The device also supplies a q-NOX index, using the same frontal channel, which aims to produce an index of depth of analgesia (Hight *et al.* 2023).

### *Non-physiological signal systems*

TIVA is an established technique that offers benefits such as reduced postoperative nausea and better control for certain surgeries. It also has significant environmental benefits. Many anaesthetists do not adopt this technique and one reason might be because there not an exact replica of the well-established endtidal volatile alarm system used in inhalational anaesthesia. EEG systems are recommended for TIVA systems, but there can be issues with these. One emerging method could be real-time monitoring of blood propofol levels as a part of a depth of anaesthesia monitor when using TIVA, or an alarm-type method. Somnus Scientific Ltd are in the process of commercialising such a real-time blood propofol monitor, which could be part of a depth of anaesthesia monitoring system.

## Artificial intelligence and depth of anaesthesia monitoring

Artificial intelligence (AI) is the capability of computer-based systems to carry out tasks and functions typically associated with human intelligence, such as problem-solving, pattern recognition and decision-making. Machine learning is a branch of AI where computer-based devices learn from large data sets to carry out pattern recognition, to make predictions or decisions, without explicit instructions being given. This can be a valuable tool to enable a more precise, accurate and personalised depth of anaesthesia monitor (Carneiro and Pereira 2025). AI and machine learning can combine EEG, AER, ECG, blood pressure, and other physiological variables. It could use other inputs such as real-time blood propofol measurements and endtidal volatile concentrations mentioned earlier. It is likely that such systems will utilise the raw EEG and AER values, such as frequency band power, amplitude, latency, etc., rather than the derived indices (which are often commercially hidden) such as BIS and PSI in their calculations. There are non-trivial challenges in using AI systems. The data used must be of excellent quality and fit for purpose. The system needs to be supported by appropriately trained personnel, and both the software and hardware.

Such AI-based systems could be transformative in depth of anaesthetic monitoring, promising more accurate and safer monitoring systems, and solving many of the limiting factors suggested in the literature (McCulloch and Sanders 2023).

## *References*

**Azzopardi, D.** (2015) Clinical applications of cerebral function monitoring in Neonates, *Semin. Fetal Neonatal Med.*, **20**, pp. 154–63.

**Bickford, R. G., Billinger, T. W., Fleming, N. I.** and **Stewart, L.** (1972) *The compressed spectral array. A pictorial EEG, Proc. San Diego Biomedical Conf. Symp. 11*, Academic Press, London, pp. 365–70.

**Bonhomme, V., Deflandre, E.** and **Hans, P.** (2006) Correlation and agreement between bispectral index and state entropy of the electroencephalogram during propofol anaesthesia, *Br. J. Anaesth.*, **97**, pp. 340–6.

**Bruhn, J., Myles, P. S., Sneyd, R.** and **Struys, M. M. R. F.** (2006) Depth of anaesthesia monitoring: what's available, what's validated and what's next? *Br. J. Anaesth.*, **97**(1), pp. 85–94.

**Carneiro, R. A. A. G.** and **Pereira, L. A. G.** (2025) Depth of anesthesia monitoring and artificial intelligence, *Curr. Anesthesiol. Rep.*, **15**(19), pp. 1–12.

**Coste, C., Guignard, B., Menigaux, C.** and **Chauvin, M.** (2000) Nitrous oxide prevents movement during orotracheal intubation without affecting BIS value, *Anesth. Analg.*, **91**(1), pp. 130–5.

**Dahaba, A. A.** (2005) Different conditions that could result in the Bispectral index indicating an incorrect hypnotic state, *Anesth. Analg.*, **101**, pp. 765–73.

**Fleming, R. A.** and **Smith, N. T.** (1979) An inexpensive device for analyzing and monitoring the electroencephalogram, *Anesthesiology*, **50**(5), pp. 456–60.

**Gentile, A.** and **Introna, A.** (2025) Interpreting heart rate variability: addressing the role of anesthesia and pain, *J. Clin. Monit. Comput.*, 39, pp. 1109–10.

**Hajat, Z., Ahmad, N.** and **Andrezejowski, J.** (2017) The role and limitations of EEG-based depth of anaesthesia monitoring in theatres and intensive care, *Anaesthesia*, **72** Suppl 1, pp. 38–47.

**Hight, D., Kreuzer, M., Ugen, G.,** ***et al.*** (2023) Five commercial 'depth of anaesthesia' monitors provide discordant clinical reommendations in reposne to indentical emergence-like EEG signals. *Br. J. Anaesth.*, **130**(5), pp. 536–45.

**Jeanne, M., Logierb, R., De Jonckheereb, J.** and **Tavernier, B.** (2009) Heart rate variability during total intravenous anesthesia: Effects of nociception and analgesia, *Auton. Neurosci.*, **147**(1), pp. 91–6.

**Johansen, J. W.** and **Sebel, P. S.** (2000) Development and clinical application of the electroencephalographic bispectrum monitoring, *Anesthesiology*, **93**(5), pp. 1336–44.

**Kreuer, S., Bruhn, J., Larsen, R., Bialas, P.** and **Wilhelm, W.** (2004) Comparability of Narcotrend index and bispectral index during propofol anaesthesia, *Br. J. Anesth.*, **93**(2), pp. 235–40.

**Litvan, H., Jensen, E. W., Revuelta, M.,** ***et al.*** (2002) Comparison of auditory evoked potentials and the A-line ARX index for monitoring the hypnotic level during sevoflurane and propofol induction, *Acta Anaesthesiol. Scand.*, **46**, pp. 245–51.

**Maynard, D. E.** and **Jenkinson, J. L.** (1984) The cerebral function analysing monitor, *Anaesthesia*, **39**, 678–90.

**Maynard, D. E., Prior, P. F.** and **Scott, D. F.** (1969) Device for continuous monitoring of cerebral activity in resuscitated patients, *Br. Med. J.*, **4**, pp. 545–6.

**McCulloch, T. J.** and **Sanders, R. D.** (2023) Depth of anaesthesia monitoring: time to reject the index? *Br. J. Anaesth.*, **131**(2), pp. 196–9.

**Mogianos, K.** and **Persson, A. K. M.** (2025) Anesthesia depth monitoring during opioid-free anaesthesia – a prospective observational study, *BMC Anesthesiol.*, **25**(1), p. 37.

**Myles, P. S., Leslie, K., McNeil, J., Forbes, A.** and **Chan, M. T. V.** (2004) Bispectral index monitoring to prevent awareness during anaesthesia: The B-aware randomized controlled trial, *Lancet.*, **363**, pp. 1757–64.

**Nishiyama, T.** (2009) Comparison of the two different auditory evoked potentials index monitors in propofol-fentanyl-nitrous oxide anesthesia, *J. Clin. Anesth.*, **21**(8), pp. 551–4.

**Pomfrett, C. J. D.** (1999) Heart rate variability, BIS and depth of anaesthesia, *Br. J. Anaesth.*, **82**, pp. 659–62.

**Rampil, I. J.** (1998) A primer for EEG signal processing, *Anesthesiology*, **89**, pp. 980–1002.

**Russell, I.** (2013) The ability of bipectral index to detect intra-operative wakefulness during total intravenous anaesthesia compared with the isolated forearm technique, *Anaesthesia*, **68**, pp. 502–11.

**Takamatsu, I.**, **Ozaki, M.** and **Kazama, T.** (2006) Entropy indices vs. the bispectral index for estimating nociception during sevoflurane anaesthesia, *Br. J. Anaesth.*, **96**, pp. 620–6.

**Viertio-Oja, H.**, **Maja, V.**, **Sarkela, M.** ***et al.*** (2004) Description of the Entropy algorithm as applied to the Datex-Ohmeda S/5 Entropy module, *Acta. Anaesth. Scand.*, **48**, pp. 154–61.

**Zhan, J.**, **Wu, Z. X.**, **Duan, Z. X.** ***et al.*** (2021) Heart rate variability-derived features based on deep neural network for distinguishing different anaesthesia states. *BMC Anesthesiol.*, **21**, p. 66.

## *Further reading*

**Hajat, Z.**, **Ahmad, N.** and **Andrezejowski, J.** (2017) The role and limitations of EEG-based depth of anaesthesia monitoring in theatres and intensive care. *Anaesthesia*, **72** Suppl 1, pp. 38–47.

**Pandit, J. J.** and **Cook T. M.** (2014) NAP5: Accidental awareness during general anaesthesia in the United Kingdom and Ireland. 5th National Audit Project of the Royal College of Anaesthetists and the Association of Anaesthetists of Great Britain and Ireland. Available at: https://www.nationalauditprojects.org.uk/downloads/NAP5%20Bulletin%20Article%20March%202012.pdf

# Chapter 20 **Pacemakers and defibrillators**

This chapter contains: pacemakers, codes, rate-responsive, interference, tachyarrhythmias; defibrillator circuits; defibrillator waveforms; biphasic defibrillators, rectilinear and truncated exponential waveforms and circuits. The chapter links with: Chapters 4, 12 and 21.

## Introduction

Cardiac pacemakers and defibrillators are used to stimulate the cardiac muscle directly. The pacemaker corrects for abnormalities in the heart rate (this can be fast or slow). Defibrillators are used to restore a fibrillating or tachycardic heart, to sinus rhythm. These are normally external, battery or mains powered, but can be internal devices, which are called *implantable cardiac devices* (ICDs).

## Pacemakers

### *Pacemakers for bradycardia*

Pacemakers that deal with bradycardia will be considered first. Normally a slow or irregular heart rhythm is caused by three types of heart block:

- First degree, where the delay at the AV junction is increased beyond the normal 0.2 s;
- Second degree, where a proportion of the depolarisation wave fails to pass through the AV junction;
- Complete block, where none of the depolarisation waves pass through the AV junction, and ventricular electrical activity is independent of supraventricular activity.

In all these cases, the ventricles will beat at a slower or irregular rate. Dizziness or loss of consciousness may occur.

### *Pacemaker components*

The simplest pacemaker consists of three major components: batteries, the pulse generator, and the electrode leads. The pulse generator is required to provide a rectangular pulse. Typical parameters are the duration of 1 ms, a voltage of 5 V and capable of delivering a current of 10 mA. The power needed per second (if the pacemaker is on all the time) would be $I^2R$ = 50 mW, for an electrode tissue resistance of 500 $\Omega$. If the pacemaker is operating at 1 Hz (60 beats per minute), then the average power consumption would be 50 $\mu$W, as the pulse width is 1 ms (the pacemaker is on for 1/1000 of a second, and so the power consumption will be divided by 1000). A typical small battery has a capacity of 1 A h, so that this battery could supply the average current (10 $\mu$A) for about 11 years. The circuitry would also absorb power so that the battery life would drop to around 5 years. The batteries used are now commonly lithium iodine. The output pulse is applied to the tissue via an electrode. The electrode tip, which can screw in (or, more unusually, sewn in), can be made of platinum, silver, stainless steel, titanium, as well as various alloys.

### *Unipolar and bipolar leads*

The electrode leads can be *unipolar*, or *bipolar*. Both type of leads can be used to *pace* (stimulate the heart) or to *sense* (receive signals from the heart). Unipolar is where one of the electrodes of the circuit is in the heart and the other part of the circuit is the pacemaker metal container. Bipolar leads are where both electrodes are contained in the chamber to be paced, about 15–30 mm apart. The unipolar leads are simpler to construct and, because there is only one lead, it can be thicker than the bipolar equivalent (two leads in the same space), and therefore will be mechanically more robust. They will be more sensitive than bipolar leads, as they are picking up signals from a wider area, but unipolar leads can also pick up far-field interference such as diathermy, domestic mains and EMG (away from the immediate sensing area). The unipolar leads can also unintentionally stimulate other areas of the heart. Bipolar leads are more selective and have a better signal-to-noise ratio. They are also more selective where they pace. However, the leads are more complex and expensive to produce.

## Simple pacemakers

The simplest type of pacemaker produces a constant stream of pulses at 70 beats per min (or whatever rate is set on the pacemaker). The heart rate is constant and will not vary in response to the patient's activity. If some heart beats do occur naturally, then competition between the heart's own pacemaker and the artificial pacemaker's pulses will occur, which will waste power (as this pacemaker beat is not needed) and can cause the heart to revert to a potentially dangerous rhythm such as tachycardia or fibrillation. The alternative to fixed rate pacing is to allow the pacemaker's electrodes to sense the activity in either the atrium or the ventricle. The pacemaker then produces a pulse in response to the detected atrial or ventricular waveform, or its absence, which will be used to stimulate the ventricle. Atrial-triggered devices produce a pulse *triggered* by the P wave of the ECG. Ventricular paced devices can be either *triggered* by the R wave or *demand* led where a pulse is only produced when there is no R wave sensed. The latter types are also labelled inhibit mode pacemakers. A block diagram of an advanced pacemaker is shown in Figure 20.1.

## Pacemaker codes

There is a lettering code to define pacemakers; either three letters or, for more complex modes, five letters. The first letter indicates which chamber of the heart is paced: A for atria, V for ventricle and D for dual (both). The second letter indicates the chamber to be sensed, with the same letters. Additionally, O indicates that the function is turned off and not used. The third letter indicates the pacing mode: I for *inhibit* or sometimes called demand mode, T for *triggered* or also called *synchronised* mode, and D for dual, where the response is either inhibition or triggering. The fourth letter indicates programmable functionality and rate responsiveness. The fifth is for anti-tachyarrhythmic functions.

In general use, five forms of pacing are likely to be used clinically, and these give an example of the use of the codes. The codes are:

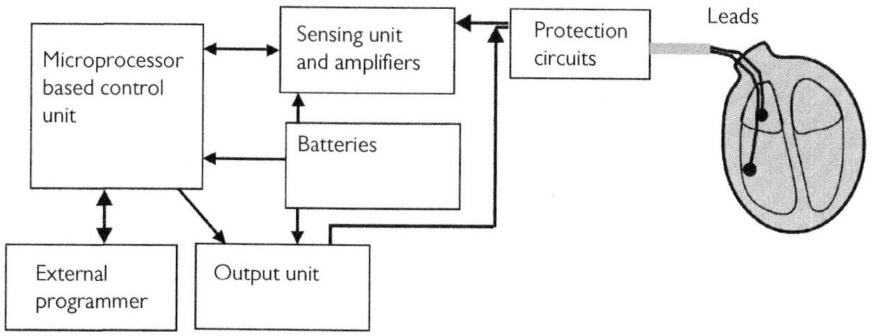


**Fig. 20.1** Block diagram of an advanced pacemaker. The external programmer communicates with the pacemaker via telemetry, using radio waves.

- VVI. This is where a single lead is placed in the ventricle for pacing and sensing. If the natural ventricular rate is above the pacemaker set rate, then pacing is inhibited. If the natural ventricular rate is below, then pacing occurs.
- AAI. This is where a single lead is in the atrium, and operation is in a similar way to the VVI mode.
- DDD. This is where leads are present in both the atrium and the ventricle. Both chambers (i.e. dual) can be paced and sensed. If activity is sensed in either chamber, then the pacing pulses will be inhibited, but if no ventricular activity follows atrial activity, then ventricular pacing will be triggered.
- AOO/VOO/DOO. These are the simplest pacing modes where no sensing occurs (and also of course no response to the sensing). This mode can be turned on temporarily using, for example, an external magnet for activation, when the sensing of external noise could lead to inappropriate lack of pacing, as described in the next section. This mode is also called asynchronous pacing.
- VDD. In this mode, only the ventricle is paced, but both chambers are sensed. Normally only one lead is used with electrodes in both chambers. This mode allows physiological pacing, described in the next section. This mode is not often used but is sometimes a simpler system alternative to DDD pacing.

### *Physiological and rate-responsive pacemakers*

Some pacemakers are *physiological*, in that sensing and pacing can be in both chambers. These devices tend to be microprocessor controlled. The pacemaker attempts to use any atrial activity to help pace the ventricles (and atria if appropriate) to produce heart-rate increases to cope with physiological demands on the body. *Rate-adaptive* pacemakers make use of other *clues* to control heart rate, when atrial information is not available to the pacemaker. For example, sensors in this type of pacemaker, such as electromagnetic or piezoelectric accelerometers, can directly detect other physiological activity. Also indirect measures can be used that rely on measurements from the body, such as respiration, intrathoracic impedance, central venous temperature, and mixed venous oxygen saturation. All these indirect measures will change in proportion to the physiological demands on the body.

### *Pacemaker interference*

In the complex pacemakers, the design must ensure that under fault conditions the pulse generator will revert to a fixed pacing rate. Also interference, such as diathermy (Goodman 1993) and drug-induced muscle movement, must be detected by the pacemaker and the device must revert to a (safe) fixed rate. Magnets are also used to put the pacemaker in a safe mode, so that when the magnet is passed over the device (by the patient or the clinician), a detector senses the magnet, and reverts the pacemaker to a fixed rate.

### *Tachyarrhythmia pacemakers*

Pacemakers can also be used to change tachyarrthymias or fast heart rates. When the heart rate is detected by the pacemaker as *too fast* by a suitable algorithm, then a specially designed sequence of pulses is fed into the ventricles. These can revert the rhythm to normal sinus rhythm. Also an electric shock can revert the rhythm back to sinus rhythm, as is used in defibrillators. Clearly pathological tachycardia must be distinguished from physiological appropriate (sinus) tachycardia (Davies *et al.* 1986).

## Defibrillators

Defibrillators are devices that are used to apply a large electric shock to the heart. They normally are standalone external devices and have three main uses:

- elective cardioversion, a synchronous shock that is applied across the chest to correct for atrial fibrillation, atrial flutter or ventricular tachycardia;

- emergency defibrillation in cases of ventricular fibrillation;
- direct defibrillation during heart surgery.

Also the devices can be implanted in the body, as *implantable cardiac defibrillators* (ICD). ICDs supply typically 25–45 J directly to the heart, and use complex algorithms automatically to detect ventricular fibrillation or ventricular tachycardia (Compton *et al.* 1995; Smith and Ideker 1999).

Both types of defibrillator are used to restore a normal sinus rhythm to a heart that is not contracting in a coordinated fashion, i.e. in fibrillation. The cause of fibrillation is commonly ischaemia of the heart conducting tissue but can also be due to electric shock (of a lower voltage and different frequency than the defibrillation voltage, e.g. domestic mains voltage), drugs, electrolyte disorders, hypoxia and hypothermia. The defibrillation shock aims to stop the heart totally and then the heart should restart in an orderly manner, returning to sinus rhythm.

## *Defibrillator waveforms*

The voltage and shape of the waveform needed to defibrillate the heart is critical. Early external defibrillators used domestic AC mains with a step-up transformer to obtain the correct voltage needed. These did not work very well because of the instantaneous power needed from the domestic mains is typically 125 kW! (50 A needed across the thorax of 50 $\Omega$, and power is $I^2R$). The maximum power from a normal mains socket is about 15 kW, which is enough to defibrillate a only a small child or animal. Defibrillators now use the charge stored in a capacitor. However, just discharging a capacitor through the thorax would result in a decaying exponential, from an initial high peak current with a very long tail. There is evidence that the high peak currents cause damage to the heart and the long tails associated with capacitor discharge could reverse the defibrillation process (Peleska 1963; Schuder *et al.* 1996). A waveform that has been used successfully in external devices is the critically damped sine wave current waveform, as shown in Figure 20.2, which has a duration of around 10 ms. The current flow from one electrode to the other is all in one direction.

This waveform has now been superseded by biphasic waveforms, which are waveforms that initially are positive, causing current to flow in one direction, and then part way through the procedure, the current waveform reverses polarity, and so the current flow changes to the opposite direction. Biphasic waveforms have been shown to be more efficient and require less energy, and have a higher success rate for first shock (Bardy *et al.* 1996). Typical values quoted are 130 joules for biphasic against 200 joules for monophasic and initial shock conversion of 97.6% for biphasic against 85.2% for monophasic (Schneider *et al.* 2000). All new external defibrillators in the UK now use biphasic waveforms. However,

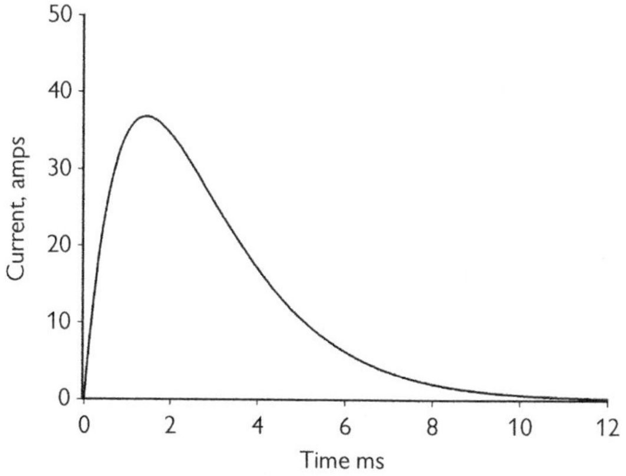


**Fig. 20.2** Critically damped waveform commonly used in the output circuits of monophasic defibrillators. The values shown are typical ones.

the circuits of monophasic defibrillators are useful to discuss, as many of the principles involved are also used in the newer biphasic devices. Also some monophasic devices are still in use in the UK and elsewhere and they are still very effective.

## *Monophasic defibrillator circuits*

The waveform for a monophasic defibrillator is produced using a circuit shown in Figure 20.3(a). The inductance in the circuit produces a resistor–inductance–capacitance (RLC) circuit and the ratio of these electrical components produces a degree of resonance and damping (as discussed at the end of Chapter 12) to optimise therapeutic performance. Changing the values of the resistance, inductance and capacitance can produce many different waveforms, from a critically damped waveform (in Figure 20.2) to an underdamped waveform shown in Figure 20.4. Biphasic defibrillators produce waveforms that could be produced by a similar circuit to that in Figure 20.3(a), but with different values of RLC circuits that produce the underdamped waveform, but in current practice the waveform is produced using more sophisticated electronic circuits as discussed in the next section.

The voltage required for defibrillation is typically 2500 V to produce a current of 50 A into 50 $\Omega$. The duration for the majority of the discharge is about 4ms and so the time constant formed by the resistor and capacitor would be 4 ms. If $R$ is 50 $\Omega$, then $C$ will be 80 $\mu$F. The energy stored when charged to 2500 V will be 0.5 ($CV^2$), which is 250 J. The delivered energy would be about 10% less. The inductance used is typically 40 mH.

The circuit described is powered by domestic mains voltage. Defibrillators can also be battery driven. The circuit shown in Figure 20.3(a) is modified in that a battery powers a high frequency oscillator as shown in Figure 20.3(b). This sine wave oscillator produces an AC output similar to the battery voltage and this is supplied to a step-up transformer as before (but the step-up in this case is much higher).

### *Biphasic waveforms*

There are now two types of biphasic waveforms in current use. One waveform is the truncated exponential biphasic waveform, shown in Figure 20.5. This waveform is again generated by the discharge of a capacitor, but the process is now controlled by electronic switches. In this process, the charged

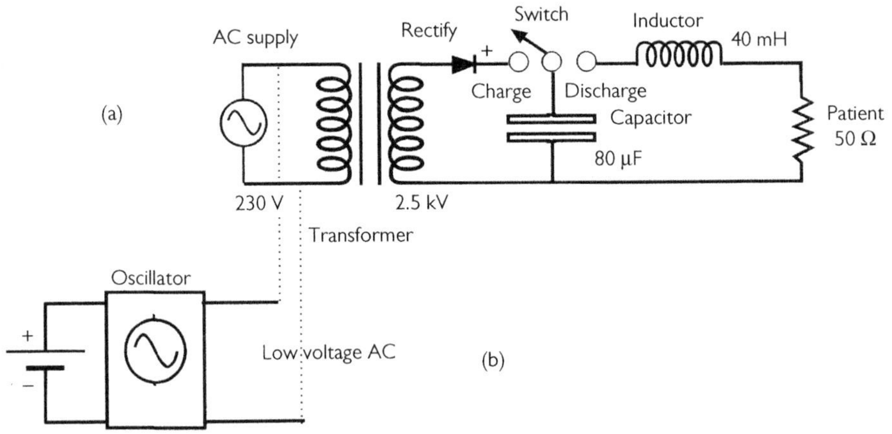


**Fig. 20.3** A typical monophasic defibrillator circuit. (a) is the mains version. The mains voltage is transformed up to a very high voltage, e.g. 2.5 kV. This voltage is rectified by a diode that only passes the positive part of the alternating cycle to the capacitor. When the switch is in the charge position, the capacitor is charged up to the supplied voltage. When the switch is passed over to discharge, it is discharged through the inductor and patient. (b) is the battery version. This part replaces the 230 V AC supply shown in (a).

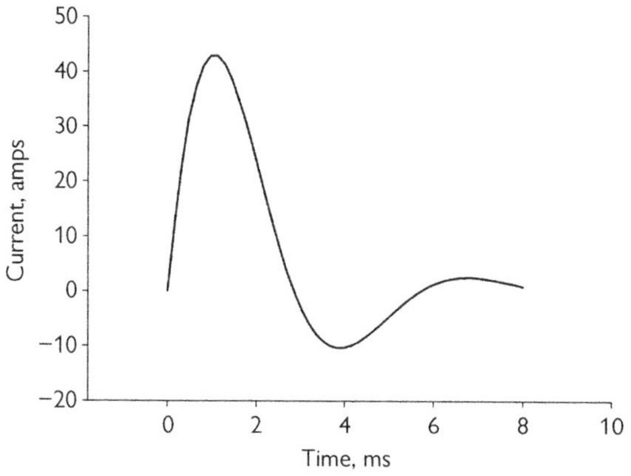


**Fig. 20.4** Underdamped biphasic waveform.

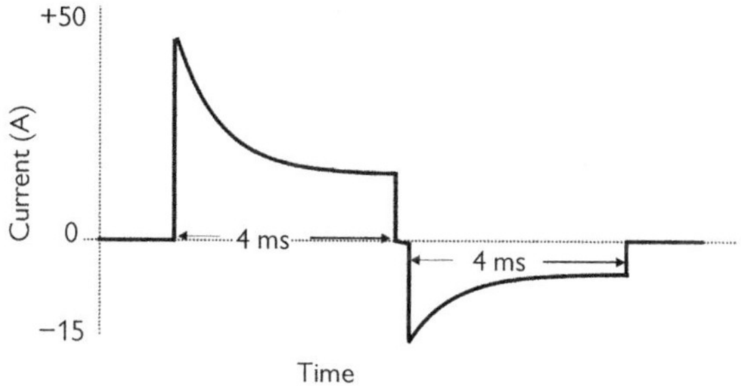


**Fig. 20.5** Diagram showing a biphasic waveform, the truncated exponential.

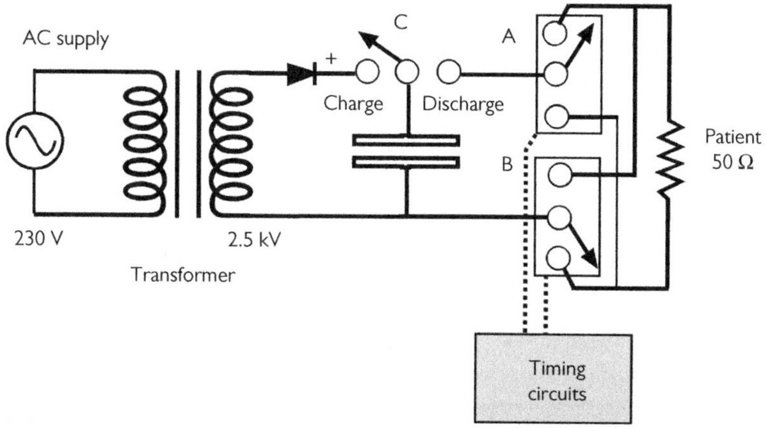


**Fig. 20.6** A typical truncated exponential biphasic defibrillator circuit. The capacitor is charged up as described in the monophasic system. When the switch C is passed over to discharge, it is discharged through the patient. After a certain time, the timing circuits switch over the electronic switches A and B, so the polarity is reversed.

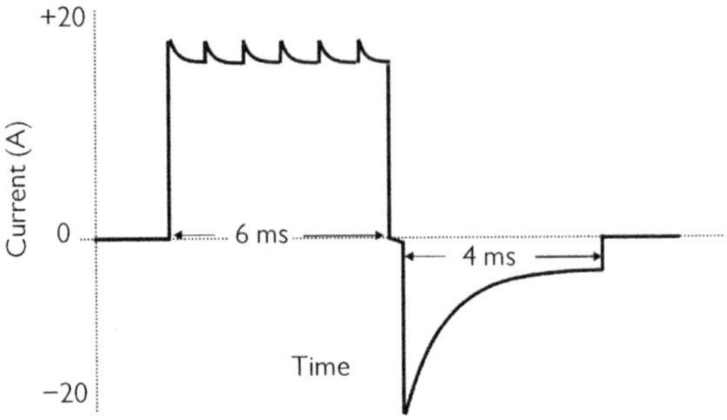


**Fig. 20.7** A typical rectilinear biphasic waveform.

capacitor is discharged through the patient, but now there is no inductance equivalent in the circuit, so there is a normal exponential decay. After typically 4 ms, the connection to the patient is broken and the capacitor connections are reversed by the equivalent of a dual-pole electronic switch, as shown in Figure 20.6, and the patient reconnected. The discharge is again programmed to be about 4 ms, but in the opposite direction. The other type of waveform used is the rectilinear biphasic waveform (Mittal *et al.* 1999), but there are many permutations of this. The circuitry required to make this waveform is more complex, but the waveform is typically a positive square wave of around 6 ms duration, followed immediately by a negative truncated exponential as before, of around 4 ms The square wave is typically produced by rapid charging and discharging of the capacitor, as can be seen by the triangular nature of the top of the square wave. An example of the waveform is shown in Figure 20.7.

## *References*

**Bardy, G. H., Marchlinski, F. E., Sharma, A. D.** ***et al***. (1996) Multicenter comparison of truncated biphasic shocks and standard damped sine wave monophasic shocks for transthoracic ventricular defibrillation, *Circulation*, **94**, pp. 2507–2514.

**Compton, A. J., Bolouri, H.** and **Nathan, A. W.** (1995) Arrhythmia recognition strategies and hardware decisions for the implantable cardioverter-defibrillator – a review, *Med. Eng. Phys.*, **17**(2), pp. 96–103.

**Davies, W., Wainwright, R., Tooley, M.** and **Lloyd, D.** (1986) Detection of pathological tachycardia by analysis of electrogram morphology, *Pacing Clin. Electrophysiol.*, **9**, pp. 200–8.

**Goodman, N. W.** (1993) Diathermy and failure of cardiac pacemakers, *Anaesthesia*, **48**(9), pp. 824–5.

**Mittal, S., Ayati, S., Stein, K. M.** ***et al.*** (1999) Comparison of a novel rectilinear biphasic waveform with a damped sine wave monophasic waveform for transthoracic ventricular defibrillation, *J. Am. Coll. Cardiol.*, **34**, pp. 1595–601.

**Peleska, B.** (1963) Cardiac arrhythmias following condenser discharges and their dependence upon strength of current and phase of cardiac cycle, *Circ. Res.*, **13**, pp. 21–32.

**Schneider, T., Martens, P. R., Paschen, H.,** ***et al.*** (2000) Multicenter, randomized, controlled trial of 150-J biphasic shocks compared with 200- to 360-J monophasic shocks in the resuscitation of out-of-hospital cardiac arrest victims, *Circulation*, **102**, pp. 1780–7.

**Schuder, J. C., Rahmoeller, G. A.** and **Stoeckle, H.** (1966) Transthoracic ventricular defibrillation with triangular and trapezoidal waveforms, *Circ. Res.*, **19**, pp. 689–94.

**Smith, W. M.** and **Ideker, R. E.** (1999) Automatic implantable cardioverter-defibrillators, Ann. *Rev. Biomed. Eng.*, **1**, pp. 331–46.

## *Further reading*

**Babbs**, **C. F.** and **Bourland**, **J. D.** (1992) Defibrillators. Chapter 3 in Cook A. M. and Webster J. G. (eds) *Therapeutic Medical Devices, Application and Design*, Prentice-Hall, New Jersey, pp. 66–85.

**Brown**, **B. H.**, **Smallwood**, **R. H.**, **Barber**, **D. C.**, **Lawford**, **P. V.** and **Hose**, **D. R.** (1999) Chapter 22, Cardiac electrical systems. In Tooley, M. A. (ed.) *Medical Physics and Biomedical Engineering*, IOP Publishing, Bristol, pp. 680–92.

**Bryant H.C.**, **Roberts P.R.** and **Diprose P.** (2016). Perioperative management of patients with cardiac implantable electronic devices. *BJA Educ.*, **16**(1), 388–96.

**Citron**, **P.**, **Duffin**, **E. G.**, **Fetter**, **J.**, **Goodman**, **L.** and **Shearon**, **L.W.** (1992) Chapter 2 in Cook, A.M. and Webster, J.G. (eds) *Cardiac Pacing: in Therapeutic Medical Devices, Application and Design*, Prentice-Hall, New Jersey, pp. 29–65.

# Chapter 21 Surgical diathermy

This chapter contains: current density; surgical effects; diathermy waveforms; electrodes, monopolar and bipolar; safety; interference.

The chapter links with: Chapters 4, 6 and 20

## Introduction

As discussed in Chapter 4, when a voltage is applied across a conductor, a current will flow. If the voltage is applied across the body via suitable electrodes, the body becomes part of the circuit (Figure 21.1) and a current will also flow, the magnitude depending on the properties of the tissues in its path, particularly the resistance. This current can cause heating or other physiological effects, depending on the *frequency* of the driving voltage. The effects of the domestic mains current flowing through the body are discussed in Chapter 6, but different effects occur as the frequency of the voltage is increased. As the frequency goes up, the heating increases but the tissue stimulation decreases and, at frequencies above 100 kHz (i.e. radio frequencies), the effect is entirely heating. This heating effect in the body by electric current is called *diathermy*, but the location, concentration and how this heat is used depend on the electrode design and the current concentration or *current density* at any point in the circuit.

## Current density

For a certain applied voltage, the *average* current throughout the circuit will be the same. The current density is the current per unit area, and so if the material in which the current passes is smaller, the heating effect increases. The resistance of the material is proportional to its size, so as the material becomes smaller, its resistance gets larger. The heating power is the product of the current squared and the resistance (*power* = $I^2 \times R$).

Surgical diathermy (or electrosurgery) is where either one or both of the electrodes are very small, and it is used to cut and coagulate tissue. The smaller electrode can be made into a pointed surgical tool and localised heating will occur at the tip of the instrument. The smaller and more pointed the instrument is, the greater the current density will be at the tip. This electrode is classified as the *active* or *live* one. The current densities around this electrode can be as much as 10 A $cm^{-2}$, and the total heating power typically around 200 W.

The other electrode in the circuit is much larger and situated on another part of the body, as shown in the Figure 21.1. This is the *passive* electrode (also called dispersive, neutral, plate, patient or indifferent) and, because of its large surface area, the current density is low, and minimal heating occurs. The current density is high only around the active electrode and quickly becomes lower in the rest of the body, as demonstrated also in the figure.

## Surgical effects and associated waveforms

### *Cutting*

Rapid heating of tissue over a very small area is produced by a fine intensity arc from the pointed active electrode. This causes boiling of intracellular fluid. The tissue is cut without heat dissipation in the

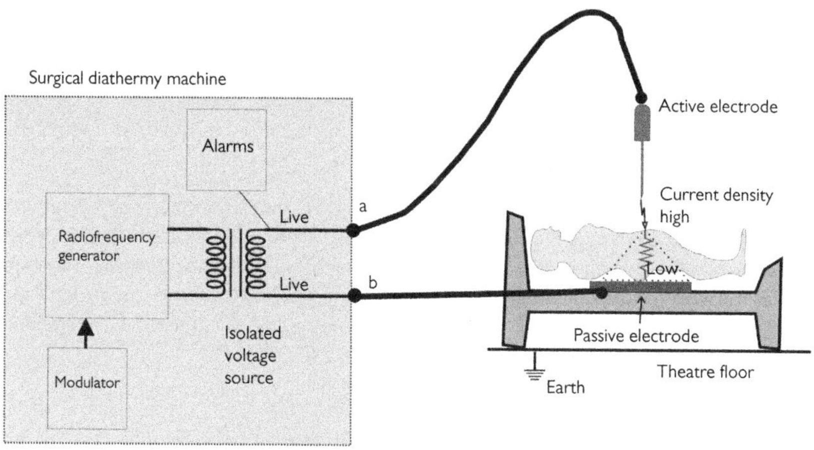


**Fig. 21.1** The set up for an isolated surgical diathermy system in the monopolar mode, showing the passive and active electrodes. a and b are the electrode connections, active and passive, respectively. (Figure adapted from Tooley (2004) with permission.)

surrounding tissue. The most efficient cutting waveform is a continuous sine wave (see Figure 21.2(a), at a voltage between 250 and 3000 V, depending on the application, the electrode and power required. Smaller voltages may be used if the tip of the electrode is pristine (the sharper the tip, the higher the current density and heating).

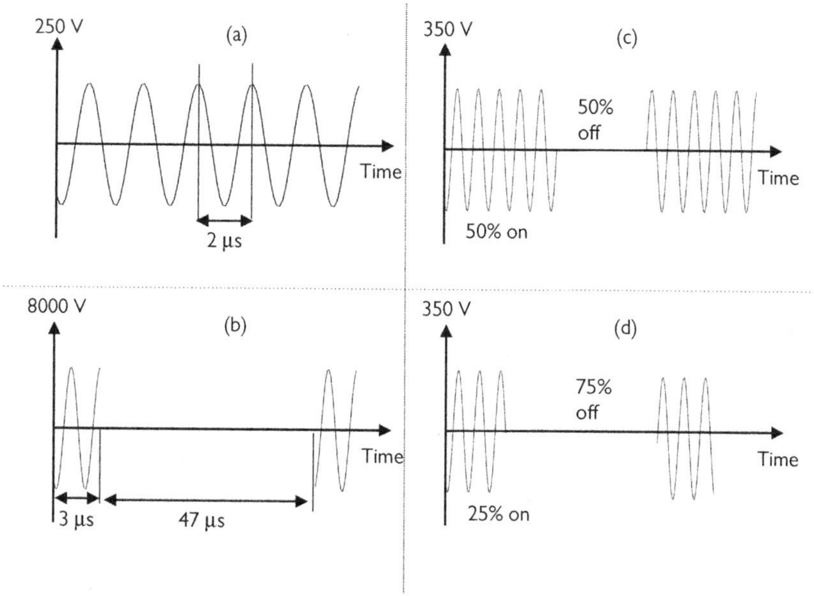


**Fig. 21.2** Different waveforms for different types of surgery. A is a continuous wave at 500 kHz at 250 V peak, suitable for cutting. B is a waveform suitable for coagulation. The time scales are expanded for clarity. C shows a 50% *on* waveform, and D shows a 25% *on* waveform. (Figure adapted from Tooley (2004) with permission.)

### Coagulation

The continuous waveform produces excellent cutting, but the edges bleed freely and hence the coagulation effect is poor. Coagulation can be provided by both *fulguration* (literally lightning!) and *desiccation* (drying).

### Fulguration

Fulguration is the destructive charring of the tissue by arcing, and is normally carried out using a flat spatula or ball shaped electrode. Blunted instruments need higher current densities for arcing, which is obtained using higher voltages, up to 9 kV. The instrument would be positioned 2–4 mm above the surgical site. The waveforms used are not necessary continuous, and the wave can be *active* for as little as 6% of the complete cycle. For example, the 500 kHz wave could be *on* (an active voltage) for 3 s and then *off* for 47 s, as shown in Figure 21.2(b).

### Desiccation

Coagulation by desiccation is the heating of tissue due to contact between the active electrode and tissue. The temperature of the tissue is increased at the point of contact and intracellular water is slowly steamed off and the tissue desiccates. The waveform shape is not critical here, and the power and voltage requirements are lower.

### Blended modes: cutting and coagulation

Modes can be *blended* as well, so that a mixture of reasonable cutting and coagulation is provided. The waves can be 50% on/50% off (Figure 21.2(c)), or 25% on/75% off (Figure 21.2(d)), and any interim range. The shorter the on-phase of the waveform, the more useful the coagulation, and vice versa (Figure 21.2(c, d)). These ratios are controlled by the *modulator*, as shown in Figure 21.1.

## Electrodes

The electrode systems used in surgical diathermy can be monopolar or bipolar. Each has different characteristics and uses.

### Monopolar electrodes

The monopolar system is the one in Figure 21.1. The power available in this mode is high, and produces efficient cutting. The active electrode is available in an assortment of tips: loops to cut and fulgurate, needles to cut and coagulate, ball electrodes for desiccation and fulguration, and blades to cut and coagulate. However, as the patient forms a major part of the electrical circuit, every precaution for safety must be taken. This mode should not be used in vicinities where the target tissue is connected to other adjoining tissue via small delicate structures. These small structures could experience high current densities and be damaged due to excessive heat transfer. If a metal prosthesis, or a pacemaker, forms part of the circuit, then this can cause problems. The device could become a major part of the circuit and some or most of the current could flow through it. The device will heat up, and any tissues joining sharp extremities of the device could become areas of high current density with the associated damage.

### Bipolar electrodes

In the bipolar arrangement both electrodes are small, forming each end of the diathermy forceps, in which high current densities are produced. The intense heating effects are the same at each electrode, and the body does not form part of the circuit. The bipolar surgical diathermy has a localised, precise effect on the tissue and suits delicate surgery such as ophthalmic surgery. The technique has good coagulation effect but less cutting ability due to the low power available. It produces less interference for pacemakers and other sensing electronic devices

# Safety of diathermy

Older diathermy machines used to have the passive electrode earthed to keep the patient earthed at zero voltage. As discussed in the Chapter 6, directly earthing of the patient is not advisable for electrical safety reasons. Modern machines have outputs isolated from earth, as shown in Figure 21.1, to minimise leakage currents from diathermy circuits to earth. To complete an electrical circuit for the maximum diathermy current to flow, the circuit must be completed from **a** (in Figure 21.1) to the active electrode, via the patient resistance, to the passive electrode, back to output **b** (in Figure 21.1). In theory, if the passive electrode were to become disconnected, no current would flow. If an earthed object (such as a drip stand) were to touch the patient, then this should have no effect, as it is not part of the return current path. However, there is also the problem of stray capacitance. This has already been mentioned in the Chapter 6, where stray capacitance exists between conductors causing leakage currents, but also stray capacitance can occur between conducting objects.

## *Stray capacitance*

As discussed in Chapter 4, capacitors allow the flow of alternating current. They can be considered as frequency dependant resistances, where the resistance deceases as the frequency increases. Capacitors can occur, for example, as the passive electrode and the ground of the theatre (which can be indirectly connected to earth). This 'capacitor' will have a low capacitance value but pass very small currents at domestic mains frequencies. However, it will present a much lower resistance at the higher diathermy frequencies and so other stray circuits can occur, which may result in burns. For example, if there is a poor connection between the passive electrode and the patient, and a sharp earthed object comes into contact with the patient (Figure 21.3), then an alternate current path could be formed for the return current. The current in this case flows from **a** (Figure 21.3) to the active electrode, into the patient, then some of current leaves by the earthed object and flows to earth. To complete the circuit back to the connection **b**, the current passes from earth to the passive electrode via the stray capacitance. Burns can arise at the connection between the sharp object and the patient, but can also arise at parts of higher

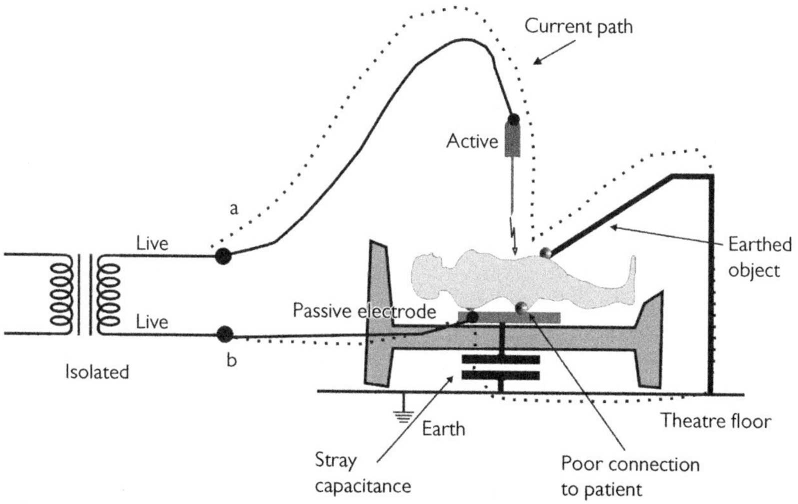


**Fig. 21.3** The diathermy circuit demonstrating stray capacitance. **a** and **b** are outputs from the diathermy machine, and the patient has a poor contact with the passive electrode. An earthed object, such as a drip stand, is touching the patient. Stray capacitance is shown between the passive electrode and the theatre floor. (Figure adapted from Tooley (2004) with permission.)

current density where only certain parts of the passive electrode are touching the patient such as an improperly applied diathermy plate. Burns can be minimised by ensuring that the passive electrode is securely and maximally attached to the patient (so that the correct circuit is the best route for the current to flow). Also it must be ensured that no other objects are touching the patient when the diathermy is on. Alarms can be installed in the equipment (Figure 21.1) to warn users that the device is active, of faulty electrode connections, and of high stray leakage currents. The stray currents gets worse with increasing frequency, so this is why modern isolated systems tend to be designed to operate at the lower frequency range of diathermy machines (500 kHz) to minimise this effect. Older machines used to operate at frequencies up to 5 MHz.

## Interference with other equipment

Surgical diathermy uses radio waves and the equipment can therefore act as a short-range transmitter, and sensitive monitoring equipment, such as ECG monitors, can be a receiver for these signals. Ideally the ECG electrodes and leads should be placed as far from the diathermy electrodes as possible, and care with interpretation must be made when diathermy is in use. Pacemakers can be similarly interfered with, and sometimes the interference can result in the pacemaker wrongly detecting a tachycardia. In these cases, the pacemaker should be put into a fixed rate mode, either automatically or by using a manual method, such as applying a magnet to the pacemaker.

### *Reference*

**Tooley, M.** (2004) Surgical diathermy, *Anaesthesia and Intensive Care Medicine*, *5*(11), pp. 369–71.

# Chapter 22 **Gas supply and the anaesthetic machine checklist**

The chapter links with: Chapters 7, 9, 11, 12, 14, 15, 16, 24, 25, 26 and 28.

## Supply of anaesthetic gases

In Europe and other advanced medical communities, medical gases are generally supplied by pipeline, with cylinders available as backup.

### *Oxygen*

Large hospitals usually have oxygen supplied and stored in liquid form, since one volume of it provides 840 volumes of gaseous oxygen at 15°C. It is stored in a secure *Vacuum Insulated Evaporator* (VIE) on the hospital site. The arrangement is shown in Figure 22.1. The VIE consists of an insulated container, the inner layer of which is made of stainless steel, the outer of which is made of carbon steel. The liquid oxygen is stored in the inner container at about –160°C (lower than the critical temperature of –118°C) at a pressure of between 700 and 1200 kPa. There is a vapour withdrawal line at the top of the VIE, from which oxygen vapour can go via a restrictor to a superheater, where the gas is heated towards ambient temperature. Where demand exceeds supply from this route, there is also a liquid withdrawal line from the bottom of the VIE, from which liquid oxygen can be withdrawn and made to join the vapour line downstream of the restrictor and pass either through the superheater or back to the top of the VIE. After superheating, the oxygen vapour is passed through a series of pressure regulators to drop the pressure down to the distribution pipeline pressure of 410 kPa. No insulation is perfect and there is a pressure relief valve on top of the VIE in case lack of demand and gradual temperature rise results in a pressure build up in the container. There is a filling port and there is usually considerable wastage in filling the VIE; the delivery hose needs to be cooled to below the critical temperature, using the tanker liquid oxygen itself to cool the delivery pipe. The whole VIE device is mounted on a hinged weighing scale and is situated outside the hospital building, protected by a caged enclosure, which also houses two banks of reserve cylinders. These take over automatically if the VIE output falls.

In a smaller hospital, in a country in which delivery of cylinders of oxygen is not a problem, banks of large cylinders can be used to deliver piped oxygen. Appropriate valves, monitoring and alarms need to be in place to ensure that the supply automatically switches to a full cylinder.

Gas pressure in a full cylinder is of the order of 135 atm (13 700 kPa); therefore, this represents the number of times the volume of the cylinder is multiplied to calculate the deliverable gas volume, remembering to use cylinder (gauge) pressure plus one atmosphere pressure to do this calculation, an application of Boyle's law.

In some countries, neither pipelines nor cylinders of oxygen are readily available and a device called an *oxygen concentrator* is useful. This takes in and compresses ambient air, which is then passed through a *zeolite* structure (Li *et al*. 1998), which adsorbs nitrogen, leaving an oxygen-rich atmosphere at the outlet. Since only nitrogen is adsorbed, leaving argon as well as oxygen in the gas, the output gas is closer to 95% oxygen than to 100%. A zeolite is often made of an aluminium hydroxide lattice, which allows nitrogen molecules to be adsorbed and trapped. Adsorption requires the device to be pressurised, and on depressurisation, the nitrogen is desorbed and released. Hence, the system also includes a compressor and, if a pair of zeolites that can be alternately compressed and decompressed is used, a

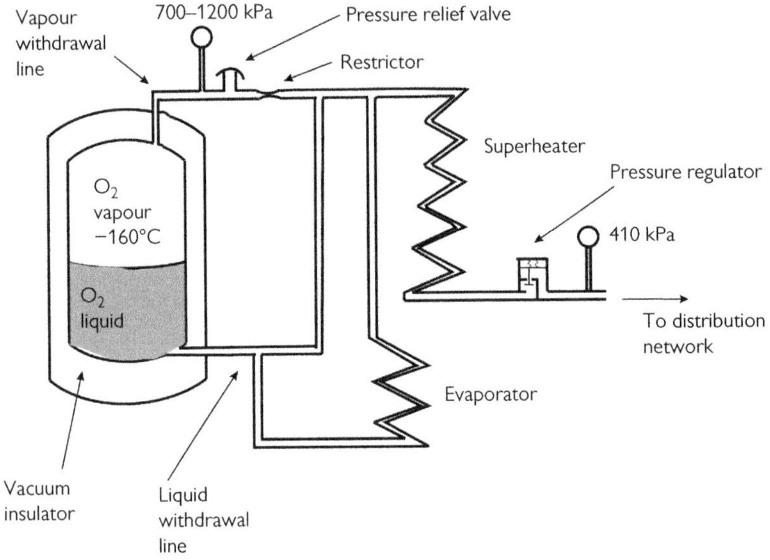


**Fig. 22.1** Vacuum insulated evaporator (VIE) for liquid oxygen supply.

relatively constant output of oxygen-enriched gas can be produced, though the devices available have their limitations (Easy *et al.* 1988, Harris and Simpson 1985). These include an efficiency limited by the pressure change available and the need to absorb water vapour from the gas first. Other methods of oxygen production, using chemical means, are available, but are intended for use in military and field anaesthesia.

## *Nitrous oxide*

Nitrous oxide has a critical temperature above room temperature in temperate climates and is therefore generally stored as a liquid in pressurised cylinders, with $N_2O$ vapour present in the space above the liquid. The actual pressure of a full cylinder is, of course, the SVP at room temperature, but generally lies between 4400 and 5000 kPa. As demand is placed on the supply, more liquid is vaporised. This vaporisation requires energy from the local environment, the latent heat of vaporisation (see Chapter 9). If the demand from the system is high, this can result in a significant fall in temperature within the cylinder's pressure regulator, thus freezing any water vapour present and causing possible obstruction of the regulator outlet. Thermostatically controlled regulators are available to prevent this.

Banks of nitrous oxide cylinders work in the same way as oxygen cylinders, with one bank of perhaps three large cylinders being the 'running' bank, the other bank being the reserve.

On-site manufacture of nitrous oxide is not yet developed for use, but could be achieved by heating ammonium nitrate. Impurities in this process include nitrogen dioxide, which must be washed out with water and sodium hydroxide before removing the water itself with aluminium silicate. Nitrous oxide is now recognised as a substance with significant global warming potential (Campbell and Pierce 2015), being 300 times as potent as $CO_2$ itself in this regard, with a molecular survival time in the atmosphere of more than a century; in addition, it depletes atmospheric ozone, thereby reducing our protection against solar ultraviolet radiation. Although most $N_2O$ pollution emanates from fertilisers in agricultural practice, of that which is used in medical practice, as much as 90% is lost to waste before being used, due to inefficient pipework and manifolds, and most of that which is delivered to patients is in the form of Entonox (Taylor-Smith and Lentzos 2023).

## Entonox

This is 50% nitrous oxide, 50% oxygen. It is used as a safe and effective analgesic gas mixture, usually in the Obstetric Delivery Suite or in the Accident Department. The gas mixture is stored in cylinders or cylinder banks and delivered to the patient using a two-stage pressure regulator, the second incorporating a demand valve, shown in Figure 22.2. If the cylinder temperature falls below -6°C, the *pseudocritical* temperature, the oxygen and nitrous oxide separate into layers, known as *lamination* or the *Poynting effect*. The effects of lamination may be minimised by two means: storing the cylinders horizontally at a temperature of 5°C or more for 24 hours allows the layers to mix. There is also a long tube from the valve housing at the top of the cylinder to a point a small distance from the bottom that prevents the withdrawal of pure $N_2O$ from the cylinder in the event of lamination. Further measures to prevent excessive cooling of the cylinder include using a number of cylinders open simultaneously, so that no single cylinder has excessive demand placed on it.

## Medical compressed air

This is more widely used in anaesthesia and intensive care than previously, as the range of intravenous anaesthetic techniques expands, and concerns about the side effects and environmental effects of nitrous oxide become apparent. Much greater purity is required from medical compressed air than from industrial compressed air. In particular, oil mist, which is often present in industrial compressed air to lubricate power tools, must be removed from medical air. This is partly because of the risk of inhalation of oil mist and partly because of the risk of explosion in an environment of raised oxygen partial pressure. Medical air for breathing devices is supplied from the pipeline at 410 kPa. When supplied at 700 kPa, it is also used for powering tools in the operating theatre, when the oil lubricant has to be added again. It is clearly important not to confuse the two sources, since, for example, ICU gas mixers are calibrated to a 410 kPa supply.

Compressed air can be supplied either by banks of cylinders or by using an air compressor. The air is drawn into such a duty compressor, with a standby compressor in reserve. The air must also be filtered and dried and regulated down to 700 kPa and 400 kPa outlet pressures. It is possible to use a small compressor for an operating or other department, to use the same compressor to run an oxygen concentrator as well, or to use a larger compressor for the whole hospital.

## Piped medical vacuum

Anybody who has used portable suction devices will know how much more efficient and readily available wall suction is. The outlet on the wall is one of many on a *ring main*, from where the pipework goes via drainage, filtering and valve mechanisms towards a vacuum reservoir. Major drainage of fluids that have been suctioned takes place and then through bacterial filters towards a vacuum pump; flexible

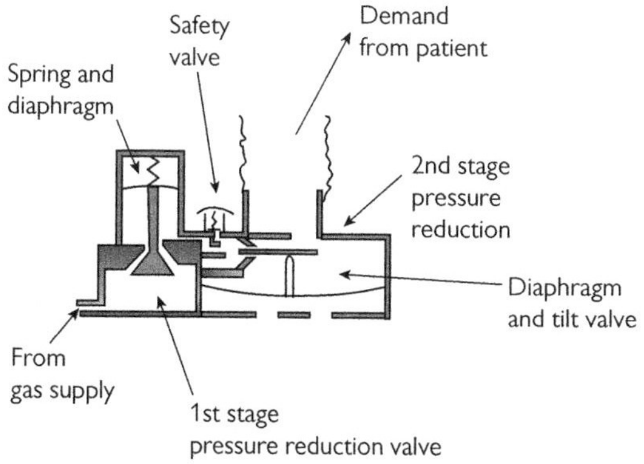


**Fig. 22.2** Two stage 'Entonox' pressure regulator and demand valve.

**Table 22.1** Medical gas cylinder nomenclature, dimensions and gas capacities

| Cylinder size | C | D | E | F | G | J |
|---|---|---|---|---|---|---|
| Dimensions, mm | 356 × 89 | 457 × 102 | 788 × 102 | 865 × 140 | 1248 × 40 | 1450 × 29 |
| Capacities, l Oxygen | 170 | 340 | 680 | 1360 | 3400 | 6800 |
| Nitrous oxide | 450 | 900 | 1800 | 3600 | 9000 | – |
| Entonox | – | 500 | – | 2000 | 5000 | – |
| Air | – | – | – | – | 3200 | 6400 |
| Carbon dioxide | 450 | 900 | 1800 | | – | – |

hoses are used for this transmission in order to reduce noise. Once again, duty and standby pumps are in the system. The pump output is passed through a silencer.

## *Gas cylinders*

Where anaesthetic gases are not supplied from one of the sources already described, they are generally supplied by cylinders. These are made from an alloy of molybdenum and steel that is resistant to corrosion.

The difference between a gas and a vapour has already been discussed (Chapter 9). Oxygen, nitrogen, air and helium are stored in cylinders as gases. Nitrous oxide, carbon dioxide and cyclopropane (which is no longer available in the UK for anaesthetic use) are stored as liquids in equilibrium with vapour at the pressures indicated on the cylinder gauges at ambient temperature. When a nitrous oxide cylinder is full, up to 0.8 of its volume contains liquid $N_2O$. The ratio of the weight of nitrous oxide the cylinder could hold to the weight of water it could hold is the *filling ratio* and this is usually 0.75 in temperate climates, 0.67 in tropical climates. The mounting of such liquid containing cylinders must be vertical. Carbon dioxide is included here, although it is no longer supplied for use in anaesthesia in many countries.

Table 22.1 and 22.2 (Medishield 1979) shows cylinder sizes, dimensions and capacities, as well as the physical properties of the relevant gases or vapours contained within them. Clearly the contents

**Table 22.2** Physical properties and colour coding of medical gases in cylinders

| | Oxygen | Nitrous oxide | Entonox | Air | Carbon dioxide |
|---|---|---|---|---|---|
| Physical state in cylinder | Gas | Liquid | Gas | Gas | Liquid |
| Pressure at 15°C, kPa | 13 700 | 4 400 | 13 700 | 13 700 | 5000 |
| Critical Temperature, °C | –118.4 | 36.5 | Separation at –7 | –140.7 | 31 |
| Critical Pressure, kPa | 5079 | 7260 | | 3773 | 7380 |
| Boiling point at 1 atm, °C | –183 | –89 | – | –194.4 | Sublimation –78.5 |
| Flammability | Supports combustion | Supports combustion | Supports combustion | Supports combustion | No |
| ISO colour coding: :body | black | blue | blue | grey | grey |
| :shoulder1 | white | blue | white | white | grey |
| :shoulder2 | white | blue | blue | black | grey |
| US colour coding | green | blue | —— | yellow | grey |

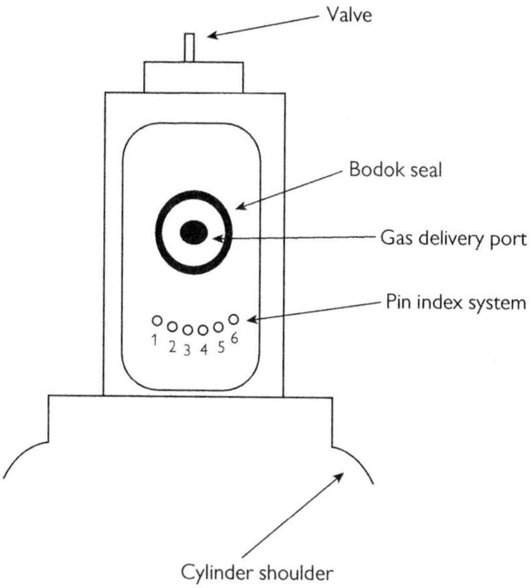


**Fig. 22.3** Cylinder valve, Bodok seal and pin index system to ensure non-interchangeability of cylinders and yokes: Pins 2 and 5 - Oxygen; Pins 3 and 5 - Nitrous oxide; Pins 1 and 5 - Air; Pins 1 and 6 - Carbon dioxide.

of a gas-containing cylinder are usefully indicated by a pressure gauge, whereas this is a less useful indicator for a liquid–vapour containing cylinder. Table 22.2 also shows the International Standards Organisation (ISO) colour coding (and that of the USA to demonstrate that even International Standards are not universal) for gases. The mechanical integrity of cylinders is tested every 5 years.

The ISO *pin index system* is a method of preventing inappropriate attachment of the wrong cylinder to the wrong yoke on the anaesthetic machine. It allows keying in of the cylinder to its own yoke. The valve block at the top of the cylinder has the pin index holes and the appropriate yoke has the mating pins. Figure 22.3 shows the pin index configuration on valve blocks to ensure unique fitting for each gas. When attaching a cylinder to an anaesthetic machine yoke, the presence of a sealing washer, the *Bodok* seal, should be noted at the point where the cylinder gas outlet attaches. If the Bodok seal is absent or in poor condition, there will not be a gas-tight fit. The valve block is fused to the cylinder by a material that melts at a relatively low temperature so that, in the event of fire, the cylinder contents can escape, thereby reducing the chance of an explosion.

## Pressure regulators, gas flow control and anaesthetic machine safety features

Gas is delivered to the anaesthetic machine from cylinders or from the pipeline at different pressures, as indicated previously. There are one or two stages of pressure reduction within the anaesthetic machine, designed to minimise the danger to patients. Between an oxygen cylinder and the anaesthetic machine, there is a reduction from 13 700 kPa to 420 kPa and on some makes (Ohmeda), a further pressure reduction to 140 kPa. Figure 22.4(a) shows a pressure reduction valve (pressure regulator) in its simplest form.

High-pressure gas, at pressure $P_H$, acts across the small cross-sectional area $a$ of the outlet nozzle from the high-pressure stage. In the low-pressure stage, the gas is at a reduced pressure $P_R$, acting across the diaphragm of larger cross-sectional area *A*. The high-pressure nozzle outlet and the diaphragm are mechanically connected by the J piece. As $P_R$ reduces, forces on the J piece open the nozzle, admitting more gas to the low-pressure side. Equilibrium of vertical forces on the J piece (using gauge pressures) gives:

$$P_H a = P_R A.$$

Hence, the pressure reduction ratio is inversely proportional to cross-sectional area ratios, and $P_R$ reduces as $P_H$ reduces, although the constant of proportionality can be reduced to a minimum as *a/A* is reduced. Figures 22.4(b) and 22.4(c) show variations on this model, with the force from a spring or the pantograph biasing the equation above and with a slightly different relationship between the forces in each case. For the example in Figure 22.4(b), the force $F_S$ from the spring, which is designed to depress the diaphragm from the outside, means the equation for equilibrium of vertical forces on the J piece now becomes

$$P_H.a + F_S = P_R.A$$

i.e

$$P_R = P_H \frac{a}{A} + \frac{F_S}{A}$$

By using a very small nozzle on the high-pressure side, and a very large diaphragm on the low-pressure side, *a/A* can be minimised, and by making the spring strong enough to make $F_S$ high, $P_R$ may be kept relatively constant, even in the face of changing $P_H$. Correct functioning of pressure regulators is essential for safe anaesthesia.

A final stage of pressure reduction is provided by a flow restrictor at the needle valve, which controls flow into the Rotameter. The performance of the needle valve is such that the mass flow through it is largely independent of downstream pressure, even if the back pressure changes, referred to in Chapter 14, cause a change in the position of the Rotameter bobbin (Hutton and Boaden 1986). In modern anaesthetic machines, Rotameters themselves no longer exist as such, but there is an electronic facsimile icon of 'Rotameters' on the monitoring screen. The mechanism for flow control is via a series of electronically controlled solenoid valves.

The pressure beyond the rotameters in the anaesthetic machine backbar ranges from 1 to 8 kPa, depending on what the gas flow rate is and whether the vaporiser, situated on the backbar, is switched on. The backbar has a pressure relief valve that activates at about 40 kPa.

Oxygen failure warning devices are activated when oxygen delivery pressure falls below 200 kPa. There are some additional safety features to minimise the possibility of delivery of an hypoxic gas mixture to the patient, apart from the rotameter bank design referred to in Chapter 14 and apart from the monitoring devices discussed elsewhere. There are means of limiting nitrous oxide flow if oxygen delivery pressure falls or fails. One is the Ohmeda chain link between the oxygen and nitrous oxide flow controls (Cicman *et al.* 1993). The other is the Draeger solution, shown in Figure 22.5. The oxygen flush button is connected directly to the high-pressure oxygen source. Modern safety dictates that the button should not be lockable in the depressed position.

## The anaesthetic machine and equipment checklist

It is mandatory for patient safety that the anaesthetist checks the anaesthetic machine and all equipment he or she is using before starting an operating list, and that a shorter check, just including the breathing system, ventilator, airway equipment and suction, must be carried out between cases (Association of Anaesthetists 2012; Weightmann *et al.* 1992; McQuillan and Jackson 1987). This is all based on the checklist recommended by the Association of Anaesthetists of Great Britain and Ireland

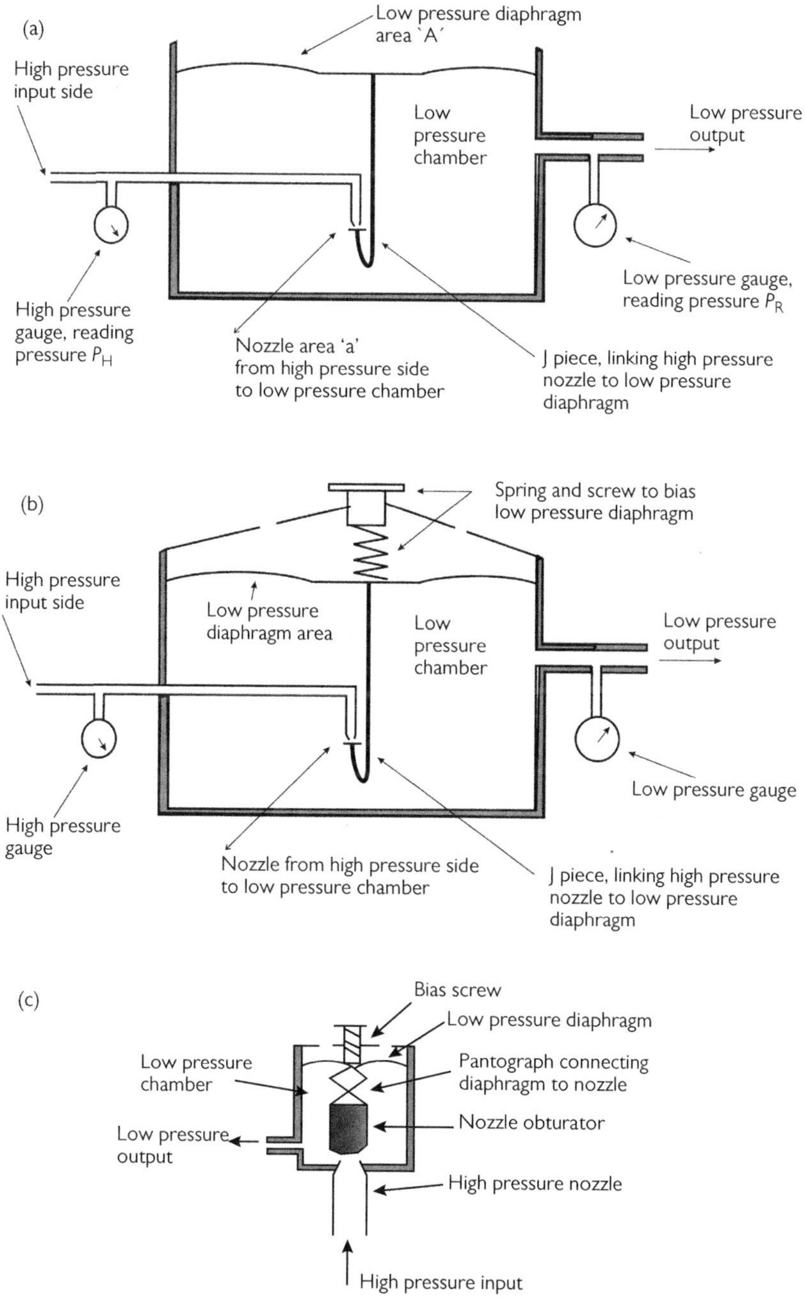


**Fig. 22.4** (a) A pressure reduction valve in its simplest form. (b) A pressure reduction valve. (c) A further example of a pressure reduction valve.

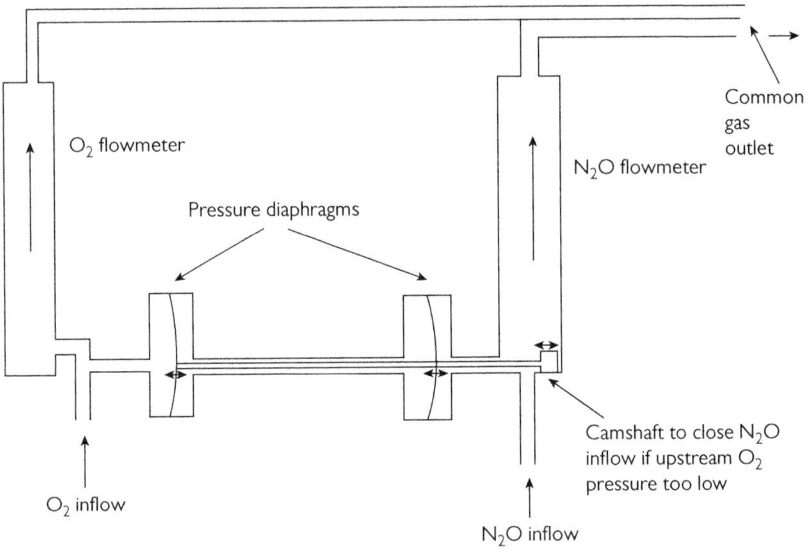


**Fig. 22.5** The Draeger anti-hypoxic mechanism.

(2012), which emphasises that anyone checking and using such equipment must be trained to do so. With advanced technology being increasingly incorporated into anaesthetic machines, an automatic machine check takes place, but this does not obviate the responsibility on the user to undertake further checks as outlined. An abbreviated copy of the checklist must be available at every anaesthetic site.

## *Anaesthetic machine*

An alternative source of ventilation must be available, together with its own supply of oxygen. The automatic machine check should be allowed to complete itself, although the user should know what this includes. The anaesthetic machine (workstation) and any attached ancillary equipment should be plugged into the mains electrical supply. Switch on the main gas supply switch and check that the system clock is set correctly

## *Gas supplies and suction*

Rather than disconnecting the gas pipelines on every occasion to test for the oxygen failure alarm, which might lead to early mechanical failure of the Schrader valve and its probe, it is recommended that a 'tug test' be done for each gas pipeline to check the integrity of attachment. It is now recommended that the oxygen failure alarm is tested on a weekly basis by disconnecting the oxygen pipeline and that a record be kept of this weekly check. The ability of the suction device to rapidly develop a negative pressure must be checked.

Having taken note of which gases are being supplied by the anaesthetic machine, and tug-tested all pipeline connections at the wall, a check should be made that the gas supply does indeed include oxygen, and that there is a spare oxygen supply from a nearby cylinder. Check that supplies of all other gases are adequate, and that all cylinders are securely seated in the manifold and switched off. Carbon dioxide cylinders should not be present, and any unoccupied yokes in the manifold should be covered by a blanking plug. Check pressure gauges from pipelines read 400–500 kPa. Check the function of the flowmeters where present, with smooth running and no sticking within the tube. If nitrous oxide is to be used, check that the anti-hypoxia device functions, by first turning on nitrous oxide flow and ensuring that at least 25% oxygen is also flowing; then turn off the oxygen and ensure that the nitrous oxide also does so; turn on the oxygen flow and ensure the oxygen analyser indicator approaches 100%. Turn off all flows (a basal supply of 300 ml/min of oxygen will continue in most modern machines). Operate the emergency oxygen bypass control valve, ensuring that flow occurs at the gas outlet without a significant reduction in pipeline pressure; ensure it cannot be 'locked on' and that the supply ceases when the control is released.

## *Breathing systems and vaporisers*

All breathing systems which are to be used must be checked, first of all by visual inspection, ensuring correct assembly of components and that connections have been secured by 'push and twist'. There must be no leaks or obstructions, and the system must be pressure tested between 20 and 60 cm $H_2O$ by occluding the patient end of the system. A 'two-bag test' should be carried out at the end of all preoperative tests. Where a Bain system or a circle coaxial breathing system is available, its integrity should be tested by occluding the inner tube (with a 2 ml syringe plunger) and checking that the pressure limiting valve can be fully opened and closed.

Testing the vaporiser on a modern machine may harm the integrity of the machine, so it is worth checking the manufacturer's manual on this matter. If vaporiser testing is permissible, check that it is firmly seated in its manifold, that it is not tilted and that it is adequately filled. Then, with the vaporiser switched off and a gas flow of 5 L/min of oxygen, the gas outlet of the machine is occluded, and there should be no leakage around the vaporiser manifold; this is repeated in turn for the other vaporisers in the manifold, and repeated again with the vaporisers switched on in turn; ensure all vaporisers are switched off at the end. If a vaporiser is exchanged intraoperatively, this test should be repeated.

Where a carbon dioxide absorber is in use, check its connections and its contents, including the colour of the absorbent.

Where an auxiliary common gas outlet is present, particular care should be taken not to connect the breathing system to it where this is not intended.

## *Ventilators*

The configuration of the ventilator should be checked as correct for its intended use, the ventilator tubing must be securely attached, and the controls should be set appropriately for use; a check should be made for the generation of adequate pressure during the inspiratory phase (Sciberras and Schembri 2016), and the pressure relief valve must function correctly at the set pressure. The configuration and function of the alarms should be checked.

## *Two bag test*

This should be performed after all the tests on individual components, outlined above, have been completed. A reservoir bag (or test lung) is attached to the patient end of the breathing system. A fresh gas flow of 5 L/min is set. The test lung is ventilated manually, ensuring the integrity of the whole, including movement of unidirectional valves, where appropriate. The pressure relief valve is tested by squeezing both bags. The ventilator should now be switched on and the whole system tested for leaks by turning off the fresh gas flow (or reducing it to a minimum) and opening and closing each vaporiser in turn.

## *Scavenging*

The scavenging system should be switched on and attached to the appropriate port of the breathing system or ventilator.

## *Monitoring*

Check that all monitors and alarms are functioning and parameters are correctly set for the intended use; sometimes alarm default settings are not appropriate and must be reset. Gas sampling tubes must be checked for patency, and attachment at both ends ensured.

## *Airway equipment*

The presence and function of bacterial filters, catheter mounts, connectors, laryngeal masks, and endotracheal tubes must be checked. The presence and function of laryngoscopes and the location of equipment for a difficult airway must also be checked.

## *Total intravenous anaesthesia*

The details of the check on such equipment are presented in Chapter 27.

## *Ancillary equipment*

Check that the patient's trolley functions as it should with access to head-down tilt. A resuscitation trolley and defibrillator must be available. The location of drugs for uncommon emergencies should be checked (e.g. malignant hyperthermia, local anaesthetic toxicity).

## *References*

**Association of Anaesthetists of Great Britain and Ireland** (2012) Checking anaesthetic equipment, *Anaesthesia*, **67**(6), pp. 660–8.

**Campbell, M.** and **Pierce, J. M. T. (**2015) Atmospheric science and the environment, *BJA Educ.*, **15**(4), pp. 174–9.

**Cicman, J. *et al.*** (1993) Oxygen failure protection device. In *Operating Principles of Narkomed Anesthesia Systems, North American Draeger*, pp. 2–17.

**Easy, W. R.**, **Douglas, G. A.** and **Merrifield, A. J.** (1988) A combined oxygen concentrator and compressed air unit with assessment of a prototype and discussion of potential applications, *Anaesthesia*, **43**, pp. 37–41.

**Harris, C. E. and Simpson, P. J.** (1985) The 'Mini-O2' and 'Healthdyne' oxygen concentrators. Performance and potential application, *Anaesthesia*, **40**, pp. 1206–1209.

**Hutton, P.** and **Boaden, R. W.** (1986) Performance of needle valves, *Br. J. Anaes.*, **58**, pp. 919–24.

**Li, Y. Y.**, **Perera, S. P. and Crittenden, B. D.** (1998) Zeolite monoliths for air separation, *Trans. I. Chem. E*, **76**(A), pp. 921–30.

**McQuillan, P. J.** and **Jackson, I. J. B.** (1987) Potential leaks from anaesthetic machines. Potential leaks through open Rotameter valves and empty cylinder yokes, *Anaesthesia*, **42**, pp. 1365–2044.

**Medishield** (1979) *General Information; Medical Gases and Cylinders*, Medishield.

**Sciberras, S. C.** and **Schembri, R.** (2016) Failure of anaesthetic machine automated self-check to detect massive leak in ventilator bellows, *Br. J. Anaesth.*, **117** Suppl. EL.14, 128.

**Taylor-Smith, R.** and **Lentzos, S.** (2023) Sustainable practice: cutting nitrous oxide loss and waste. *BMJ.*, **383**, p. e076649.

**Weightmann, W. M. *et al.*** (1992) Functionally crossed pipelines. An intermittent condition caused by a faulty ventilator, *Anaesthesia*, **47**, pp. 500–2.

# Chapter 23 Airway management devices

The chapter links with: Chapters 7, 22, 24, 25 and 26.

## Introduction

The most important interface between the breathing system and the patient's lungs is an *airway management device* (AMD). Postoperatively it can be considered to be a means of delivering oxygen-enriched air to the patient. Intraoperatively it is intended to secure the patient's airway, which might otherwise obstruct due to deep anaesthesia, to provide a reasonably gas-tight seal to ensure accurate delivery of anaesthetic gases and, if necessary, to protect the lungs against aspiration of gastric contents. Postoperatively, the AMD can be nasal prongs or a variable performance mask, whose efficiencies may be variable (Wagstaff and Soni 2007). Intraoperatively it might be an artificial airway with a facemask (though rarely in the UK these days), a supraglottic airway of one of the many types available or an endotracheal tube (ETT). A supraglottic airway is one that sits in the pharynx or larynx above the vocal cords and is usually a laryngeal mask airway (LMA) of the numerous types now used, or a cuffed oropharyngeal airway (COPA), or a Combitube. The LMA types available consist of: the classical LMA; the flexible (reinforced) LMA with a flexible tube to the breathing system; the 'Proseal', which has a gastric drainage tube as well as a gas transport tube; the intubating LMA, a device with a rigid right-angled tube that acts as a ventilation conduit in the usual way, but through which an endotracheal tube may also be blindly introduced into the trachea; the 'I-gel' which has a gastric and a respiratory port as does the Proseal, but is more rigid and less bulky, and whose bowl does not require inflation with air, but is filled with a gel that expands with body heat to form a seal. These days, almost all devices are made of material that excludes latex, but care should be taken to ensure this is indeed the case when there is a latex-sensitive patient. Depending on the exact surgical and anaesthetic circumstances, the anaesthetist's experience and equipment availability, a choice is made between these devices to secure the airway for a given operation. Additionally, there are other devices available to assist in securing the airway, such as the laryngoscope, the fibre optic bronchoscope and the cricothyrotomy tube.

## The artificial airway

This is often an oropharyngeal device, shown in Figure 23.1, designed to prevent the tongue from obstructing the pharynx, to provide an elliptically shaped patent airway for gases to flow and to provide a route for suction of the pharynx. It is important that a suitable size is chosen for efficacy, from size 000 (smallest for neonates), through sizes 00, 0, 1, 2, 3, to size 4 (biggest for adult males). Its use does not preclude the need for effective manual airway management. It is usually made of a polyvinyl chloride (PVC) and problems with the Guedel airway include damage to bridged or capped teeth and intolerance in a patient with inadequately attenuated upper airway reflexes. Some oropharyngeal airways are designed to allow the introduction of a fibre optic bronchoscope into the mouth (see Chapter 24); they are also constructed as two longitudinally separable halves, so that an endotracheal tube can be subsequently introduced over the fibre optic bronchoscope into the trachea.

Alternatively, a nasopharyngeal airway can be inserted through the nose. It is of circular cross-section, made of soft polyurethane, and its tip reaches the pharynx (Figure 23.2). Usually, one size down from the equivalent endotracheal tube size is used, e.g. size 6 or 7. Epistaxis is a potential problem. Artificial airways are usually used in conjunction with a facemask.

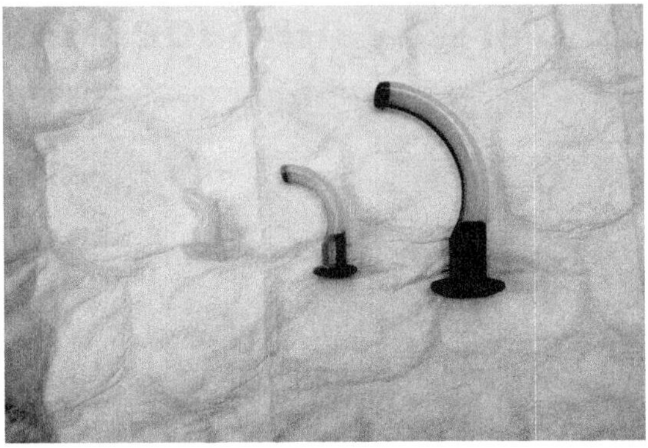

**Fig. 23.1** The Guedel oropharyngeal airway; sizes 0, 1 and 4 are shown.

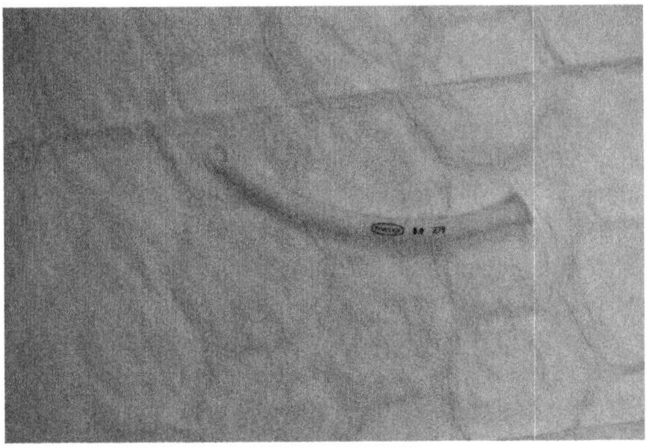

**Fig. 23.2** A nasopharyngeal airway.

# The facemask

These days, the facemask is used for pre-oxygenation prior to securing the airway more formally, rather than for the duration of the surgery. It is designed to fit snugly over the patient's face around the nose and mouth, and the freedom from gas leak is maintained by an adjustable air-filled cushion around its edge. The mask body is made of a rigid PVC, often transparent to allow visualisation of the exhaled breath, secretions or vomit. The apex of the mask contains the means of connecting the catheter mount or angle piece for connecting the mask to the breathing system. Some facemasks have a separate or combined port to allow introduction of a fibre optic laryngoscope during anaesthesia. In an anaesthetic setting, the mask is usually applied gently but efficaciously to the patient's face. In neonatal and paediatric facemask anaesthesia, it is necessary to use a mask which is designed to minimise the dead space.

As indicated earlier, masks for use in the recovery ward or on other wards do not attempt to have a gas-tight seal, rather the reverse. A 3 l $min^{-1}$ supply of oxygen can be delivered to the mask, which then acts as an oxygen reservoir, but it also has some holes in the side, which entrain air during peak inspiration and allow excretion of alveolar gas during exhalation. This is a variable performance device, since the precise inhaled concentration of oxygen depends on the patient's peak inspiratory flow. A slightly more accurate variant on this is the *Venturi mask*, which allows a precise amount of air to be entrained through a manually adjustable orifice, which will yield a more accurately metered level of inspired oxygen. There is a choice of devices for managing the airway in the immediate postoperative phase, in order to optimise oxygenation. These include the laryngeal mask airway (LMA) itself, which can be left *in situ* postoperatively until the patient wakes up, the MC facemask, and nasal prongs, all of which are capable of providing adequate oxygenation (Peyton *et al.* 2000; Martins and Brimacombe 1997). Extreme care must be taken when connecting a high-pressure oxygen source to any device attached to the patient's airway to ensure there is a low impedance conduit for exhalation. High flow nasal oxygen may also be used in recovery and is proving popular and efficacious in ICU in post-extubation patients with respiratory failure (Renda *et al.* 2018).

## The laryngeal mask airway

The laryngeal mask airway (LMA) provides a means of securing the patient's airway, leaving the anaesthetist's hands free from holding a facemask, without the need for endotracheal intubation. The functionally important part of the device is an oval bowl-shaped structure with an inflatable cuff around the rim, which is introduced into the pharynx. The cuff ensures that the pharyngeal structures remain open and that the airway is surrounded by a relatively gastight seal, although that is not guaranteed. The cuff at the tip of the LMA sits over the oesophagus, partially occluding it. The fenestrated lumen in the centre of the bowl on its concave, ventral side, which sits over the glottis, is continuous with a tube connecting the bowl to the outside of the mouth; the tube is the means of introducing the LMA through the mouth and of connecting the LMA to the breathing system. LMAs come in sizes 1 (neonates to 6.5 kg), 1½ (infants to 10 kg), 2 (children to 20 kg), 2½ (to 30 kg), and 3, 4 and 5 (small adults to large adults). Each size requires a maximum volume of air to be inflated into the cuff of $10(n - 1)$ ml, where $n$ is the LMA size; the exception to this is size 1, which requires 4 ml of air, although cuff pressure measurement is encouraged. Inserting the LMA is achieved by sliding the device through the mouth with the cuff deflated, maintaining bowl contact with the palate while doing so. Sometimes the tip of the cuff gets caught at the right-angled turn of the pharynx, or the insertion process allows the epiglottis to become folded down to obstruct the glottis. Otherwise, there is no positive endpoint to indicate successful insertion, other than watching the quality of the ensuing spontaneous or manual ventilation. If there is any doubt about the success of the insertion, there should be a low clinical threshold for removing the LMA and trying again. The LMA lends itself to the introduction of a fibre optic laryngoscope into the tube to just beyond the bowl in order to inspect the glottis. An example of the LMA is shown in Figures 23.3(a) and (b).

There are variations on the standard LMA. The *reinforced LMA* (flexible LMA) has a wire-reinforced tube, which is rather narrower than the tube on the classical LMA, and which provides greater flexibility while preventing the tube from kinking. This is useful when the operative site is in or near the mouth itself. However, these LMAs may require temporary reinforcement of the tube to aid LMA insertion. Such a tube can be used for airway laser surgery (Lockey and Woodward 1997).

The *intubating LMA* (ILMA) (Baskett *et al.* 1998; Brain *et al.* 1997) is a device with a rigid right-angled tube attached to the bowl, shown in Figure 23.4. The tube is made of low-friction metal, so that an endotracheal tube can be introduced inside the tube and inserted through the glottis (Asai *et al.* 1993).

The *Proseal LMA* (Brain *et al.* 1995) essentially has two tubes in the same mould connected to the bowl; one has a fenestrated lumen in the centre of the bowl on its concave, ventral surface, that sits opposite the glottis for ventilation as normal; the other tube has a lumen that goes to a point on the tip of the cuff, to sit opposite the oesophagus and allow gastric drainage while the cuff seals the glottis. This makes the Proseal a rather bulkier device to insert than the classic LMA, and it usually needs a metal scoop to aid insertion. The device is shown in Figures 23.5(a) and (b).

The LMA is often used for patients breathing spontaneously, although there is some increase in airway resistance (Righini *et al.* 1997) compared with a facemask. However, it can also be used for artificial ventilation, although it should not be assumed to provide the same protection against aspiration of gastric contents as an endotracheal tube, even if a Proseal is used. Furthermore, the seal provided by the bowl cuff may not be adequate to ventilate the patient if airway pressures are high, such as

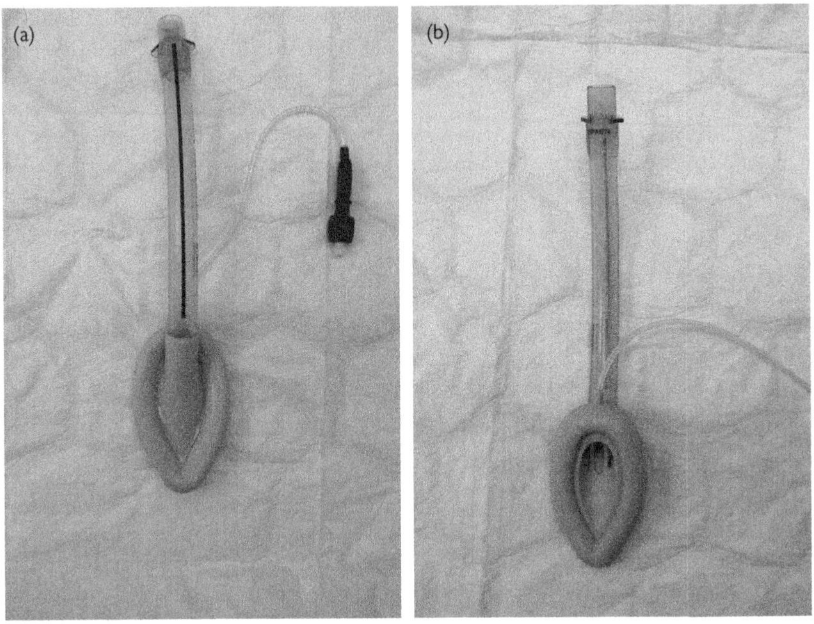


**Fig. 23.3** The classical laryngeal mask airway (LMA): (a) dorsal view; (b) ventral view.

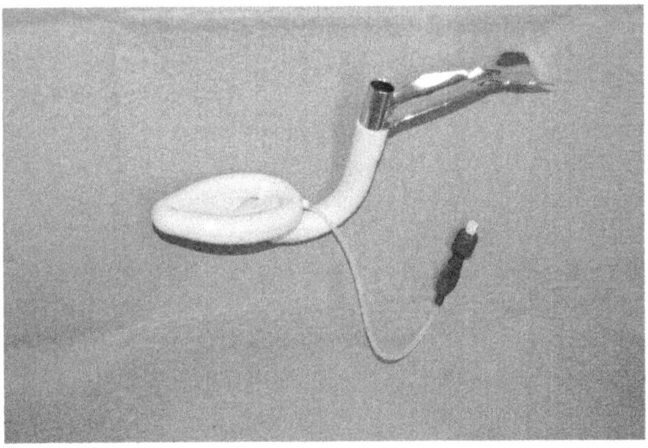

**Fig. 23.4** The intubating LMA (ILMA), lateral view.

during laparoscopic surgery. XIIth cranial nerve damage from the cuff has been reported (King and Street 1994).

## The I-gel

The I-gel is a device that is functionally like a Proseal in that it acts like an LMA, sitting in the oropharynx, and also has a gastric drainage port, shown in Figure 23.6(a) and (b). It is of a more compact and rigid construction than a Proseal, and can be introduced without the aid of a scoop. In particular, its sealing cuff does not require inflation, but contains a gel within it that expands on exposure to body heat, resulting in an effective seal for positive pressure ventilation where moderate pressures are involved

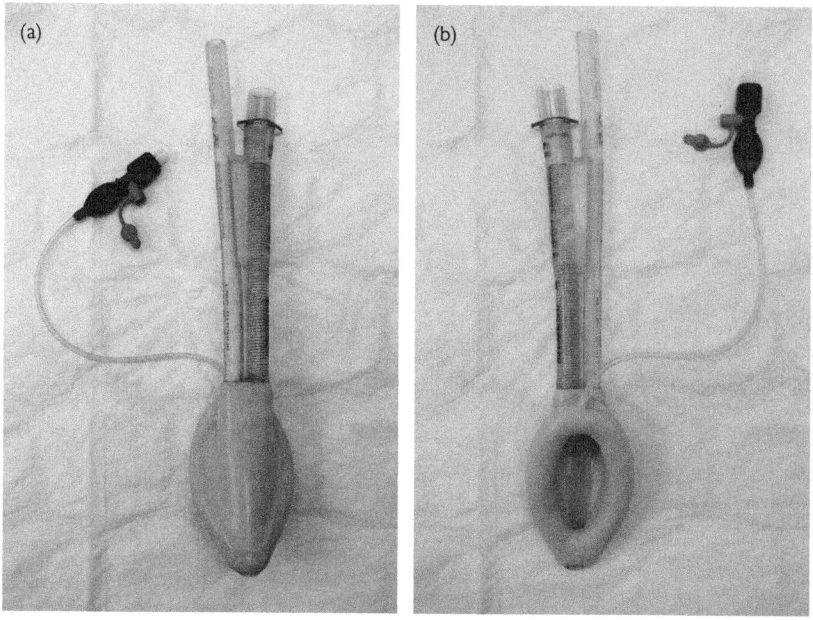


**Fig. 23.5** The Proseal LMA: (a) dorsal view; (b) ventral view.

(Uppal *et al.* 2009). In many departments its use, and that of other second-generation, single-use supraglottic airway management devices, now supercedes that of the classical LMA and other earlier generation devices for safety, ease of insertion and with the benefit of less of a post-operative sore throat (Cook and Kelly 2015; de Montblanc *et al.* 2014).

## The cuffed oropharyngeal airway

These are devices with some functional similarities to the classic LMA and Proseal LMA. The cuffed oropharyngeal airway (COPA) (Rees and Gabbott 1999) consists of a ventilating tube, introduced into the pharynx through the mouth; it has a single circumferential cuff to keep it centrally placed over the glottis.

The *Combitube* (Hartmann *et al.* 2000) is a double-lumen, double-cuff device, designed with one lumen at its tip and the other lumen being circumferentially placed around the tube, near, but not at its tip; the two lumina are functionally separated on the outside of the device by the distal cuff. The proximal cuff is to keep the tube approximately in the middle of the pharynx. The tube is inserted and if the distal lumen goes into the glottis, the circumferential lumen can be used for gastric aspiration. If the distal lumen ends up in the oesophagus, the distal cuff functionally separates the oesophagus from the glottis and the proximal lumen can be used to ventilate the patient; a gastight seal for this purpose is assured by the proximal cuff. Some device for detecting which tube was fulfilling which function would be required, such as a Wee oesophageal detector (see later section).

## The endotracheal tube

Despite the greatly increased use of supra-glottic devices described earlier, when absolute security from gastric aspiration (Oikkonen and Aromaa 1997), or muscle relaxation and artificial ventilation are required, endotracheal intubation is often still the preference of anaesthetists. Endotracheal tubes

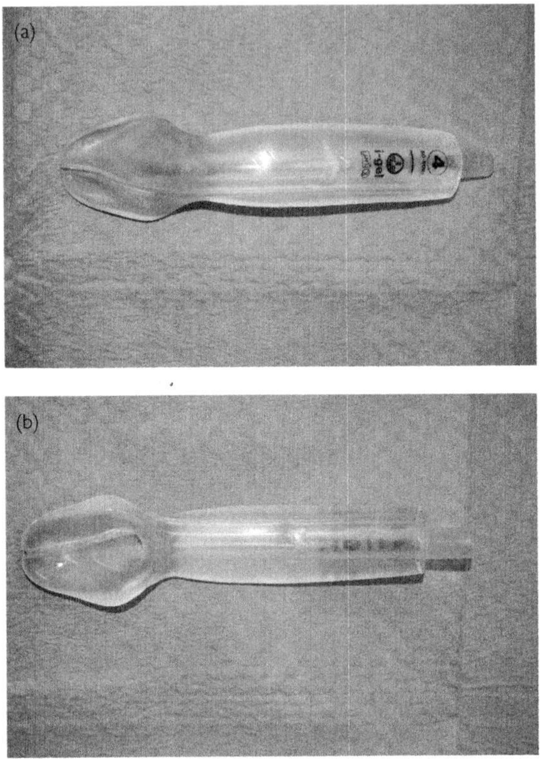

**Fig. 23.6** The I-gel airway: (a) dorsal view; (b) ventral view.

(ETTs) are introduced through the mouth or the nose, invariably using a laryngoscope. The orotracheal tube is usually about 30 cm long if left uncut; these days, it is disposable and made from clear PVC rather than red rubber, with a curvature down its length that corresponds to the anatomical curvature from the mouth to the trachea, as shown in Figure 23.7(a). The tip has a left-handed bevel to allow easier visual insertion and there may be an additional lumen on the opposite side, a *Murphy's eye*, to ensure that gas can pass through the tube if the bevelled end is obstructed. The size by which the tubes are described is the internal diameter in cm and ranges from 2.5 cm for a neonatal patient to 9.0 cm for a large male patient, although these days larger diameter tubes are avoided to reduce tracheal trauma. The size necessary for a given patient is dictated by the need to pass the tube easily through the narrowest part of the airway, which is the glottis in an adult and the cricoid cartilage in a child. The larger the tube used, the lower the resistance to gas flow through the tube, but damage to the vocal cords and the tracheal mucosa must be avoided. In general, cuffed tubes are used in adults to ensure a leak free seal to the airway, and uncuffed tubes are used in neonates and infants to avoid tracheal mucosal damage (Figure 23.8).

In children over 2 years of age, the tube size is given by (*age*/4)+4.5 cm internal diameter, with sizes between 3.0 and 4.5 for younger infants according to weight . In neonatal anaesthesia, or where there is a need to use a particularly narrow ETT in an adult, such as a micro-laryngeal tube in pharyngoscopy, thought must be given to the fact that the airway resistance down such a tube is extremely high, being inversely proportional to the fourth power of the radius (see Chapter 7). In such a situation, tube design is very important and adequate time must be given to allow for full expiration of the tidal volume; furthermore, it should be recognised that high peak measured airway pressure does not necessarily mean

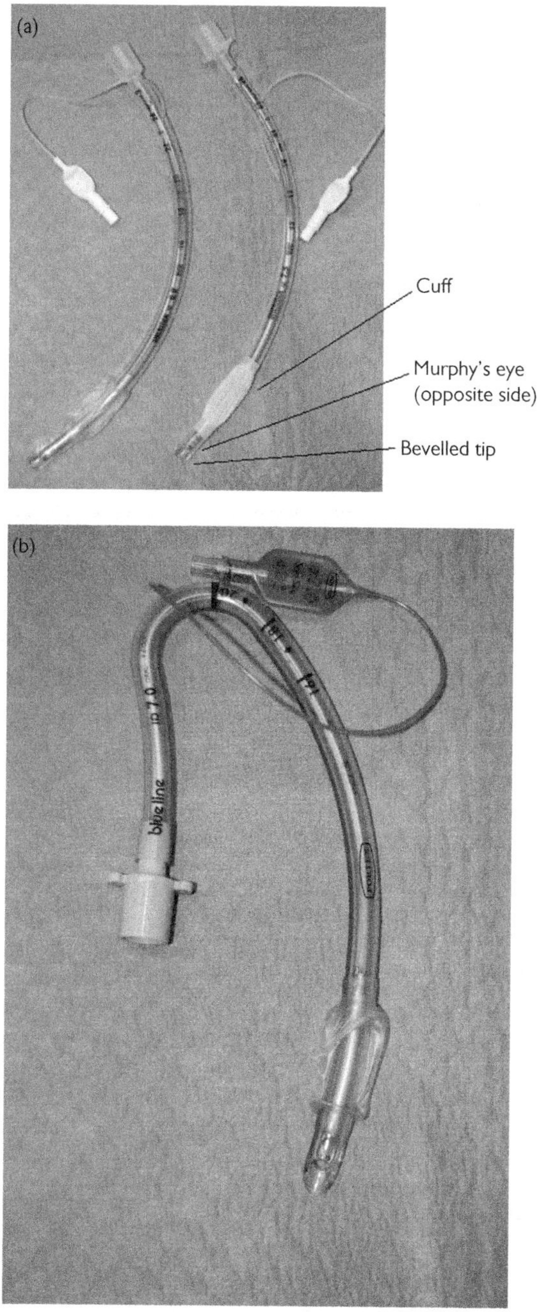


**Fig. 23.7** (a) The standard cuffed, adult endotracheal tube; (b) the preformed, downward facing Rae tube.

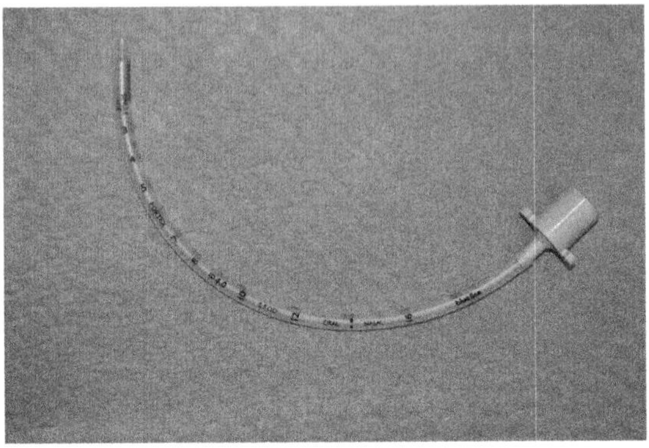

**Fig. 23.8** Uncuffed paediatric endotracheal tubes.

high alveolar pressure. Similarly, if any sort of device is introduced down the length of an ETT, such as a fibre optic bronchoscope or a suction catheter, there will be a dramatic increase in airway resistance (Magee 2008).

The wish to avoid causing ischaemic damage to the tracheal mucosa is the reason that a leak is tolerated around the tubes used in neonates and children. However, in recent years there has been an increasing use of cuffed endotracheal tubes in children. A reliable seal with lack of stridor due to tracheal mucosal oedema after extubation has been demonstrated (Weiss *et al.* 2009a, 2009b). In adults, an inflatable cuff around the distal end of the ETT is always used to ensure freedom from gas leak and absolute security from gastric contents entering the trachea. Old red rubber tubes had low-volume high-pressure cuffs, which had a small area of contact with the trachea and might therefore have caused high contact pressures, particularly if the cuff was over-inflated. When autoclaved multiple times, the old cuffs also had a tendency to herniate and obstruct the end of the ETT. Modern ETTs have large-volume low-pressure cuffs, designed to have large contact areas and low contact pressures with the mucosa, although these too can cause damage if over-inflated (Messahel *et al.* 1994). Ideally the cuff pressure should be measured, monitored and maintained at no more than 2.5 kPa (25 $cmH_2O$) (Miller 1992). Automatic cuff pressure controllers that make rapid changes to cuff pressure have been found to reduce the integrity of the seal (Weiss *et al.* 2009a, 2009b). The cuffs are normally filled with air through a narrow cuff inflation tube that also has a pilot balloon, but will enlarge if nitrous oxide is absorbed into the cuff volume, unless it is prefilled with nitrous oxide instead (Karasawa *et al.* 2001). Another problem with air-filled ETT cuffs is the change in their volume according to Boyle's law with a change in altitude when an intubated patient is being transported by air. A solution to both these problems is to fill the cuff with saline (Smith and McArdle 2002) or to use a foam-filled cuff (Power 1990). This is also a solution to prevent an airway fire during airway laser surgery. There are ETTs whose pilot balloons have a secondary latex pilot balloon within them; these provide an extra reservoir for additional gas being absorbed within the cuff, thereby preventing the ETT cuff from enlarging excessively.

The length of an ETT is dictated by the need for the tip to reach into the trachea, but to avoid being so long as to enter a main bronchus, usually the right, and also to avoid adding unnecessarily to airway resistance. The correct length of tube is judged visually on laryngoscopy. In adults the correct length of the tube in the trachea is usually between 20 and 25 cm. As a guide, the length of an ETT in children is given by

$$\frac{age\ yr}{2} + 12.0\,\text{cm}$$

However, the adequacy of ventilation in both lungs should be checked visually, by testing the quality of manual inflation pressure, by auscultation, and by the presence of an adequate $CO_2$ trace.

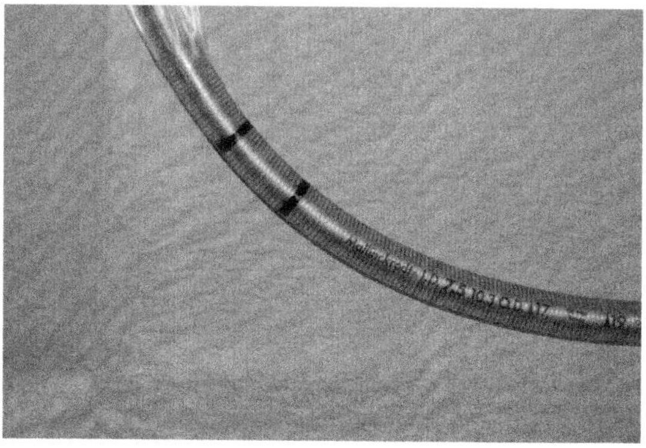

**Fig. 23.9** A flexo-metallic endotracheal tube for use in the presence of lasers.

Nasotracheal tubes are naturally longer than orotracheal tubes, and the tubes are often made of soft polyurethane or silicone rubber in order to cause less trauma to the nasal mucosa. It is usually necessary to use a nasal tube one size smaller than the equivalent oral tube.

Any PVC ETT can kink as it heats up to body temperature. Care must be taken in securing the tube to a catheter mount to avoid this and this connection should be visible where possible. There are preformed, specially shaped ETTs to try to minimise the chance of kinking, such as RAE tube (see Figure 23.7(b)). Alternatively, the ETT can be reinforced with a wire coil down its length.

Methods of confirming correct placement of an ETT include visual and auscultatory; the $CO_2$ analyser, pulse oximetry, pH indicator (Gedeon *et al.* 1995) and the Wee detector (Wee 1988), which consists of a tube attached at one end to a large rubber bulb. The bulb is initially squeezed to evacuate it and when the other end is attached to the visible end of the ETT, if the bulb reinflates, the ETT is in the trachea; if it remains deflated, it is in the oesophagus. Another detection device is the SCOTI device (*S*onomatic *C*onfirmation of *T*racheal *I*ntubation), which differentiates the acoustic properties of the trachea and the oesophagus (Nandwani *et al.* 1996). A comparative study showed the Wee device to be more reliable than the SCOTI (Lockey and Woodward 1997).

Other ETTs for special circumstances include tubes for use in airway laser surgery, which have a metallic surface incorporated in the wall in order to reflect the laser beam away from the tube and prevent the tube material from igniting in the oxygen or nitrous oxide environment (Hunton and Oswal 1988; Pandit *et al.* 1997), see Figure 23.9; there are often two cuffs in case one is damaged and rendered useless by the laser.

Tracheostomy tubes are much shorter than ETTs and have a non-bevelled end, with the cuff closer to the end, and a right-angled bend. It is possible to use a percutaneous dilatational technique to insert a tracheostomy tube in the ICU (Oldroyd and Bodenham 1995). A variant, used for emergency access to the airway through the tracheal wall, is the cricothyrotomy tube (Patel and Frerk 2008). However, care must be taken in ventilating patients through high-pressure oxygen sources, that surgical emphysema is not inadvertently caused by malposition of the cricothyrotomy needle. Care must also be taken to ensure that there is an open pathway for expiration if pulmonary barotrauma is to be avoided.

Double-lumen tubes, for use in thoracic surgery where the two lungs need to be functionally separated, are made to be right or left sided, have a tracheal lumen and an endobronchial lumen and a carinal hook to aid correct placement. The right-sided tubes have an additional bronchial opening to ensure adequate ventilation of the right upper lobe of the lung. Because the two lumina are constructed back-to-back, they are D-shaped and the sizes are described in French gauge, usually available from FG 35 to 41 (see Figure 23.10) Each lumen has different flow characteristics (Chiaranda *et al.* 1989). When inserting a double-lumen tube, the tube must be inserted with the endobronchial end facing forward

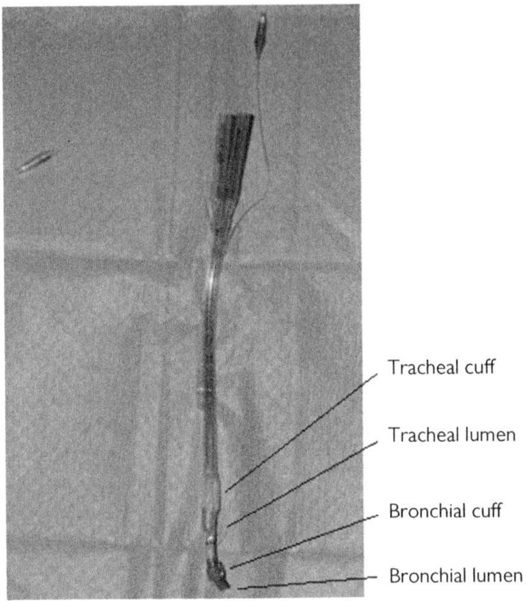


**Fig. 23.10** A typical left-sided double-lumen tube, ventral view.

initially, then rotated appropriately. Then the cuffs must be inflated separately and sequentially and finally together to confirm each lumen is where it is intended to be. Fibre optic bronchoscopy is the best method to confirm the appropriate placement of a double-lumen tube. Excessive inflation of the bronchial cuff can be a cause for concern. In order to isolate one of the lungs for surgery, clear testing procedures for knowing which lung is being ventilated and which is being blocked must be in place (Patel *et al*. 2023).

## *References*

**Asai, T.**, **Latto, I. P.** and **Vaughan, R. S.** (1993) Distance between the grill of the LMA and the vocal cords, *Anaesthesia*, **48**, pp. 667–9.

**Baskett, P. J. F.**, **Parr, M. J. A.** and **Nolan, J. P.** (1998) The intubating laryngeal mask. Results of a multicentre trial of experience of 500 cases, *Anaesthesia*, **53**, pp. 1174–9.

**Brain, A. I. J.** ***et al.*** (1997) The ILMA: development of a new device for intubation of the trachea, *Br. J. Anaesth.*, **79**, pp. 699–703.

**Brain, A. I. J.**, ***et al.*** (1995) A new laryngeal mask prototype; a preliminary evaluation of seal pressures and glottic isolation, *Anaesthesia*, **50**, pp. 42–8.

**Chiaranda, M.** ***et al.*** (1989) Measurement of flow resistive properties of double lumen bronchial tubes in vitro, *Anaesthesia* **44**, 335–40.

**Cook, T. M. and Kelly, F. E.** (2015) Time to abandon the 'vintage' laryngeal mask airway and adopt second generation supraglottic airway devices as first choice, *Br. J. Anaesth.*, **115**(4), pp. 497–9.

**de Montblanc, J.** ***et al.*** (2014) A systematic review and meta-analysis of the I-gel vs the LMA in adults, *Anaesthesia*, **69**, pp. 1151–62.

**Gedeon, A.**, **Knill, P.** and **Mobius, C.** (1994) A new colorimetric breath indicator. A comparison of the performance of two $CO_2$ indicators, *Anaesthesia*, **49**, pp. 798–803.

**Hartmann, T.** ***et al.*** (2000) The oesophageal-tracheal Combitube small adult. An alternative airway for ventilatory support during gynaecological laparoscopy, *Anaesthesia*, **55**, pp. 670–5.

**Hunton, J.** and **Oswal, V. H.** (1988) Anaesthesia for $CO_2$ laser laryngeal surgery in infants, *Anaesthesia*, **43**, pp. 394–6.

**Karasawa, F.** ***et al.*** (2001) An assessment of a method of inflating cuffs with a nitrous oxide gas mixture to prevent an increase in intracuff pressure in five different tracheal tube designs, *Anaesthesia*, **56**, pp. 155–9.

**King, C.** and **Street, M. K.** (1994) Twelfth cranial paralysis following use of the laryngeal mask airway, *Anaesthesia*, **49**, pp. 786–87.

**Lockey, D. J.** and **Woodward, W.** (1997) SCOTI versus Wee. An assessment of two oesophageal intubation detection devices, *Anaesthesia*, **52**, pp. 242–3.

**Magee, P. T.** (2008) A study of gas flow in coaxial tubes *Anaesthesia*, **63**, pp. 905–6.

**Martins, J. and Brimacombe, J. R.** (1997) Oxygen enrichment during emergence with the LMA-T-Bag vs. T piece *Anaesthesia*, **52**, 1195–8.

**Messahel, B. F.** ***et al.*** (1994) Total tracheal obliteration after intubation with low pressure cuffed endotracheal tube, *Br. J. Anaesth*, **73**, 697–9.

**Miller, D. M.** (1992) A pressure regulator for the cuff of a tracheal tube, *Anaesthesia*, **47**, 594–6.

**Nandwani, N.** ***et al.*** (1996) Configuration of the SCOTI device with different tracheal tubes, *Anaesthesia*, **51**, pp. 932–4.

**Oikkonen, M.** and **Aromaa, U.** (1997) Leakage of fluid around low-pressure tracheal tube cuffs, *Anaesthesia*, **52**, pp. 567–9.

**Oldroyd, G. J.** and **Bodenham, A. R.** (1995) An evaluation of a new percutaneous tracheostomy kit, *Anaesthesia*, **50**, pp. 49–51.

**Pandit, L. J., Chambers, P.** and **O'Malley, S.** (1997) KTP laser resistant properties of the reinforced LMA, *Br. J. Anaesth*, **78**, pp. 594–600.

**Patel, B.** and **Frerk, C.** (2008) Large bore cricothyrotomy devices, *Br. J. Anaesth. Continuing Education Series*, **8**(5), pp. 157–60.

**Patel, M., Wilson, A.** and **Ong, C.** (2023) Double lumen tubes and bronchial blockers, *BJA Educ.*, **23**, (11), pp. 416–42.

**Peyton, P., Cowie, D.** and **Howard, W.** (2000) Supplementary oxygenation with the LMA: a comparison of four devices, *Anaesthesia*, **55**, pp. 992–9.

**Power, K. J.** (1990) Foam cuffed tracheal tubes. Clinical and laboratory assessment, *Br. J. Anaesth.*, **65**, pp. 433–7.

**Rees, S. G. O.** and **Gabbott, D. A.** (1999) Use of the oropharyngeal airway for manual ventilation by non-anaesthetists, *Anaesthesia*, **54**, pp. 1089–93.

**Renda, T., Corrado, A., Iskander, G.** ***et al.*** (2018) High flow nasal oxygen therapy in intensive care and anaesthesia, *Br. J. Anaesth.*, **120**(1), pp. 18–27.

**Righini, E. R.** ***et al.*** (1997) Additional inspiratory resistance imposed by the LMA: in vitro vs. in vivo comparison, *Anaesthesia*, **52**, pp. 872–8.

**Smith, R. P. R.** and **McArdle, B. H.** (2002) Pressure in cuffs of tracheal tubes at altitude *Anaesthesia*, **57**, pp. 374–8.

**Uppal, V., Fletcher, G. and Kinsella, J.** (2009) Comparison of I-gel with a cuffed endotracheal tube during pressure-controlled ventilation, *Br. J. Anaesth.*, **102**, 264–8.

**Wagstaff, T.** and **Soni, N.** (2007) Performance of six types of oxygen delivery devices at varying respiratory rates, *Anaesthesia*, **62**, pp. 492–503.

**Wee, M. Y. K.** (1988) The oesophageal detector device. Assessment of a new method to distinguish oesophageal from tracheal intubation, *Anaesthesia*, **43**, pp. 27–9.

**Weiss, M., Dullenkopf, A., Fischer, J.** ***et al.*** (2009a) Prospective randomised controlled multi-centre trial of cuffed or uncuffed endotracheal tubes in small children, *Br. J. Anaesth.*, **103**, pp. 867–73.

**Weiss, M., Doell, C., Koepfer, N.** ***et al.*** (2009b) Rapid pressure compensation by automated cuff pressure controllers worsens sealing in tracheal tubes *Br. J. Anaesth*, **102**, pp. 273–8.

# Chapter 24 **Aids to intubation**

The chapter links with: Chapter 23.

## The laryngoscope

This device was invented by Sir Ivan Magill and Sir Robert Macintosh to visualise the vocal cords to aid intubation. The curved blade of the Macintosh laryngoscope is still popular as the standard and its design has been reshaped in recent years to reduce the biomechanical forces on the teeth (Bucx *et al.* 1994). The handle has a battery and a light source in it, and the light is transmitted by a fibre optic cable to the tip of the blade, which is usually at right angles to the handle. There are many different-shaped blades to suit different circumstances, particularly to visualise the anatomically different airway of the neonate. Other variants to aid difficult intubations include the Polio laryngoscope, in which the angle between the handle and the blade is an obtuse one and the McCoy laryngoscope, which has a lever to manipulate the tip of the laryngoscope blade to improve the view of the vocal cords (McCoy and Mirakhur 1993); some of these devices are shown in Figure 24.1.

In recent years a new range of laryngoscopes has been introduced with fibre optic systems that allow indirect visualisation of the vocal cords via an eyepiece or a small video screen. These devices clearly improve access to the airway where there would otherwise be a laryngoscopic view with a high Cormack-Lehane score. They currently include the McGrath (Ray *et al.* 2009), the Glidescope, the Airtraq (Lange *et al.* 2009) (shown in Figures 24.2(a) and (b)), the C-MAC (McElwain *et al.* 2010 and others). As with all new devices, their efficacy depends on the skill and training of the user, and sometimes the familiar device is better to use than a newer one (Powell *et al.* 2009).

With the emergence of Jakob–Creutzfeldt disease and the recognition of the infectious risk of prions from tonsillar tissue on laryngoscope blades, a range of disposable paediatric blades has been produced, with variable quality of mechanical flexibility and light quality (Goodwin *et al.* 2006).

Where the surgical procedure itself is laryngoscopy and the airway must be ventilated by a jet attached to the side of the laryngoscope, the laryngoscope is designed to allow a jet of high-pressure oxygen at its proximal end to entrain a much larger volume of air into the lungs, which may or may not be by the Venturi effect, depending on the precise design of the attachment (see Chapter 7). This is usually done manually by the anaesthetist.

## Fibre optics

Optical fibres can be used with lasers (see Chapter 29) to direct the beam, but they are also used in the design of endoscopes and bronchoscopes to permit the clinician to see around corners. Another medical use is for electrical isolation of the patient (as discussed in Chapter 6) and interference-free transmission of signals, for example, from an electroencephalogram (EEG) head box to the main amplifier via an optical fibre link. In these cases, the electrical signals are converted to modulated light via a photodiode, sent down the fibre and then converted back via a detector.

The fibre is shown in Figure 24.3. The light propagates along the fibre by the process of total internal reflection.

(a)

(b)

(c)

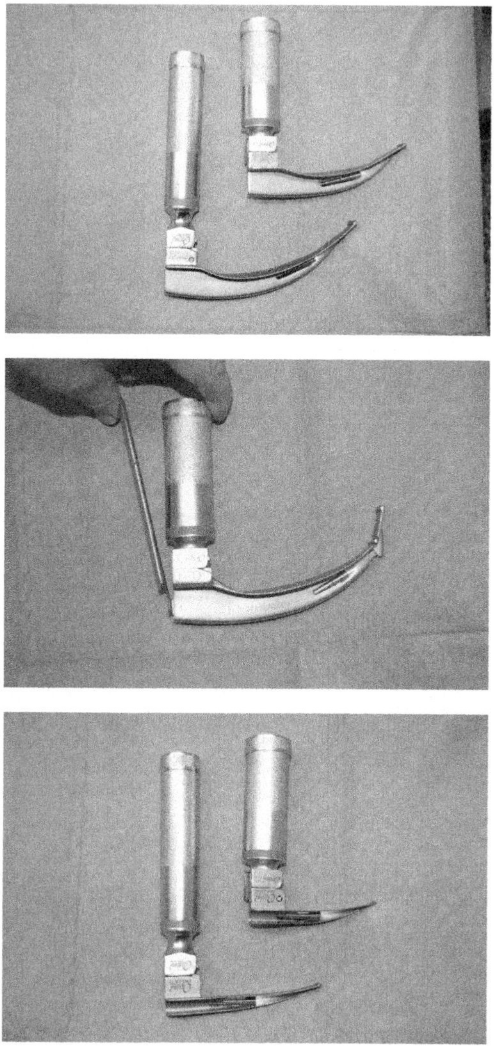

**Fig. 24.1** Some different laryngoscopes and blades to aid endotracheal intubation; (a) Standard MacIntosh laryngoscopes, medium and long blades; (b) McCoy laryngoscope with adjustable blade tip; (c) two variants of blade for paediatric laryngoscopy.

## *Reflection and refraction of light*

When light travelling in a transparent material meets the surface of another transparent material, two things happen: some of the light is reflected, and some of the light is transmitted into the second transparent material.

The light which is transmitted usually changes direction when it enters the second material (e.g. the glass cladding of the optical fibre). This bending is called refraction and it depends upon the fact that

(a)

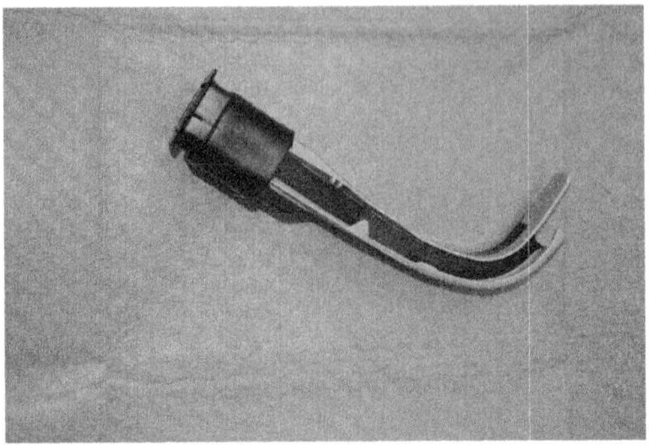

(b)

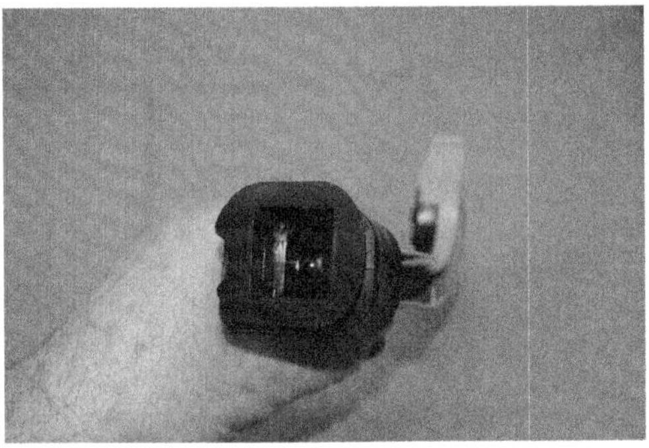

**Fig. 24.2** Airtraq optical laryngoscope: (a) lateral view showing gutter for endotracheal tube placement; (b) proximal end showing optical eyepiece.

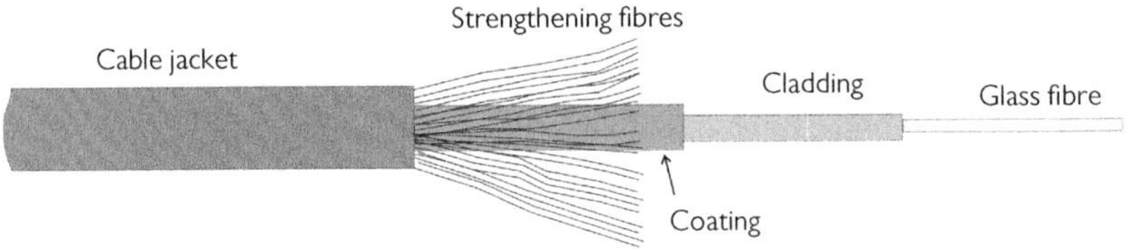


**Fig. 24.3** The fibreoptic cable showing the coating, cladding and core.

light travels at one speed in one material and at a different speed in another. Therefore, each material (glass core, cladding) has its own refractive index. In this case the light goes from a higher index (glass core) to a lower one (cladding). In Figure 24.4 $\theta_2$ is always greater than $\theta_1$, and as $\theta_1$ increases, at the critical angle $\theta_c$, all the light will be reflected. As long as the angle of incidence is greater than the critical angle (which is set by the smallness of the glass core), then total internal reflection will occur. Even if the optical fibre is bent (to certain limits), then light will be transmitted along the tube as demonstrated in Figure 24.5.

## Videolaryngoscopy

In recent years, videolaryngoscopy (VL) has become more popular to help anaesthetists acquire a better view of what might otherwise be a difficult larynx to visualise in order to access and secure. It incorporates a high-resolution video camera in the laryngoscope blade, whence the view is relayed either

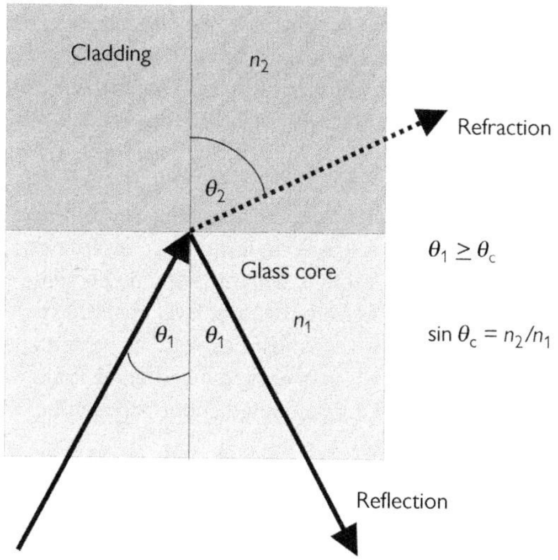


**Fig. 24.4** Diagram showing angle of incidence, reflection, refraction and critical. $n_1$ and $n_2$ are the refractive index in the glass core and cladding, respectively.

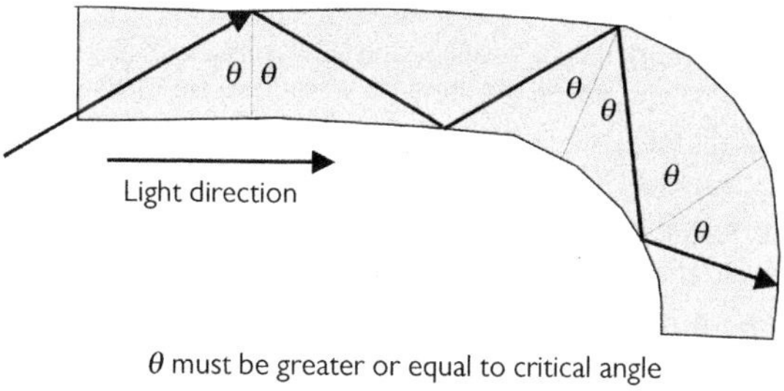


**Fig. 24.5** The bending of optical fibres.

electronically (e.g. C-MAC) or optically (e.g. Glidescope) to a screen on the handle or to a screen more remotely placed in order to aid training. The blade is either a MacIntosh-shaped blade (e.g. C-MAC, Glidescope) or hyperangulated (C-MAC D-blade). It allows a view 'around a corner' of the pharynx, and a better view of the larynx with less local trauma. It also allows laryngoscopy with reduced movement of the head and neck, important sometimes. Clearly the laryngoscopist must be trained in its use, and it is better if a whole department undergoes training and acceptance in its use, both in the operating theatre and the intensive care unit (Cook *et al.* 2018). However, being an expert with a standard MacIntosh laryngoscope or with one type of VL does not equate to expertise with another type of VL (Kelly and Cook 2016). Furthermore, although a good camera view of the larynx is usually obtained with VL, it does not follow that intubation will always be easy, so there may yet be a need for a bougie, and an appropriate choice of VL must be made in advance.

## *Fibre optic intubation*

The use of a fibre optic scope to aid awake intubation is well established. Where there is some doubt about the ability to visualise the vocal cords with orthodox laryngoscopy, or to maintain the integrity of the airway following intravenous induction of anaesthesia, awake intubation using an endotracheal tube railroaded on to the fibre optic laryngo- or broncho-scope is an extremely valuable technique.

Fibreoptic visualisation of the trachea and bronchi is also helpful following insertion of a double-lumen tube to ensure correct positioning. It can also be used through an intubating or classical LMA or an I-gel to visualise the state of the glottis prior to intubation in an anaesthetised patient, and subsequently to access the trachea with a railroaded endotracheal tube (de Lloyd *et al.* 2010).

## *Bougies and catheters*

These simple devices as aids to intubation should not be forgotten in the quest for technology. Frequently, when the view of the glottis is impaired, it is easy to insert a bougie into the trachea, over which the endotracheal tube can be railroaded, when there may be some difficulty inserting a tube directly. The bougie must be relatively new, with the right level of stiffness along its length, with an adjustable tip, which may even be steerable. Care must be taken not to damage mucosa as it is inserted. A Cook catheter is like a hollow bougie, which is easy to insert and through which the patient may be ventilated while awaiting the insertion of the railroaded endotracheal tube.

## *References*

**Bucx, M. J. L.**, **Sniders, C.**, **van Geel, R. T. M.** ***et al.*** (1994) Forces acting on the maxillary incisor teeth during laryngoscopy using the McIntosh laryngoscope, *Anaesthesia*, **49**, pp. 1064–70.

**Cook, T. M.**, **Boniface, N. J**, **Seller, C.** ***et al.*** **(**2018) Universal videolaryngoscopy: a structured approach to videolaryngoscopy for all intubations in an anaesthetic and an intensive care department, *Br. J. Anaesth.*, **20**(1), 173–80.

**de Lloyd, L., Hodzovic, I., Voisey, S.** ***et al.*** (2010) Comparison of fibrescope guided intubation via the classic laryngeal mask airway and I-gel in a manikin, *Anaesthesia*, **65**, pp. 36–43.

**Goodwin, N.**, **Wilkes, A. and Hall, J.** (2006) Flexibility and light emission of disposable paediatric Miller 1 laryngoscopic blades, *Anaesthesia*, **61**, pp. 792–9.

**Kelly, F. E.** and **Cook, T. M.** (2016) Seeing is believing: getting the best out of videolaryngoscopy. *Br. J. Anaesth.*, **117**, Suppl 1, pp. 19–113.

**Lange, M., Frommer, M., Redel, A.** ***et al.*** (2009) Comparison of Glidescope and Airtraq optical laryngoscopes in patients undergoing direct microlaryngoscopy, *Anaesthesia*, **64**, pp. 323–8.

**McCoy, E. P. and Mirakhur, R. K.** (1993) The levering laryngoscope, *Anaesthesia*, **48**, 1993, pp. 516–519.

**McElwain, J., Malik, M., Harte,** B. ***et al.*** (2010) Comparison of the C-MAC videolaryngoscope with the MacIntosh, Glidescope and Airtraq laryngoscopes in easy and difficult laryngoscopy scenarios in manikins, *Anaesthesia*, **65**, pp. 483–9.

**Powell, L.**, **Andrzejowski, J.**, **Taylor, R.** and **Turnbull, D.** (2009) Comparison of four laryngoscopes in a high fidelity simulator using normal and difficult airway, *Br. J. Anaesth.*, **103**, pp. 755–60.

**Ray, D. C.**, **Billington, C.**, **Kearns, P. K.** ***et al.*** (2009) A comparison of McGrath and Macintosh laryngoscopes in novice users: a manikin study, *Anaesthesia*, **64**, pp. 1207–10.

# Chapter 25 **Breathing systems**

The chapter links with: Chapters 7, 11, 14, 15, 16 and 26.

## Introduction

An anaesthetic breathing system is a means of transferring the breathing gas mixture from the anaesthetic machine common gas outlet to the patient. It is also the means of transferring the exhaled gas from the patient to the outside world, usually via a scavenging system. Alternatively, after the carbon dioxide is absorbed from the exhaled gas, the unused fresh gas components of the exhaled gas are recirculated back to the patient. In general, a breathing system consists of a fresh gas limb, an inspiratory and expiratory limb, an expiratory valve, a reservoir bag and it may also consist of one or more unidirectional valves and a $CO_2$ absorber. The simpler devices have fewer components and usually involve some rebreathing of expiratory gas, depending on the level of fresh gas flow. The ability to minimise rebreathing at as economical a fresh gas flow as possible is a measure of the breathing system's efficiency. Depending on the precise design of the breathing system, such efficiency will vary depending on whether the patient is breathing spontaneously or is undergoing controlled artificial ventilation (see Chapter 26). The more complex systems ensure minimum rebreathing by the use of unidirectional valves and $CO_2$ absorption systems; in this way, the additional complexity allows more economical use of fresh gas and volatile agent.

The systems that use higher fresh gas flows (FGF) and involve some rebreathing were classified in 1954 by Professor Mapleson, according to their behaviour in terms of the FGF requirement to prevent $CO_2$ rebreathing (Mapleson 1954). At the time and for three decades beyond, they were the most popular breathing systems in UK anaesthetic practice. The *Mapleson Classification* of rebreathing systems is shown in Figure 25.1.

## The Mapleson classification of semi-closed rebreathing systems

### *Mapleson A systems*

The *Magill* breathing system was invented by Sir Ivan Whiteside Magill in the early twentieth century. As shown in Figure 25.1A and Figure 25.2, the system is characterised by having the expiratory valve close to the patient and the fresh gas inflow at a distance from the patient, but close to the reservoir bag. Because of this particular configuration, the system is very economical in spontaneous breathing. On inspiration fresh gas from the gas supply and that already stored in the reservoir bag travels down the tubing towards the patient. The expiratory valve is closed at this point of the respiratory cycle and the deadspace of the system contains a small amount of alveolar ($CO_2$ containing) gas from the previous exhaled breath; the system deadspace lies between the patient's mouth and the expiratory valve. This is the first gas to be inhaled on the next inspiration. The last gas to be inhaled on inspiration is fresh gas, which therefore resides in the patient's own deadspace and becomes the first gas to be exhaled on expiration. On early expiration the pressure in the breathing system has not risen adequately for the expiratory valve to open and the fresh gas from the patient's deadspace is stored in the tubing. As expiration proceeds, the expiratory valve opens and alveolar gas is preferentially exhaled. In the meantime, fresh gas from the gas supply is being stored in the tube and reservoir bag. This means that relatively low fresh gas flows can be used while keeping rebreathing to a minimum, which also reduces the

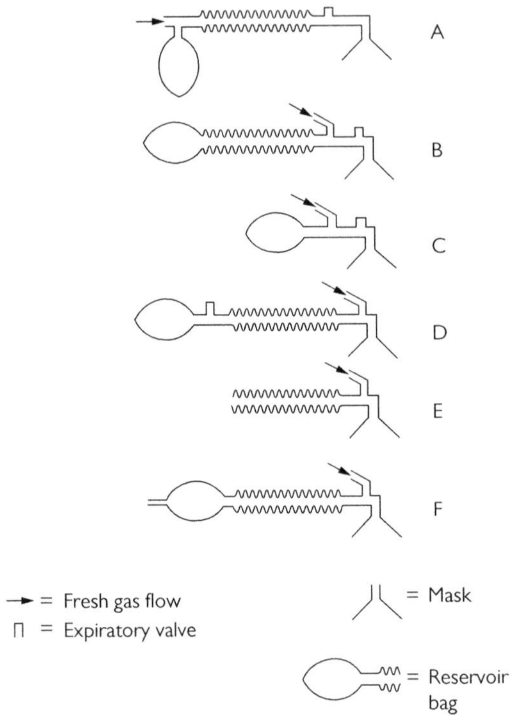


**Fig. 25.1** The Mapleson classification of semi-closed rebreathing systems.

likelihood of spilling fresh gas from the valve. In fact, no significant rebreathing occurs when the FGF falls to as low as 70% of the patient's minute ventilation, and this efficiency is unrelated to the respiratory pattern (Cook 1996a, b). If the FGF falls any lower, then more of the expired alveolar gas is stored in the tubing for subsequent rebreathing. Figure 25.2 shows the distribution of fresh gas, deadspace gas and alveolar gas in early and late expiration, at low and high FGFs. The system also imposes minimum respiratory work on the patient (Ooi *et al.* 1993b).

A modern variant of the Magill system is shown in Figure 25.3; it is known as the *Lack* breathing system. It consists of two concentric tubes, inspiration occurring down the outer, expiration down the inner. The expiratory inner tube must therefore be of sufficient diameter in order not to create significant resistance to expiration and it must be accommodated within the inspiratory outer tube. Therefore, the concentric Lack is 30 mm in diameter, wider than the standard 22 mm tubing. If it is compared with the Magill system, it can be seen that the Lack system is functionally identical to the Magill, and is probably as efficient as the MaGill (Miller *et al.* 1989). The expiratory outlet from the common part of the system is close to the patient, although the valve itself is at some distance and the fresh gas inlet and reservoir bag are distant from the patient. There is also a version called the *parallel Lack* system, where the tubes lie side by side rather than concentrically and may superficially resemble a circle system (Ooi *et al.* 1993a).

If such Mapleson A systems are used for controlled ventilation, the efficiency of the gas usage is relatively poor. The design, which preferentially excretes alveolar gas and stores fresh gas in spontaneous breathing, does the opposite when positive pressure breathing is applied. To facilitate inspiration, if the reservoir bag is squeezed, or if a bellows is applied to the reservoir limb, the pressure in the system increases, the partially closed expiratory valve near the patient opens and the fresh gas stored in the tube is preferentially excreted, although some will go to the patient. On expiration, the system preferentially

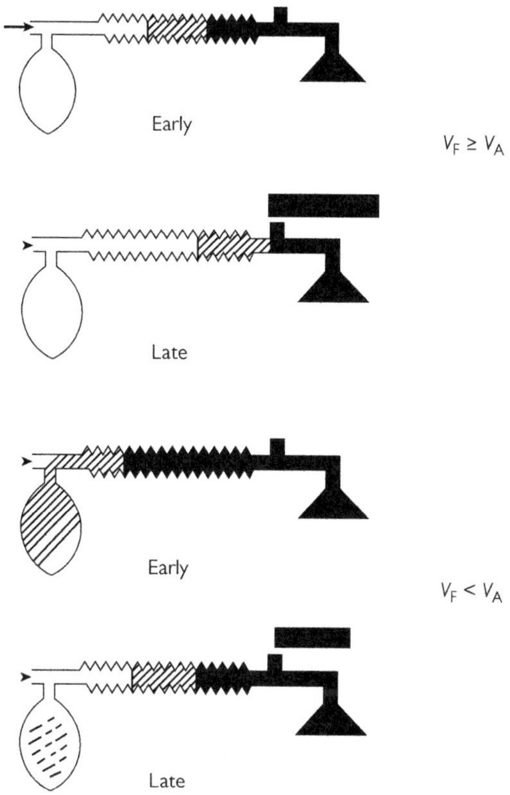


**Fig. 25.2** Distribution of gas in a Mapleson A (Magill) breathing system in early and late expiration at FGFs at least equal to (top pair) and greater than (bottom pair) alveolar ventilation ($V_A$); white is fresh gas; hatched is deadspace gas, black is alveolar gas.

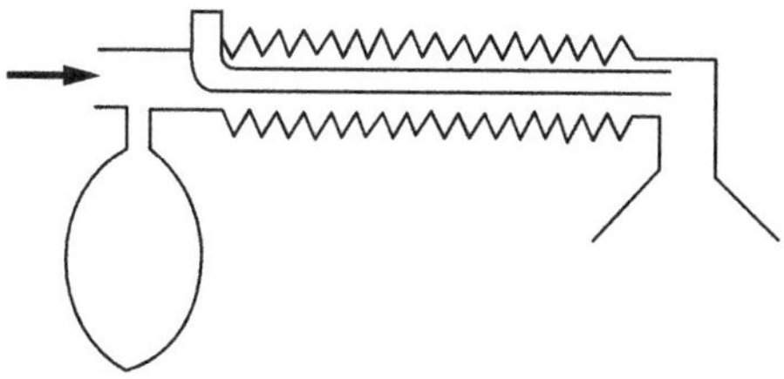

**Fig. 25.3** The coaxial Mapleson A (Lack) breathing system.

fills with alveolar gas, partly because of the partially closed valve, and it is ready to be rebreathed on the next inspiration (Waters and Mapleson 1961). Mapleson A systems are the least appropriate systems for controlled ventilation and a FGF of four times minute ventilation, with an expiratory time of four times inspiratory time, is required to prevent rebreathing (Tyler *et al*. 1989).

The efficiency of the Mapleson A system in controlled ventilation could be improved if the escape of fresh gas during inspiration could be prevented. Figure 25.4 shows such a modification, known as the

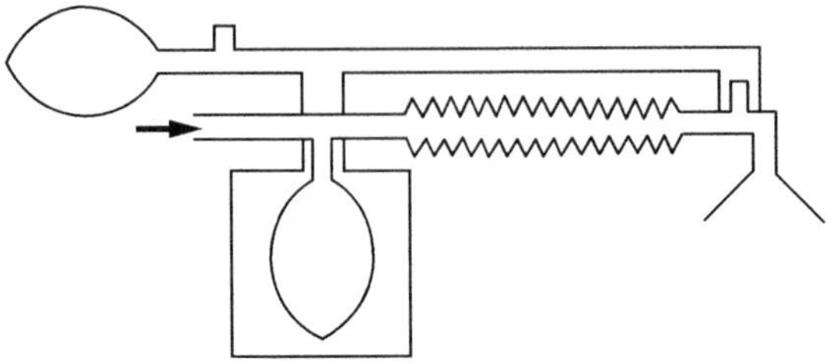

Fig. 25.4 The Miller modification (Enclosed MaGill) breathing system.

*Miller modification* (Miller and Miller 1988,). One study has demonstrated a greater efficiency of the enclosed Mapleson A in controlled ventilation than the Mapleson D (Tham *et al.* 1993). The generic term for the Miller modification is the *enclosed afferent reservoir system* (EAR) and has been shown to minimise rebreathing at a FGF of at least 80 ml $kg^{-1}$ $min^{-1}$ (Jennings *et al.* 1992).

## Mapleson B and C systems

These are shown in Figure 25.1B and C for historical interest only, since they were once commonly used in UK anaesthetic rooms. A version of the Mapleson B forms the basis of modern mask-bag-valve resuscitators (Lee and Yip 2023).

## Mapleson D, E and F systems—T pieces

These are shown in Figure 25.1D, E and F and are otherwise known as *T pieces*, because the fresh gas is delivered to the system at a T junction close to the patient. This feature is common to all T pieces, whether the rest of the system has merely tubing or an open tailed reservoir bag and an expiratory valve. Functionally, T pieces have a common mode of performance, due to the close proximity of the fresh gas delivery close to the patient end of the system, which ensures preferential delivery of fresh gas. Figure 25.5 shows a sinusoidal inspiratory waveform and a constant FGF. In the early part of inspiration, the FGF exceeds the inspiratory requirement. Area 'A' represents fresh gas that could be stored in the system for later use; area 'B' represents a time when the inspiratory requirement exceeds the FGF; if B ≤ A, then the gas rebreathed from the system consists solely of stored fresh gas, providing it has

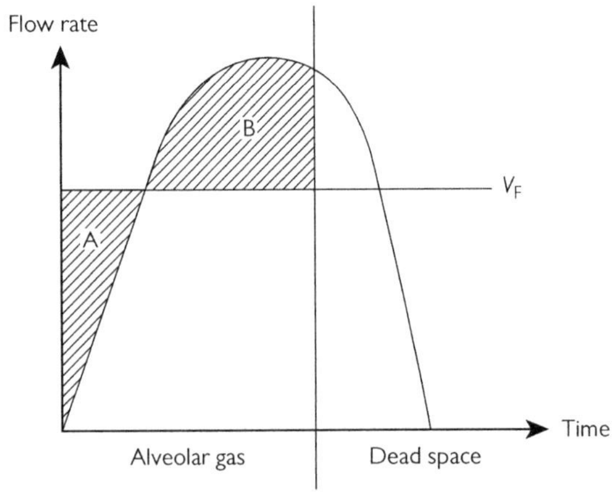


Fig. 25.5 The functional gas storage property of T pieces; by storing the fresh gas and deadspace gas in the reservoir of a T piece, rebreathing can be avoided at FGFs less than peak inspiratory flow rate.

remained unmixed with alveolar gas. T pieces need a higher FGF than Mapleson A systems to minimise rebreathing in spontaneous rebreathing, but are more efficient than Mapleson A in controlled ventilation. A FGF of about twice the minute ventilation is needed, but the exact FGF required depends on the inspiratory flow waveform, $V_D$ to $V_T$ and $I$ to $E$ ratios (Mapleson 1954; Mapleson 1958). The performance of these systems is highly dependent on a long expiratory pause (Cook 1996a, b).

### *Mapleson D*

This system has a reservoir bag and expiratory valve distant from the patient. In spontaneous breathing, the patient inspires fresh gas from the T junction and some alveolar gas from the previous exhaled breath from the tubing and reservoir bag. On expiration, the anatomical deadspace fresh gas is lost to the system, alveolar gas follows and it is eventually excreted from the distant expiratory valve. As fresh gas continues to be supplied during expiration, it too is stored in the tubing. The higher the fresh gas flow, the greater will be the ratio of fresh gas to alveolar gas stored in the tubing for the next inspiration, and the more quickly will alveolar gas be excreted. In controlled ventilation, squeezing the reservoir bag in inspiration uses the column of stored gas (alveolar and fresh) in the tubing to push a bolus of relatively pure fresh gas into the patient. Expiration follows the same pattern as in spontaneous breathing. It can be seen from Figures 25.1D and 25.5, that factors that exacerbate rebreathing in this system are a low FGF and an inadequate length of tubing: the tubing should generally be about 1 m long.

Figure 25.6 shows a latter variant of the Mapleson D, known as the *Bain system*, designed by Bain and Spoerel in 1972 (Bain and Spoerel 1972). It is a system of concentric tubes and superficially resembles the Lack. However, the FGF is delivered down the relatively narrow bore inner tube, which delivers the gas close to the patient (as a T piece). Expiration occurs down the standard diameter outer tube towards a distant reservoir bag and expiratory valve. Care must be taken with this, as with all coaxial systems, that the inner coaxial tube does not become detached at either end or the system's deadspace become much larger (Heath and Marks 1991). There are two tests for the integrity of such a system before use: in one an obturator is applied to the inner tube to ensure its integrity from leakage; in the other, on passing a high flow of oxygen through the inner tube, collapse of the reservoir bag must be observed to demonstrate its continuity from one end to the other. Coaxial systems should not be used with intermittent flow anaesthetic machines, since the narrow inner tube does not allow the patient's inspiratory effort to be transmitted to the demand valve of the machine.

In spontaneous breathing, a FGF of between 2.5 and 3 times the patient's minute ventilation (Conway *et al.* 1977) is required to prevent rebreathing. Any reduction in this value leads to a sudden increase in rebreathing or ventilation or both. The coaxial T piece may not be as efficient as the orthodox Mapleson D because the coaxial arrangement at the patient end of the system may encourage gas mixing.

Figure 25.7 shows graphs of FGF delivery plotted against patient minute volume required for controlled ventilation from T pieces in adults for different values of $P_{ECO_2}$. Generally, a FGF of between 70 and 100 ml kg$^{-1}$ min$^{-1}$ is sufficient for normocapnia, providing minute ventilation is kept sufficiently high at between 120 and 150 ml kg$^{-1}$ min$^{-1}$ (Bain and Spoerel 1973).

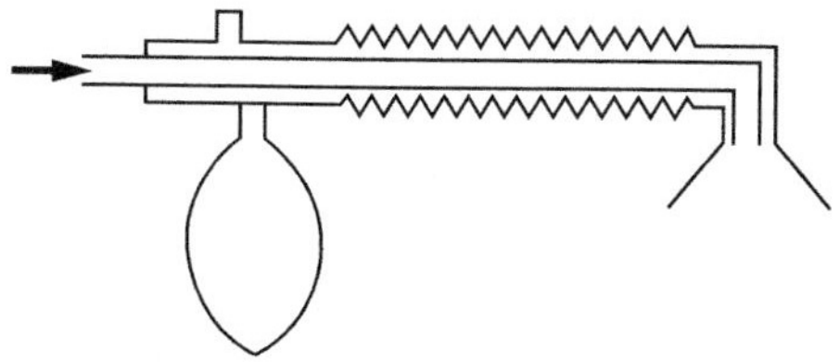

**Fig. 25.6** The coaxial Mapleson D (Bain) breathing system.

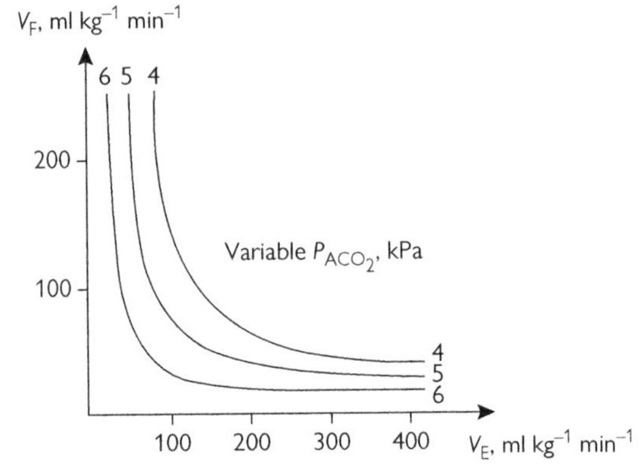


**Fig. 25.7** A graphical aid to estimating alveolar $P_{CO2}$ ($P_{ACO2}$) in kPa, from a given combination of FGF ($V_F$) and minute ventilation ($V_E$).

With the advent of the need to ventilate patients from a distance in an MRI scanner, the long Bain breathing system has been introduced. The additional length increases the compliance of the system such that smaller tidal volumes and higher end expiratory pressures result (Sweeting *et al.* 2002).

## *Mapleson E and F*

These systems are otherwise known respectively as the *Ayre's T piece* and with its *Jackson Rees modification*, shown in Figure 25.1E and F. The Ayre's T piece was invented by Phillip Ayre in 1937 for use in cleft lip and palate surgery in children. In deciding on the length of the reservoir tube, too long a tube would add unnecessary deadspace, which might permit rebreathing; too short a tube would allow dilution of fresh gas with air. A tube of a volume one third that of the patient's tidal volume is the optimal length (Ayre 1956). The valveless system is simple and provides low resistance to spontaneous breathing for small children (Hatch 1987), although there are now some variants with an overflow valve. Jackson Rees' modification is the addition of an open tailed reservoir bag to allow visible monitoring of breathing, as well as a means of manual controlled ventilation. The FGF required to avoid rebreathing is twice the child's minute ventilation, $V_{min}$:

$$V_{min} = V_T \times f,$$

where $V_T$ is tidal volume and *f* is respiratory rate = 7 ml kg$^{-1}$ body weight × (15–30 breaths min$^{-1}$).

**Table 25.1** Fresh gas flow requirements for children per minute using a T piece under controlled ventilation

| | Patient weight, kg | | |
|---|---|---|---|
| Rosea and Froese | | Predicted $PaCO_2$kPa | |
| | | 4.9 | 4 |
| | 10.0-30.0 | 1000 ml + 100 ml kg$^{-1}$ | 1600 ml + 100 ml kg$^{-1}$ |
| | >30 | 2000 ml + 50 ml kg$^{-1}$ | 3200 ml + 50 ml kg$^{-1}$ |
| Hatch | | Measured $PECO_2$ = 4.5 kPa, $PICO_2$ < 0.5 kPa | |
| | 3.0–20.0 | 1000 ml + 200 ml kg$^{-1}$ | |

Table 25.1 shows some suggestions for the FGF for this particular T piece for controlled ventilation in children and these techniques have been confirmed in clinical use (Park *et al.* 1998). However, the reader is encouraged to check current paediatric practice in this regard in specialist paediatric anaesthetic texts.

## Humphrey ADE system

This system was designed in 1983 by Humphrey in South Africa, so that, at turn of a lever, a system with Mapleson A characteristics could be used for spontaneous ventilation, and a system with D and E characteristics was available for controlled ventilation (Humphrey *et al.* 1986) and can be used for paediatric patients as well (Orlikowski *et al.* 1991).

## Venturi systems

A Venturi can be incorporated into a Bain system to deliver fresh gas and entrain expiratory gas that has had its $CO_2$ absorbed by a soda lime canister, to reduce the FGF requirements to 30 ml kg$^{-1}$ min$^{-1}$ (Jörgensen and Hansen 1985). However, care must be taken in its design if adequate inspired oxygen concentrations are to be preserved (Campbell and Fairfield 1996; Magee 2014). A similar device has been incorporated into a Magill system to reduce FGF requirements to 40 ml kg$^{-1}$ min$^{-1}$ (Jakubazsko *et al.* 1989).

## The circle system

This is altogether a more complex system in which exhaled gas is recirculated, but is the system in most common use today. It incorporates unidirectional valves and a means of absorbing carbon dioxide. Its advantage is the ability to use low, very low or minimal FGF (Virtue 1974), which is appropriate with the use of expensive modern volatile agents. Its disadvantage is its complexity; there are many

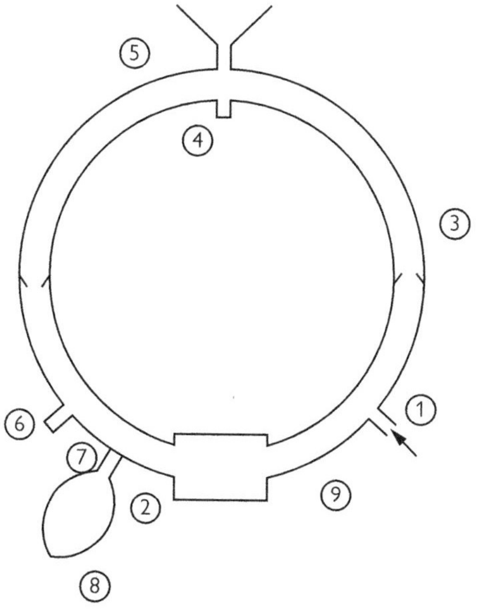


**Fig. 25.8** Arrangement of components of a circle system. See text for referral to numbered points.

components and connections and the inspired gas concentrations are not closely related to the concentrations dialled up on rotameters or the vaporiser, particularly at low FGFs. Therefore, in the modern era, sophisticated gas monitors are needed and have become the required standard.

In deciding where to place the various components of a circle system, shown in Figure 25.8, Eger (Eger 1974) suggested three rules:

- there must be a unidirectional valve between the reservoir bag and the patient, on both the inspiratory and expiratory sides;
- fresh gas must not enter the system between the patient and the expiratory valve;
- the overflow valve must not be placed between the patient and the inspiratory unidirectional valve.

Different configurations of circle systems have different efficiencies, as defined by fresh gas utilisation (Zbinden *et al.* 1991). Figure 25.9 shows three configurations of the system, A, C and H, that obey these rules and that otherwise have slightly different characteristics (Eger and Ethans 1968). In evolving circle system designs, it was found that the greatest efficiency in spontaneous breathing occurred where the overflow valve is close to the patient (cf. the Magill system); this arrangement is least efficient in controlled ventilation, except when both unidirectional valves are also close to the

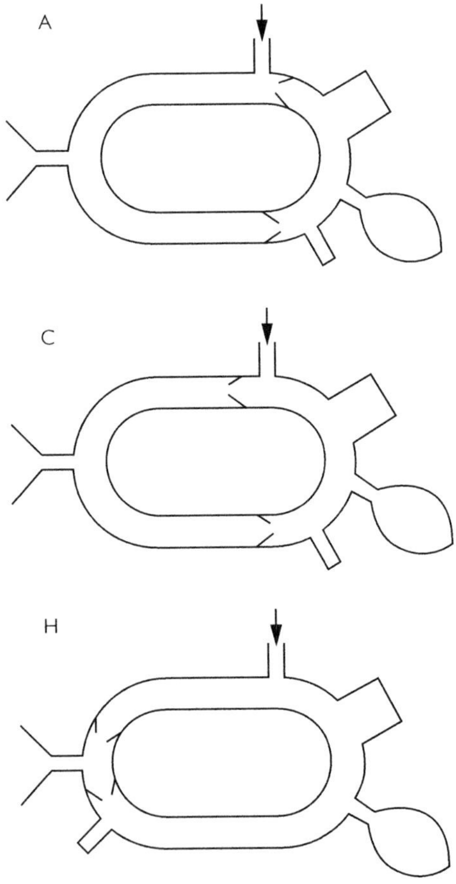


**Fig. 25.9** Three arrangements of the circle system with different behavioural characteristics.

patient (system H). The differences between systems are not great, but become accentuated as FGF is reduced.

Referring again to Figure 25.8, in deciding where to put the FGF inlet, the best compromise is achieved in position 1, just downstream of the $CO_2$ absorber. Fresh gas can collect retrogradely in the absorber and reservoir bag, pushing expired gas back towards the overflow valve. At low flows, the vented alveolar gas will not yet have passed through the absorber, thus economising on its use. As the FGF is increased, so does the likelihood of venting expired gas that has already passed through the absorber, as well as venting fresh gas itself. Placing the FGF inlet at position 2, upstream of the absorber, could help humidify the fresh gas, but may also cause unnecessary venting of fresh gas and venting of absorbent dust into the inspiratory limb, as well as preventing retrograde flow of recently exhaled alveolar gas.

During controlled ventilation, gas spills out of the overflow valve during inspiration. In order to minimise the chance of this being fresh gas, the best position for the overflow valve is at 6 or 7 as shown in Figure 25.8, which will preferentially allow for venting of alveolar gas before it has reached the absorber.

Equal efficiency can be obtained during spontaneous and controlled ventilation with the reservoir bag in positions 8 or 9. If the bag is downstream of the absorber at position 9, then in controlled ventilation a squeeze of the bag forces retrograde flow of gases already cleared of $CO_2$ back through the absorber. Placing the bag upstream of the absorber in position 8 allows retrograde filling of the bag with fresh gas and this is the most common position of the reservoir bag. A modern development of circle system structure is characterised by a coaxial inspiratory limb (Cook and Chakrabati 1996); such a modification improves the response time at low FGFs to step changes in fresh gas concentrations.

A most critical part of the circle system is the $CO_2$ absorber, which has to be designed to allow low resistance to flow and to avoid *channelling*, where gas flows through the absorbent crystals along paths of least resistance, thus avoiding contact with the absorbent in other parts of the absorber. Although absorbent canisters have traditionally been large and arranged in two halves to allow partial change of absorbent, modern canisters are smaller and anticipate more frequent exchange of crystals (Shaw and Scott 1998).

Two absorbents in common use are soda lime and Baralyme. Soda lime consists of 4% sodium hydroxide, 1% potassium hydroxide, 14–19% water and the rest as calcium hydroxide (Dorsch *et al.* 1984). Additionally, there are small amounts of silica for drying, kieselguhr for hardening and dye indicators to show when the crystals are spent. The water is essential for the reaction, which occurs as:

$$CO_2 + H_2O \Leftrightarrow H_2CO_3$$

$$2NaOH + 2H_2CO_3 + Ca(OH_2) \Leftrightarrow CaCO_3 + Na_2CO_3 + 4H_2O.$$

These reactions occur with the liberation of heat and water, both of which are useful by-products in the context of heat and humidity preservation of the patient.

Baralyme is a mixture of 20% barium hydroxide, 80% calcium hydroxide and some potassium hydroxide. The water for the reaction is present as the octahydrate of barium hydroxide.

In all cases the monovalent hydroxides are more reactive than the divalent $Ca(OH)_2$. Where crystals have been allowed to dry out, such as leaving the gas flowing through the canister overnight, these highly reactive monovalent hydroxides can also produce significant amounts of carbon monoxide and even formaldehyde. An absorbent consisting of only $Ca(OH)_2$ (Amsorb, Belfast) has been produced to counteract this (Bedi 2001).

As well as absorbing $CO_2$, the absorbents also tend to absorb volatile agents; this is generally acceptable, though wasteful, with a major exception: when the volatile agent *trichloroethylene* reacts with soda lime, it produces dichloroacetylene gas, otherwise known as phosgene, a neurotoxic agent. When Sevoflurane was being developed, it was thought to react with soda lime to produce a renally toxic agent, *Compound A*; this was not found to be of clinical significance (Baxter *et al.* 1998) although in the USA the Federal Drug Administration recommends keeping the FGF at more than 3 $L min^{-1}$ under these conditions. Soda lime that is allowed to dry out has been found to encourage carbon monoxide formation (Harrison *et al.* 1996). Indicators added to the absorbent show when it needs replacing. Ethyl violet is a commonly used example, although its usefulness can be impaired by photo deactivation by fluorescent lighting (Andrews *et al.* 1990).

The purpose of using a circle system is to use low FGF in order to economise on the consumption of increasingly expensive volatile agents and minimise pollution; an agent concentration on the vaporiser of 1% of a low FGF uses much less agent than 1% at a high FGF. At the start of an anaesthetic, none of the body tissues contains anaesthetic agent. To enhance anaesthetic uptake and excretion of nitrogen, high FGF is generally used at the start (Mapleson 1998). When clinically desirable levels are reached in relevant tissues, these FGF's can be reduced, theoretically to metabolic $O_2$ consumption rate, say 250 ml $min^{-1}$, assuming no gas leakage and no further uptake by tissues or tubing. In reality both exist and some nitrous oxide and volatile agent is also switched on. The response time of the system is inversely proportional to the difference between gas inflow and tissue uptake and directly proportional to system volume (Conway 1986). At high FGF, gas concentrations delivered to the circle system from the anaesthetic machine are nearly equal to those received by the patient. As FGF becomes a significantly smaller part of what the patient receives, the majority being recirculated gas, the gas concentrations received by the patient bear significantly less resemblance to those delivered by the anaesthetic machine (Mapleson 1960). At the beginning of an anaesthetic, when anaesthetic gas uptake by the patient from the alveoli to the tissues is high (oxygen uptake being relatively constant), alveolar $O_2$ concentrations appear higher than expected and this effect becomes very marked as FGF is reduced. As the anaesthetic proceeds and tissues become saturated, less anaesthetic gas is absorbed from the system, alveolar $O_2$ concentrations are lower than expected and this effect also becomes more marked as FGF is reduced (Conway 1981). This degree of uncertainty means that $O_2$, volatile agent and $N_2O$ monitoring, with gases sampled from the patient end of the system, are highly desirable, possibly mandatory. The capital cost of such monitoring is offset within a short time against the revenue savings on volatile agent. Furthermore, the oxygen consumption of patients can vary, as can the rate of uptake of anaesthetic agents. There are coaxial versions of circle systems available, which have similar performance to the standard version (Magee 2014). The whole matter of the use of nitrous oxide and volatile agents is currently under scrutiny, as they are greenhouse gasses and $N_2O$ depletes the ozone layer (Campbell and Pierce 2015). To this end, the use of total intravenous anaesthesia (TIVA) is being encouraged, even though these gaseous and volatile agents remain clinically useful (Buhre *et al.* 2019).

Circle systems can be used for paediatric anaesthesia, using a 1 L reservoir bag and smaller bore tubing. Despite the presence of valves, the work of breathing has been found to be acceptable (Conterato *et al.* 1989).

## References

**Andrews, J. J., Johnston, R. V., Bee, D. E.** and **Arens, J. F.** (1990) Photodeactivation of ethyl violet: a potential hazard of Sodasorb, *Anesthesiology*, **72**, pp. 59–64.

**Ayre, P.** (1956) The T-piece technique, *Br. J. Anaesth.*, **28**, pp. 520–3.

**Bain, J. A.** and **Spoerel, W. E.** (1972) A streamlined anaesthetic system, Canad. *Anaesth. Soc. J.*, **19**, pp. 426–35.

**Bain, J. A.** and **Spoerel, W. E.** (1973) Flow requirements for a modified Mapleson D system during controlled ventilation, *Canad. Anaesth. Soc. J.*, **20**, pp. 629–36.

**Baxter, A. *et al.*** (1998) Formation of carbon monoxide from difluoro-methyl ether anaesthetics, *Anesthesiology*, **89**, pp. 937–40.

**Bedi, A.** (2001) The in vitro performance of carbon dioxide absorbent with and without strong alkali, *Anaesthesia*, **56**, pp. 546–50.

**Buhre, W., Disma, N., Hendricx, J. *et al.*** (2019) European Society of Anaesthesiology Task Force on Nitrous Oxide: a narrative review of its role in clinical practice, *Br. J. Anaesth.*, **122**(5), pp. 587–604.

**Campbell, D. J.** and **Fairfield, M. C.** (1996) The delivery of oxygen by a venturi T-piece, *Anaesthesia*, **51**, pp. 558–60.

**Campbell, M.** and **Pierce, M. J. T.** (2015) Atmospheric science, anaesthesia, and the environment, *BJA Educ.*, **15**, 173–9.

**Conterato, J., Lindahl, S. G., Meyer, D. M.** and **Bires J. A.** (1989) Assessment of spontaneous ventilation in anesthetised children with use of a pediatric circle or a Jackson-Rees system, *Anesth. Analg.*, **69**, pp. 484–90.

**Conway, C. M., Seeley, H. F.** and **Barnes, P.K.** (1977) Spontaneous ventilation with the Bain anaesthetic system, *Br. J. Anaesth.*, **49**, pp. 1245–9.

**Conway, C. M.** (1981) Alveolar gas relationships during use of the circle system with carbon dioxide absorption, *Br. J. Anaesth.*, **53**, pp. 1135–46.

**Conway, C. M.** (1986) Gaseous homeostasis and the circle system; factors influencing anaesthetic gas exchange, *Br. J. Anaesth.*, **58**, pp. 1167–80.

**Cook, L. B.** (1996a) Respiratory pattern and rebreathing in the Mapleson A, C and D systems with spontaneous ventilation. A theory, *Anaesthesia*, **51**, pp. 371–85.

**Cook, L. B.** (1996b) The importance of the expiratory pause. Comparison of the Mapleson A, C and D rebreathing systems using a lung model, *Anaesthesia*, **51**, pp. 453–60.

**Cook, L. B**. and **Chakrabarti, M. K.** (1996) Circle systems with a coaxial inspiratory limb, *Anaesthesia*, **51**, pp. 247–54.

**Eger, E. I. II** and **Ethans, C. T**. (1968) The effects of inflow, overflow and valve placement on the economy of the circle system, *Anesthesiology*, **29**, pp. 93–100.

**Eger, E. I. II** (1974) *Anesthetic systems: construction and function. Chapter 13 in Anesthetic Uptake and Action*, Williams & Wilkins, Philadelphia, PA, pp. 206–27.

**Harrison, N., Knowles, A. C.** and **Welchew, E. A.** (1996) Carbon monoxide within circle systems, *Anaesthesia*, **51**, pp. 1037–40.

**Hatch, D. J.** (1987) Paediatric anaesthetic equipment, *Br. J. Anaesth.*, **57**, 672–84.

**Heath, P. J.** and **Marks, L. F.** (1991) Modified occlusion tests for the Bain breathing system, *Anaesthesia*, **46**, pp. 213–16.

**Humphrey, D., Bock-Utne, J. G.** and **Downing, J. W.** (1986) Single lever Humphrey ADE low flow universal breathing system: Part I: comparison with dual lever ADE, MaGill and Bain systems in spontaneously breathing adults. Part II: Comparison with Bain system in anaesthetised adults during controlled ventilation, *Canad. Anaesth. Soc. J.*, **33**, pp. 698–718.

**Jakubazsko, J., Christensen, P. and Jorgensen, S.** (1989) The MaGill–Venturi attachment: studies in volunteers and patients, *Acta Anaesthesiol. Scand.*, **33**, pp. 422–5.

**Jennings, A. D. *et al.*** (1992) Physical characteristics of the EAR breathing system, *Br. J. Anaesth.*, **68**, pp. 625–9.

**Jorgensen, S. and Hansen, L. K.** (1985) The Venturi anaesthetic circuit. 1. An all purpose breathing system for anaesthesia, *Acta Anaesthesiol. Scand.*, **29**, pp. 269–72.

**Lee, C. P.** and **Yip, Y. Y.** (2023) Understanding your bag-valve-mask resuscitator. *BJA Educ.*, **23**(6), pp. 208–11.

**Magee, P.** (2014) The mathematical modelling and clinical testing of low flow breathing systems, *University of Bath*, PhD thesis Ch. 8, pp. 127–70.

**Mapleson, W. W.** (1960) The concentration of anaesthetics in closed circuits, with special reference to halothane. I. A theoretical study, *Br. J. Anaesth.*, **32**, pp. 298–309.

**Mapleson, W. W.** (1954) The elimination of rebreathing in various semi-closed anaesthetic systems, *Br. J. Anaesth.*, **26**, pp. 323–32.

**Mapleson, W. W.** (1998) The theoretical ideal FGF sequence at the start of low flow anaesthesia, *Anaesthesia*, **53**, pp. 264–72.

**Mapleson, W. W.** (1958) Theoretical considerations of the effects of rebreathing in two semi closed anaesthetic systems, *Br. Med. Bull.*, **14**, pp. 64–8.

**Miller, D. M.** and **Miller, J. C.** (1988) Enclosed afferent reservoir breathing systems, *Br. J. Anaesth.*, **60**, pp. 469–75.

**Miller, S. W., Barnes, P. K., Soni, N**. and **Tennant, R.** (1989) Comparison of the MaGill and Lack anaesthetic breathing systems in anaesthetised patients, *Br. J. Anaesth.*, **62**, pp. 153–8.

**Ooi, R., Lack, J. A., Soni, N., Whittle, J. and Pattison, J.** (1993a) The parallel anaesthetic Lack breathing system, *Anaesthesia*, **48**, pp. 409–14.

**Ooi**, R., **Pattison**, J. and **Soni**, N. (1993b) Additional work of breathing imposed by Mapleson A systems, *Anaesthesia*, **48**, pp. 599–603.

**Orlikowski**, C. E., **Ewart**, M. C. and **Bingham**, R. M. (1991) The Humphrey ADE system: evaluation in paediatric use, *Br. J. Anaesth.*, **66**, pp. 253–7.

**Park**, J. W. ***et al.*** (1998) Predictable normocapnoea in controlled ventilation of infants with the Jackson-Rees or the Bain system, *Anaesthesia*, **53**, pp. 1180–4.

**Shaw**, M. and **Scott**, D. H. (1998) Performance characteristics of 'to and fro' disposable soda lime canister, *Anaesthesia*, **53**, pp. 454–60.

**Sweeting**, C. J., **Thomas**, P. W. and **Sanders**, D. J. (2002) The long Bain system: an investigation into the implications of remote ventilation, *Anaesthesia*, **57**, pp. 1183–6.

**Tham**, E. J. ***et al.*** (1993) Efficiency of breathing systems A and D in the Carden Ventmasta ventilator, *Br. J. Anaesth.*, **71**, pp. 741–6.

**Tyler**, C. K. G., **Barnes**, P. K. and **Rafferty**, M. P. (1989) Controlled ventilation with a Mapleson A (MaGill) breathing system: reassessment using a lung model, *Br. J. Anaesth.*, **62**, pp. 462–6.

**Virtue**, R. W. (1974) Minimal flow nitrous oxide anesthesia, *Anesthesiology*, **40**, pp. 196–8.

**Waters**, D. J. and **Mapleson**, W. W. (1961) Rebreathing during controlled ventilation with various semi-closed anaesthetic systems, *Br. J. Anaesth.*, **33**, pp. 374–81.

**Zbinden**, A. M., **Feigenwinter**, P. and **Hutmacher**, M. (1991) Fresh gas utilization of eight circle systems, *Br. J. Anaesth.*, **67**, pp. 492–9.

# Chapter 26 **Artificial ventilators**

The chapter links with: Chapters 3, 4, 7, 11, 14, 15, 16, 22, 23, 24 and 25.

## Respiratory mechanics during ventilation

When pressure is applied by the ventilator to drive gas into the lungs, energy is expended to overcome airway resistance *R* to gas flow in the airways, in order to store gas in the alveoli, whose readiness to have their volume increased is represented by the concept of compliance, *C*. The storage of gas within individual compliances represents potential energy storage (see Chapter 3).

At conventional ventilation frequencies, the system behaves like a flow resistor in series with a compliance. These variables determine the pressure and volume changes that take place within the lung. As ventilation frequency increases into the high range, inertance (resistance to accelerative forces) becomes significant and the frequency response of anatomical structures becomes important, with phase differences between pressure and volume signals occurring (Lin *et al.* 1989), much as occurs between current and voltage in electrical circuits. Mechanical resistance, *R*, in the system is largely due to resistance to gas flow down airways and is defined as pressure change per unit flow $\Delta P/Q$, typically $4cmH_2O.\ l^{-1}\ s.$ at $0.5\ l\ s^{-1}$. However, there is a contribution from viscous resistive forces in the lung and chest wall tissues. High resistance may require long inspiratory times, while expiratory times that are too short may lead to gas-trapping in alveoli. Excessive resistance may mean that the power required to ventilate the patient exceeds that available to the ventilator.

Compliance, *C*, is a measure of the capacitative properties of the alveoli and is defined as volume change per unit pressure change $\Delta V/\Delta P$. It is not uniform throughout the respiratory cycle and has values in the range 0.05–0.10 L $(cmH_2O)^{-1}$. Dynamic compliance is the value given to this variable throughout the inspiratory period to the end of inspiration, when airway pressure is highest. During the inspiratory pause, airway pressure falls to a plateau during which the so-called static compliance can be measured, which is greater than the dynamic compliance. Compliance differs between these two parts of inspiration, because of the redistribution of gas between the lung units during the pause and because of a degree of stress relaxation in the elastic tissues of the lung. Such a phenomenon leads to hysteresis in the pressure–volume curve, shown in Figure 3.2. If compliance is low, short inspiratory times may result in inadequate lung filling; if compliance is high, normal driving pressures may be high enough to cause barotrauma.

## Ventilator mechanics

### *Ventilator classification*

Modern ventilators are very flexible in function due to fast-responding solenoid valves and sophisticated electronic controls, but some basic mechanical principles apply to all of them. Numerous methods of classifying artificial ventilators evolved, but Mapleson's classification (Mushin *et al.* 1980) has remained the most useful, defining ventilators as pressure generators (often considered as low-power ventilators) or flow generators (high power). Modern ventilators can function as both types of generator under different conditions, depending on the settings of the electronic systems which control their function, and providing there is enough pneumatic power to drive the required function. The basic classification is shown in Figure 26.1, which also shows that the ventilator has to carry out an inspiratory phase, a change from inspiration to expiration, an expiratory phase and a change from expiration to inspiration.

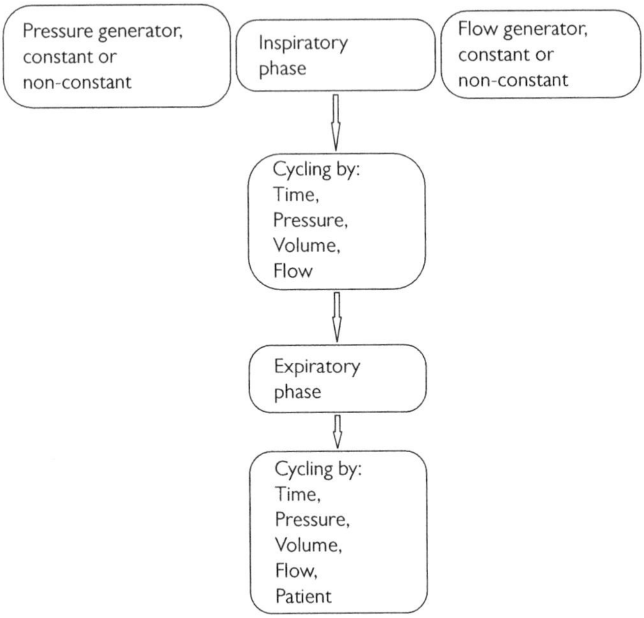


**Fig. 26.1** Ventilator classification and cycling modes.

The consideration of a ventilator as a pressure generator or a flow generator applies during the inspiratory phase, when it may be a constant or non-constant pressure or flow generator, and possibly during the expiratory phase. Cycling, the change from inspiratory to expiratory phase and vice-versa, is according to one of the variables shown in Figure 26.1, namely, time, volume, pressure, flow or patient triggering.

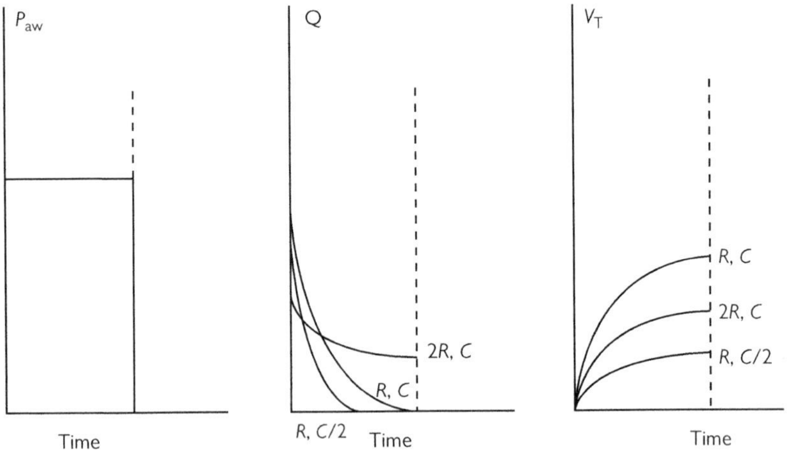


**Fig. 26.2** Effects on flow and tidal volume of altered airway resistance and lung compliance when using a constant pressure generator.

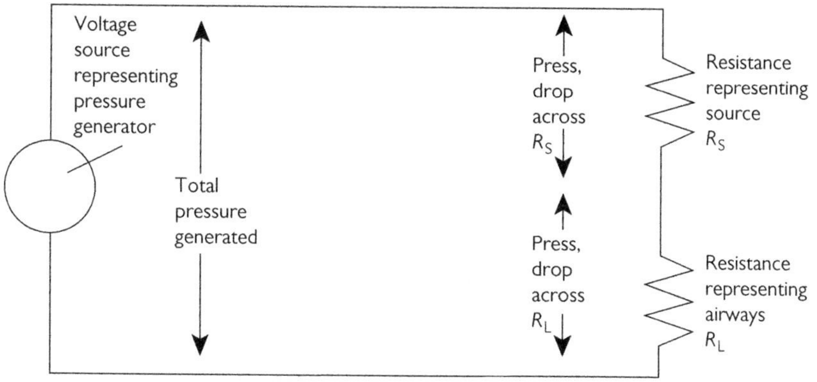


**Fig. 26.3** Electrical analogue of a constant pressure generator.

An ideal pressure generator maintains a preset pressure, $P_{aw}$, at its output, which is then delivered to the patient. The flow, $Q$, generated in the airways depends on the resistance and compliance of the respiratory system, which in turn determines the tidal volume, $V_T$, delivered to the lungs. Figure 26.2 shows the curves for $P_{aw}$, $Q$ and $V_T$ under these conditions. It also shows that, in the presence of reduced compliance or increased airway resistance, the rate of fall of $Q$ varies.

Conceptually, a constant pressure generator consists of a weighted bellows; if these bellows are spring loaded, the generator is a decreasing pressure generator, which can be thought of as a discharging compliance. A flow generator with a leak takes on the characteristics of a pressure generator in series with a resistance. These pneumatic definitions have analogies in electrical circuits (see Chapter 4).

A pressure generator delivers gas through its own internal resistance and through the resistance of the tubing. It can be thought of as generating a pressure, which is dropped across this *source resistance* $R_S$, and the series airway resistance $R_L$, shown in Figure 26.3. The presence of $R_S$ reduces the pressure available to $R_L$, which may reduce tidal volume, $V_T$. Therefore, an ideal pressure generator should keep internal and connecting tubing resistance as low as possible. The electrical analogy is of a voltage source in series with resistances $R_S$ and $R_L$. Although mechanically simpler, pressure generators may not be able to deliver adequate $V_T$ if lung $R$ and $C$ are unfavourable.

Ideal flow generators determine the preset flow pattern (constant, ramp, decelerating) that is delivered to the patient. This preset flow is maintained whatever the patient's airway resistance or lung compliance may be. Changes in patient $R$ and $C$ do not affect $Q$, but $P_{aw}$ may change under these circumstances, which, if unfavourable, may result in a rise in $P_{aw}$, high enough to cause barotrauma. Figure 26.4 shows graphs of $Q$, $P_{aw}$ and $V_T$ under conditions of constant $Q$ and the way in which low lung compliance $C$ and high airway resistance $R$ alters $P_{aw}$ is also shown.

Conceptually, constant flow generation is achieved by delivering a high generated pressure through a nozzle or high source resistance, which is how a constant current generator works in the electrical analogy. Thus, a continuum of behaviour of ventilators has now been considered, despite the initial discrete separation of flow and pressure generators. Indeed, many practical ventilators have characteristics of both, depending on the circumstances of use. Sinusoidal or other positive displacement pumps generate variable but predictable flow. Gas injectors do not necessarily produce constant flow but, as indicated, have characteristics of constant pressure generators in series with high source resistance.

The loss of gas volume $V_S$, from a flow generator to a patient's respiratory system can be thought of as an internal or source compliance $C_S$, in parallel with the lung compliance $C_L$, as in Figure 26.5. Thus, delivered tidal volume $V_T$ is the sum of $V_S$ and patient tidal volume $V_L$. The electrical analogy is of a current source connected to two parallel capacitors, $C_S$ and $C_L$. Parallel compliance becomes

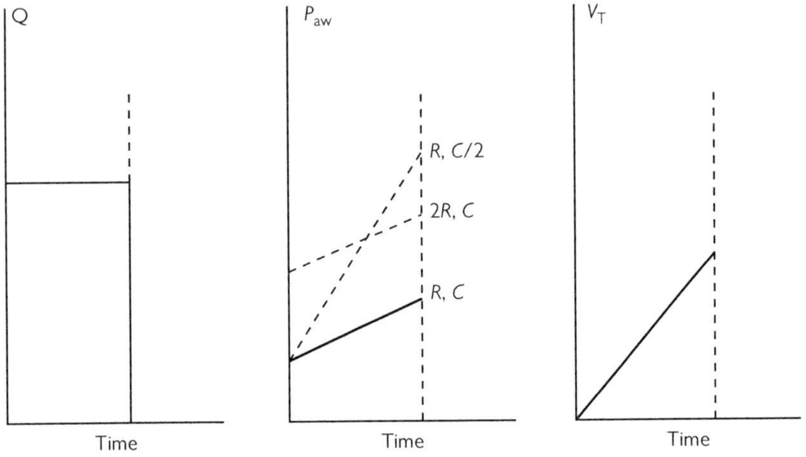


**Fig. 26.4** Effect on airway pressure and tidal volume of altered airway resistance and lung compliance when using a constant flow generator.

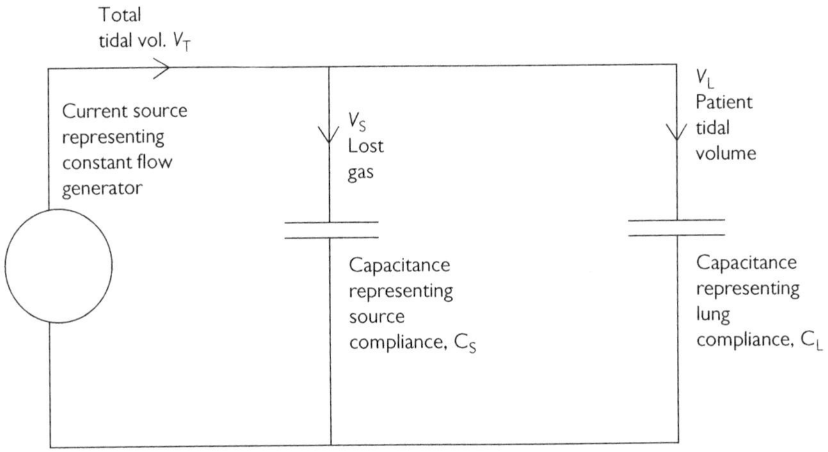


**Fig. 26.5** Electrical analogue of a constant flow generator.

significant at high ventilation frequencies and in patients with low lung compliance, such as infants. Source compliance should be minimised, but this implies narrow rigid tubing, which is not ideal if the patient is to spontaneously breathe through the same tubing, unless adequate bias flow is also present.

## Power

This is required to drive the ventilator during the active part of the inspiratory phase and, in selecting a ventilator, thought should be given to its power requirement and whether this will be adequate for the intended use. Required power can be estimated from the product of airway pressure and flowrate and a typical value is 20 W. Peak power production is likely to be the limiting variable in a ventilator and must be greater than the peak airway pressure times peak flowrate plus the energy losses described earlier. A high proportion of the required power is in overcoming the internal resistance of the ventilator; this can be as much as 200 W if the device is a flow generator, where internal resistance is high. Although more flexible, this aspect makes flow generators mechanically less efficient than pressure generators. The power provided may be from the fresh gas flow itself in minute volume dividers (e.g. the *Manley* ventilator), electrical power or compressed gas, usually oxygen.

## *Cycling*

Cycling is according to one of the variables shown in Figure 26.1; the ventilator incorporates a device to cycle at a predetermined value of those variables. Many ventilators require careful inspection to determine which variable is being used at a given moment.

In cycling from inspiration to expiration, time cycling implies that the inspiratory phase is determined solely by the ventilator and not by the characteristics of the lungs. $V_T$, $P_{aw}$ and $Q$ are all free to vary and the value at the moment of cycling depends on the effect on the lungs of the generator of flow or pressure. The mechanism is usually electronic or fluidic gating, an electromechanical device such as a solenoid, or a pneumatic spool valve. In volume cycling, $P_{aw}$ and inspiratory time vary depending on lung characteristics, but the variation is small in a constant flow (high pressure) generator. In a constant (low) pressure generator, if lung compliance is too low, $V_T$ might never be delivered and the ventilator might never volume cycle. The volume cycling device is usually a concertina bellows, whose volume can be mechanically or electrically preset. In pressure cycling, the inspiratory time alters when $R$ and $C$ vary and usually takes the form of a diaphragm toggle. Usually, a ventilator that can be triggered by a patient's breath cycles using this mechanism.

Table 26.1 summarises the effects on $V_T$ of the different forms of cycling.

## *Expiration*

This phase is generally passive and is usually a matter of discharging the gas stored in the lungs under compliance C, through airways and tubing resistance R to atmosphere. There are times when it is clinically useful to raise the expiratory pressure above atmospheric pressure in order to increase FRC and improve oxygenation; this is known as PEEP, positive end expiratory pressure. This can be done either by retarding expiratory flowrate via an expiratory limb resistor, or by using a threshold resistor that closes below a preset pressure in the expiratory limb. The methods include a flow restrictor, an underwater blow-off or a pressure sensitive solenoid valve. Negative end expiratory pressure (NEEP) is no longer used because it may induce premature airway closure.

## *Safety features*

In inexperienced hands a ventilator can be a dangerous device. All users should have a low threshold of suspicion for fault finding and be familiar with its use. Numerous variables are monitored on a ventilator (see below) and there should be appropriate alarms on these monitors so that inadequate or excessive volume or airway pressure can be detected before the patient is harmed. Safe ventilators have evolved by design and experience, but there are still potential and real problems.

**Table 26.1** Effect on tidal volume of altered airway resistance and lung compliance for different cycling modes when using ventilators with different generation characteristics.

| **Cycling mode >** | **Time** | | | **Pressure** | | | **Volume** | | |
|---|---|---|---|---|---|---|---|---|---|
| Lung/airway state > | Normal | *2R* | *C/2* | Normal | *2R* | *C/2* | Normal | *2R* | *C/2* |
| Pressure generator | $V_T$– normal | $V_T$↓ reduced | $V_T$↓ reduced | Not | possible | | $V_T$– | Cycling volume may not be reached | |
| Flow generator | $V_T$– normal | $V_T$– normal | $V_T$– normal | $V_T$– normal | $V_T$↓ reduced | $V_T$↓ reduced | $V_T$– normal | $V_T$– normal | $V_T$– normal |

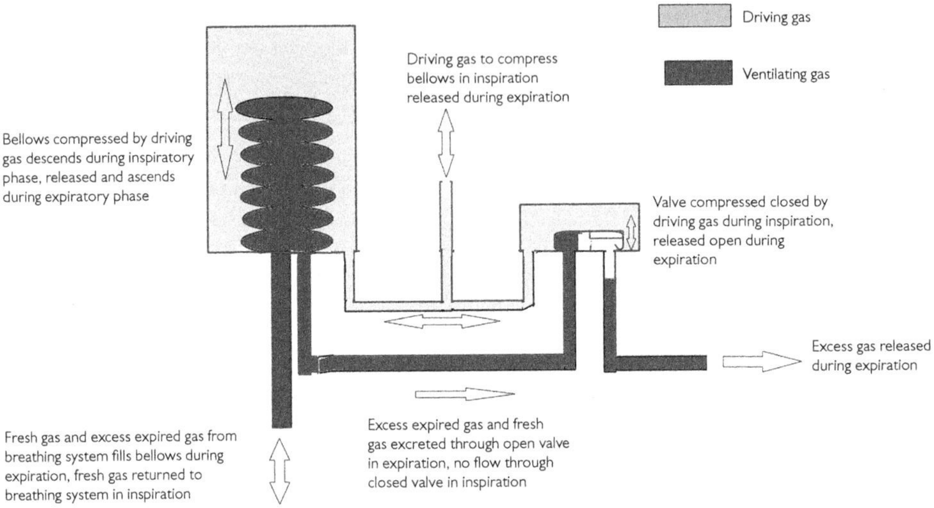


**Fig. 26.6** The functional parts of a bag-in-bottle ventilator of the ascending bellows type.

For example, some ventilators used to be of the descending bellows type; in the case of a patient becoming disconnected from the ventilator, gravity would continue to expand the bellows, drawing in room air; subsequent compression of the bellows in the inspiratory phase would generate adequate pressure to fail to trigger a disconnection alarm. In a modern ventilator of the ascending bellows type shown in Figure 26.6, a patient disconnection would cause the bellows to collapse and pressure and volume alarms would annunciate. Pressure-sensitive alarms that are inappropriately used may fail when used with ventilators, which can be thought of as 'discharging compliances' such as the Manley MP3 ventilator (Campbell *et al.* 1996). Other mechanical causes of hypoventilation or excessive airway pressure due to bad design have been reported (Schreiber 1985; Roth *et al.* 1986; Sara and Wark 1986; Pryn and Crosse 1989) and include blocked expiratory valves and misconnected tubing.

# Testing

Before being put into clinical use, all ventilators are rigorously tested on a lung model containing a variable R and a variable C. Testing according to an ISO (International Standards Organisation) standard ISO 80601-2-12:2023; ISO 19223:2019(en) includes endurance, waveform and volume performance tests, internal compliance testing and many other aspects.

## Special features of paediatric ventilators

Ventilators used for babies and children need far more flexibility in some respects than adult ventilators. Respiratory rate needs to be in the range 15 to 40 breaths minute$^{-1}$, deliverable tidal volume may need to vary from 16 to 500 ml. Lung compliance of babies can vary from 2.5 to 30 ml (cm $H_2O$)$^{-1}$ and airway resistance from 2 to 30 cm$H_2O$ L$^{-1}$. For neonates the respiratory time may need to be as short as 0.5 seconds, inspiratory flow as low as 2Lmin$^{-1}$ and peak airway pressure limited to 6–7 cm $H_2O$, even in the presence of an uncuffed endotracheal tube. As mentioned earlier, source-compliant $C_S$ (Figure 26.5) can become significant under these conditions and it is preferable that neonatal and infant ventilators are valveless (Chakrabarti 1990), so that the infant can breathe without doing excessive respiratory work. Ventilators such as the *Bear Cub* and *Sechrist* function by intermittently occluding gas escape to the atmosphere from a T piece during the inspiratory phase. However, it has been shown that some infant ventilators do not successfully limit peak inspiratory pressure reliably, resulting in possible barotrauma (Kirplani *et al.* 1988). The combination of short inspiratory times and small-diameter endotracheal tubes may mean that there is a significant difference between indicated airway pressure and alveolar pressure, while short expiratory times may lead to incomplete expiration (Tipping and Sykes 1991). Appropriate alarms should be available and used to respond to the tight constraints of excessive or inadequate measured values of preset variables. Adequate humidification is mandatory, as in adult ventilation.

## Some ventilator types

A few examples of mechanisms of ventilators will be given here, but the list is by no means complete. Although they are not necessarily the most modern, they are still widely used and the principles of their structure and function are relevant to all ventilators.

### *Minute volume dividers*

These devices do not have separate driving gas and breathing gas supplies. The only gas supply to the ventilator is from the common gas outlet of the anaesthetic machine, and it both drives the mechanism and supplies the patient with breathing gas. During inspiration, a preset tidal volume of ventilating gas, previously stored inside the main ventilating bellows, is delivered to the patient, while a separate reservoir fills with fresh gas; during expiration, the patient's tidal volume is passively released to waste, as the ventilating bellows are refilled by the reservoir with its stored supply of fresh gas. There is a pair of toggled valves in the system which ensures that the reservoir and the bellows are functionally separated and connected as appropriate during the two halves of the respiratory cycle. With tidal volume preset, the respiratory rate is governed by the fresh gas flow, since it all goes to the patient. Despite its limitations, the advantage of this type of ventilator is its non-dependence on any driving source of power except the ventilating fresh gas itself. Historically the most well-known of this type was the Manley series (Classic Paper, *Br. J. Anaesth*. 1995).

### *The bag-in-bottle ventilator*

Most modern anaesthetic machines have an integrated ventilator that appears as a bellows which is visible inside a Perspex cylinder. It is clear from observation that the bellows is compressed by a pressurised driving gas source inside the cylinder (but outside the bellows) to facilitate inspiration of the patient's lungs, and is allowed to expand by being passively filled with breathing gas, while passive expiration occurs. The generic name for this type of ventilator is the 'bag-in-bottle', and the bellows is usually of the ascending type, as alluded to earlier, in order that a leak in the breathing system would immediately become visible by the collapse of the bellows under its own weight. This configuration provides a small amount of inherent PEEP, although it may also add some expiratory resistance. A descending bellows arrangement is seldom seen these days. Note that in both cases, the driving gas is separated from the breathing gas by the bellows; if the bellows itself develops a leak, the breathing gas inside it is contaminated by the driving gas, usually oxygen. The mechanism to intermittently power the driving gas to compress the bellows can either be by a piston, an electric motor driving a cam, or by an electronically controlled flow valve.

An example of a 'bag-in-bottle' ventilator would be of the sort found integrated into a modern anaesthetic machine. It is usually a volume preset, time cycled ventilator with pneumatic power and an ascending bellows, as shown in Figure 26.6, which acts as a pressure generator in the inspiratory phase. Respiratory frequency and I:E ratio (inspiratory to expiratory time ratio) are preset; the ventilator can be set to be volume controlled (when it acts primarily as a flow generator) when the volume is preset; or it can be set to be pressure controlled (when it acts as a pressure generator) and the peak pressure is preset. A smaller bellows can be inserted if tidal volumes of smaller than 200 ml are required. Figure 26.6 shows that during inspiration the driving gas passes into the cylinder and compresses the bellows, which thus delivers breathing gas to the patient's breathing system. It can be seen that the driving gas pressure also keeps the overflow valve of the breathing system closed during this phase of the ventilatory cycle. In expiration the driving gas pressure reduces to a minimum, the bellows expands, admitting a mixture of fresh breathing gas and mixed expired gas, and the overflow valve is allowed to open so that any excess gas may be expired to atmosphere. The driving gas flowrate adjusts itself to deliver the preset variables according to the ventilator's setting as a pressure or volume-controlled device. A modern version of this ventilator (e.g. Datex-Ohmeda AS5) also compensates the tidal volume setting for different fresh gas flows and for the system's compressible volume.

## Intermittent blowers

These devices are also driven by a separate driving gas source, usually air or oxygen pressurised to between 250 and 400 kPa. Prior to the advent of microprocessor control of ventilators, the most important component of this type of ventilator for anaesthetic use was the control module, described in the example below and shown in Figure 26.7, which consists of a pneumatically controlled spool valve and an inspiratory and expiratory timer; such a device does not require electrical power and divides the breathing gas into tidal volumes controlled by adjusting the timers. Figure 26.7a shows the inspiratory phase, when the driving gas enters the valve at (1), and divides into three directions: one part enters the valve housing containing the spool (2), the other two parts enter the two pneumatic timing chambers, inspiratory (3) and expiratory (4). The position of the spool valve shown in Figure 26.7a, towards the left, allows the gas in the valve housing to pass through towards the patient's breathing system (5); note that this position of the spool valve also allows gas to pass freely through the expiratory timing chamber (4), as pressure builds up in the inspiratory timing chamber (3). This pressure builds up at a rate determined by the inspiratory timer setting (6), and at a certain point the spool is pushed across the valve housing towards the right-hand side, thus determining the tidal volume delivered; this allows the expiratory phase to start, and the gas supply to the valve is blocked; gas to the inspiratory timer pathway is allowed to flow through the valve, while pressure now builds up in the expiratory timing chamber at a rate determined by the expiratory timer setting (7). The driving gas, usually oxygen or air, going to the breathing system must be kept separate from the fresh gas to the patient by an adequate length of tubing. More sophisticated intensive care ventilators in this class use an electrically switched magnetic field in a coil to displace an iron core to open a valve that is otherwise held closed by a spring. It may be designed to open and close the valve, or to allow a variable flow through the valve, depending on the electric current flowing through the coil (solenoid) when it is a proportional flow valve (see later). This system works well with a short response time in a high-pressure, low-compliance system using a small valve aperture. The same mechanism operates to close a PEEP valve when used in a low-pressure system with a large-aperture valve, otherwise kept open by a light spring. On modern ventilators microprocessors control the electrical signal to a proportional flow valve to provide a range of ventilator modes and variables.

The Penlon Nuffield 200 ventilator is a relatively compact and versatile ventilator in this class, and can be thought of as a time-cycled flow generator. As such, it is versatile enough to be used with patients of a wide range of size, airway resistance and lung compliance. When used for adults it is volume preset, and when used for babies, it is pressure preset. It can be used with different breathing systems, ones which lend themselves to controlled ventilation. The driving gas and the breathing gas are separated pneumatically, hence, the tubing connecting the breathing system to the ventilator must be of sufficient volume (a tidal volume at least) and length (1 m) to ensure continuous separation of these two gas flows, otherwise dilution of the breathing gas can occur. The control module, accessible to the user, has an airway pressure gauge, an on–off switch, a flow control knob and controls for inspiratory and expiratory times.

The control module for the portable paediatric ventilator, the Pneupac, is almost identical to that of the Penlon Nuffield. The additional piece of technology that the Pneupac has is its patient valve, shown in Figure 26.8, which can be compared to those in manual resuscitators (see

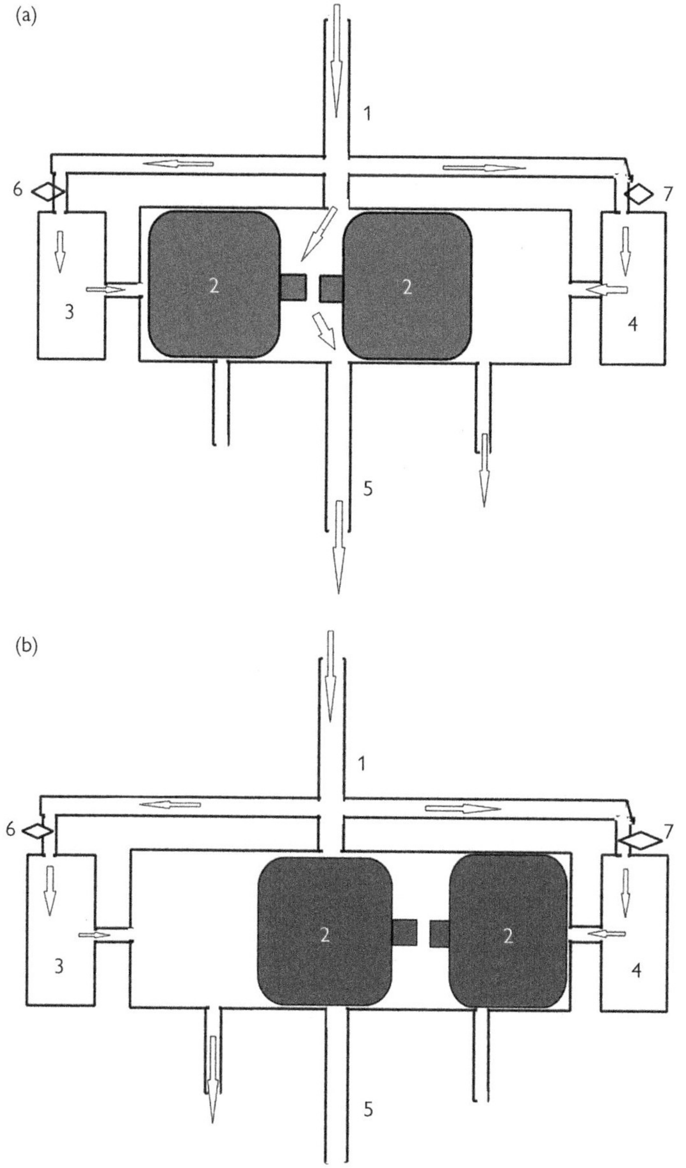


**Fig. 26.7** A pneumatically controlled spool valve: (a) inspiratory phase, (b) expiratory phase. (1) Fresh gas entry; (2) spool valve; (3) inspiratory timing chamber; (4) expiratory timing chamber; (5) outlet to breathing system; (6) inspiratory timer setting; (7) expiratory timer setting.

next). The Pneupac Ventipac ventilator is a useful device for ventilating paediatric patients during transfer, but ideally it needs an additional means of confirming delivered tidal volume (McCluskey and Gwinnutt 1995). Both these ventilators have been modified for use in a hyperbaric chamber, when such a facility is needed to care for a critically ill diver, for example (Lewis *et al.* 1991; Spittal *et al.* 1991).

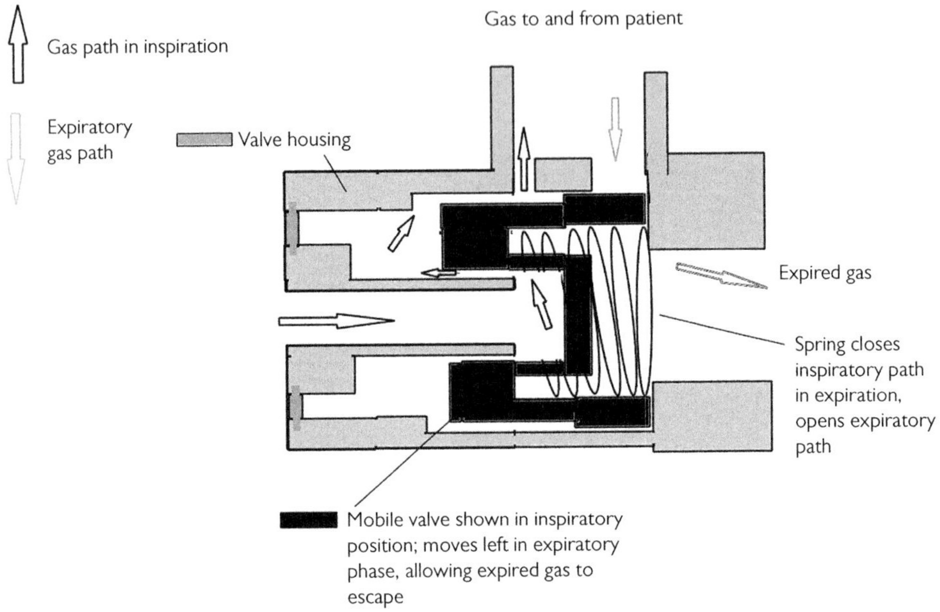


**Fig. 26.8** Pneupac type portable ventilator patient valve shown in the inspiratory position.

## Intensive care ventilators

Ventilators for use in intensive care have a more complex task than those for use in anaesthesia (Davey 2012) . They are required to ventilate patients of all sizes, and lungs with a wider range of compliance, often through airways of increased resistance. They must provide a wide range of respiratory support to accommodate the patient's changing dependence on such support, from intermittent positive pressure ventilation with positive end expiratory pressure (BiPAP), volume or pressure-assisted ventilation to augment or supplement the patient's own efforts where appropriate, and other modalities. This range of operation is afforded by microprocessors for electronic control of function, and by proportional flow valves to accurately control gas flowrates. This allows the patient adequate ventilation with more complexity and more flexibility than the anaesthesia ventilators described hitherto, although there is now considerable overlap between the two classes of ventilators. These days more ventilation is carried out by mask or hood in non-intubated patients, so the ventilators have to accommodate significant leakage (Bauchmuller and Glossop 2016). Testing, even for new generation ventilators, sometimes reveals that not all aspects of the ventilation performances are fulfilled in terms of delivered tidal volume with changes in fresh gas flow (Wallon *et al.* 2013) or in the presence of leakage (Garnier *et al.* 2015).

An intensive care ventilator is a complex machine, which usually needs to be powered in one of a number of ways, and yet be able to function independently of that power source in an emergency. The power source might be an electric motor driving an intermittent blower, which produces large volumes of gas, or it might drive a gas compressor, which provides high pressure, both of which can be manipulated pneumatically downstream. Alternatively, these gas modalities can be supplied pneumatically without the use of a motor. The ventilator consists of a pneumatic flow system and an electronic control system. The pneumatic flow system consists of an air–oxygen pressure regulator and gas mixer, a gas reservoir, a servo-controlled flow proportional flow valve, a patient overpressure valve, an ambient air inlet, a flow sensor, an expiratory valve and a pressure source for a nebuliser. The electronic control system is used to check the pneumatic flow system and consists of an analogue valve control, pressure

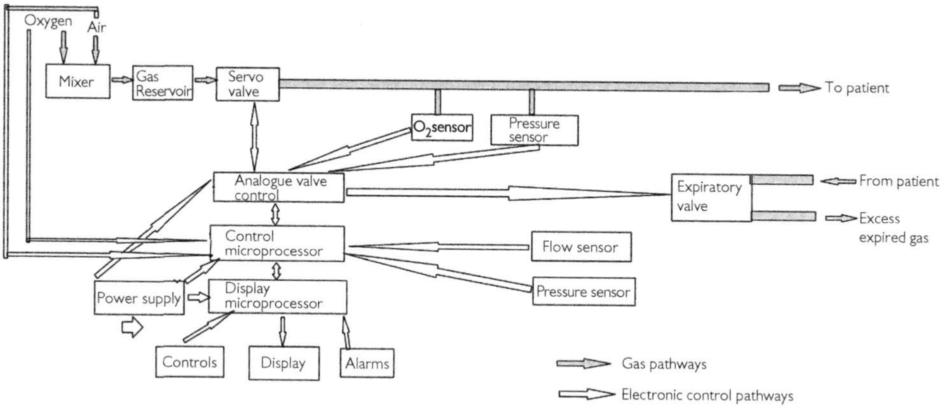


**Fig. 26.9** Functional diagram of the microprocessor control system in an intensive care ventilator.

sensors. The function of the whole system is continually checked by the two microprocessors, one of which is linked to the display system, the other of which is linked to the control valve system, but which in any case cross-check each other's outputs. Figure 26.9 shows the microprocessor controls and their connections.

Pneumatic flow system, air and oxygen, at pressures of between 2 and 8 bar are delivered to the ventilator; the gases then pass one-way valves to the gas pressure regulators, which drop gas pressures to 1.5 bar. The gas mixer allows manual adjustment of the oxygen concentration. The gas mixture enters the gas reservoir, which holds a gas volume of 8 L, compressed to 350 $cmH_2O$ pressure, which means that the gas delivery to the patient can be largely independent of supply flow rate. The reservoir has an added safety valve to prevent overpressure.

The servo-controlled flow valve: Figure 26.10 shows this high-speed device, a solenoid valve that is able to deliver flows in the range 20 to 300 ml $s^{-1}$ with precision. The valve uses an electrodynamic motor, an electromagnetic device similar to a solenoid, such as is found in a loudspeaker, to move a vertical piston. The piston is connected by a rod to a small cylindrical-shaped plunger that has a triangular-shaped orifice on two sides. The rod is also connected to a high-precision linear potentiometer, as in

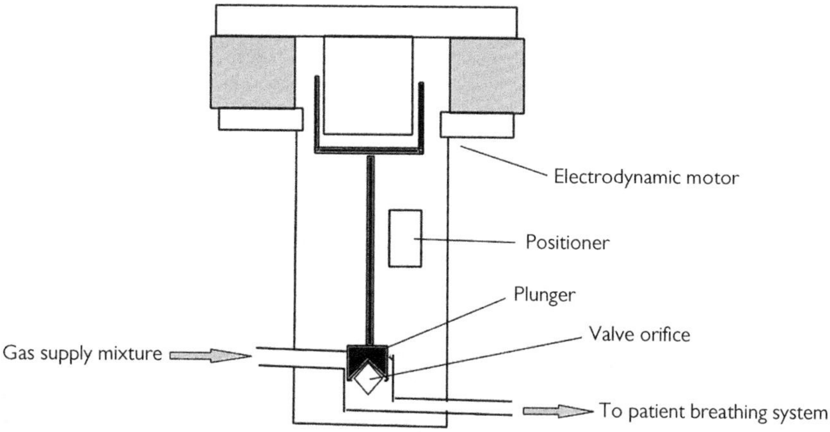


**Fig. 26.10** An inspiratory servo-controlled valve.

a control system. The motor raises the plunger and allows gas flow through the valve to the patient. The triangular-shaped orifice in the plunger outlet allows a precise relationship between the triangular height, the pressure differential across the plunger orifice and the flowrate; an electronic servo control loop is driven by this relationship. Depending on the ventilator control settings, the control microprocessor determines the correct signal to send to the motor to raise the plunger. The analogue valve controller compares the perceived flow, determined by the actual height of the plunger from the information provided by the potentiometer, to the pressure drop across the plunger. The plunger in this case acts as a flowmeter, the actual flow rate being proportional to the measured pressure drop. The analogue valve controller then readjusts the current to the motor to deliver the flow needed. The response time of this system is less than 100 ms, due to the precision of the control loop and the small system deadspace. It allows precise control of tidal volume, with any desired flow pattern and at any pressure, with an accuracy of 5%, regardless of back pressure. Because of frequent checking of measured flow against plunger height and motor current, the microprocessor assures accurate function under all conditions. Numerous alarm systems back up this function. In spontaneous modes of ventilation, the valve acts as a demand valve, matching desired flow and pressure.

The flow sensor: This is incorporated within the patient breathing system, using the principle of measurement of pressure differential across a variable orifice in the form of a fine Mylar membrane. The pressure transducer thus formed is an accurate, differential electronic device. This arrangement gives a linear relationship between $Q$ and $\Delta P$ over a range of 200 to 3000 ml s$^{-1}$ (see Chapter 7). However, further electronic linearisation can allow flow measurement down to 30 ml s$^{-1}$, maintaining a ±5% accuracy, which is only marginally affected by humidity or nebulised drugs. The flow sensor is used to provide information on flow, volume and timing of the respiratory cycle to the alarm systems, but is not used to control inspiratory and expiratory valves.

The expiratory valve: This consists of a large surface area silicone rubber membrane inside a plastic housing. Occlusion of the membrane against the patient expiratory tubing during the inspiratory phase, or partial closure during PEEP or CPAP, occurs by the action of a solenoid, which closes the valve. During expiration, the current to the motor is off and a spring opens a valve to allow expiration to occur. Although the valve housing and silicone rubber membrane are labelled, it is unfortunately still possible to place the membrane back into the housing back-to-front after cleaning.

The electronic control system: This is divided into two independent systems, controlled by two separate microprocessors, operating in parallel and simultaneously; in addition, each microprocessor checks the other.

The display processor: This manages control settings and alarms, determining the setting of every control knob and sending the relevant information to the control processor. All monitored data are displayed, alarm conditions are determined and identified and internal circuits and voltage levels are all checked by this processor.

The control processor: This controls inspiratory and expiratory valves via the analogue valve control. It also contains *A to D* (ADC) and *D to A* (DAC) converters for flow and pressure control. It integrates flows to give tidal volume, calculates all pressure values and determines a number of alarm conditions.

## COVID-19 and ICU ventilator development

In 2020–21 the COVID-19 pandemic, there was real concern that there would not be enough ventilators in the country for all the patients who would need them. The notion of 'ventilator sharing' between patients was considered, despite the obvious difficulties; engineers came up with some ingenious solutions to sharing a ventilator between two patients with different physiological requirements in terms of airway resistance and lung compliance discussed above. Ways were found of splitting the flow (Arellano *et al.* 2022), preferentially restricting the flow to one patient (Plummer *et al.* 2020). Looking to the future of ventilator development, it is one area where artificial intelligence (AI) could benefit patient care, providing appropriate algorithms could be developed and rigorously tested (Gallifant *et al.* 2022).

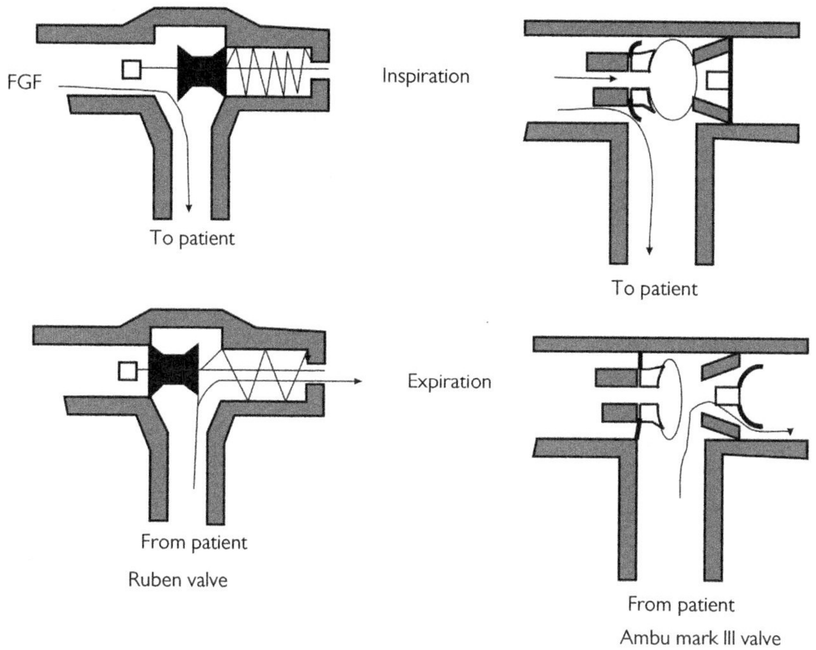


**Fig. 26.11** Two examples of patient valves in manual resuscitators.

# Manual resuscitators

On occasions, a very much simpler device is needed to allow ventilation by hand (Lee and Yip 2023). This consists basically of a self-inflating reservoir bag with a supply of fresh gas, and a non-rebreathing valve. The design of this valve is crucial to the successful function of the resuscitator and two examples of its design are shown in the diagram in Figure 26.11.

# Portable ventilators

There are now numerous compact ventilators on the market, which are useful for transporting patients. They are usually powered by a cylinder of oxygen, which is also the source of the gas to be delivered to the patient. Their mechanisms of action are similar to those of some ventilators already described. All have limitations of performance, but are adequate for short-term use (Attebo *et al.* 1993; Heinrichs *et al.* 1989; Wong and McGuire 2000; Fludger and Klein 2008).

# Other methods of gas exchange

## *High-frequency ventilation*

High-frequency ventilation (HFV) is a term used to describe artificial ventilation at frequencies ranging from 1 to 20 Hz, depending on the mode of application (Chang and Harf 1984; Crawford 1986). It uses tidal volumes, which are often smaller than the patient's deadspace volume. First used with some enthusiasm in the 1980s, it was initially thought to result in lower mean airway pressures than conventional ventilation. However, this subsequently proved not to be the case (Sherry *et al.* 1987), although the method has applications where conventional ventilation is inconvenient (e.g. chest surgery), or where each lung has different ventilatory requirements. Under these conditions, HFV is applied to one lung, while IPPV (BiPAP) is applied to the other (Raphael and Atkinson 1995).

High-frequency positive-pressure ventilation: High-frequency positive-pressure ventilation (HFPPV) is administered by a positive-pressure device, with either a timed solenoid valve or a mechanically driven rotating valve. An ordinary endotracheal tube is used and the ventilation frequency is usually 1–2 Hz.

High-frequency jet ventilation: High-frequency jet ventilation (HFJV) is widely used where bronchoscopic work is being carried out. A high velocity jet of gas, usually oxygen, attached to the inside of a rigid bronchoscope or endotracheal tube, results in air or gas entrainment, which provides an adequate inspired volume. The jet is sometimes manually controlled, or sometimes the frequency is controlled by a solenoid valve, when the frequency may be 2–10 Hz. Precise positioning of the gas injector is important if a wide variation in performance of the device is to be avoided.

High-frequency oscillation: High-frequency oscillation (HFO) (Kolton 1984) uses a reciprocating mechanism, usually a piston pump, to produce an oscillatory gas flow. Unlike the other methods, expiration is not passive, but a well-defined negative pressure change. A steady bias FGF is also required to maintain appropriate oxygen and carbon dioxide transfer gradients. The frequency of HFO is 3–50 Hz.

High-frequency chest wall oscillation: High-frequency chest wall oscillation (HFCWO) means that rapid reciprocating chest wall compression allows gas flow to occur to and from the lungs without tracheal intubation. This is usually achieved by applying a gas-tight cuirass to the chest wall and applying a reciprocating pressure waveform to its inner surface. The Hayek oscillator is the modern development of this method (Petros *et al.* 1995).

## *Mechanisms of gas transport in HFV*

With high frequencies and small tidal volumes, gas transport by normal convective mechanisms plays some part (Scherer *et al.* 1989), but this cannot be the only mechanism. This is particularly true where

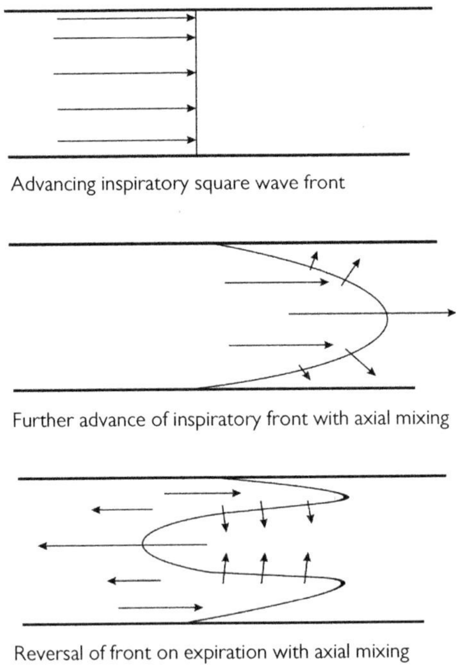


**Fig. 26.12** Axisymmetric velocity profiles and axial gas mixing contribute to convective gas transport in high frequency ventilation (HFV).

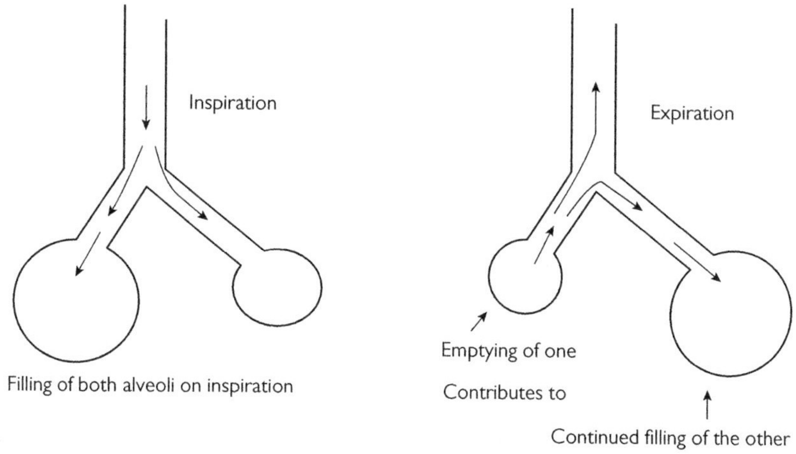


**Fig. 26.13** Pendelluft as a mechanism of gas transport in HFV.

different lung units have different time constants and where gas acceleration and inertance become significant variables. The presence of axisymmetric velocity profiles, shown in Figure 26.12, also contributes to convective gas transport in HFV; around bifurcations, inspiratory velocity profiles are peaked and expiratory profiles are flattened (Crawford 1986; Haselton *et al.* 1982), allowing oxygen transport to occur towards the periphery of the lung and carbon dioxide transport to occur from the periphery to the central bronchial tree. Another mechanism of transport in the convective range is *Pendelluft*, where gas is transported between lung units with different time constants, out of phase with the ventilatory cycle, shown in Figure 26.13.

Secondary mechanisms of transport (Smith 1990) may include:

- resonance – the frequency of ventilation approaches the natural resonant frequency of the structures of the lungs and chest wall, leading to volume amplification (Bourgain *et al.* 1994).
- Taylor dispersion – convection and radial dispersion;
- turbulence in the upper airways, which abolishes radial gas concentration gradients;
- laminar flow in the smaller, peripheral airways, where radial gas concentration gradients are preserved, which allows radial mixing to occur along the airway long axis; it can be calculated and confirmed that overall gas transfer is proportional to $frequency \times (V_T)^2$;
- molecular diffusion at alveolar level.

## *Extracorporeal membrane oxygenation (ECMO)*

There are occasions when the lung needs to be rested at FRC and oxygenation of the blood stream is achieved by a membrane oxygenator, much like those used in cardiac surgery (Martinez and Vuylstecke 2012). It is also possible to facilitate carbon dioxide removal by an extracorporeal membrane and to oxygenate with reduced IPPV via the lungs. Clearly, in either case, vascular access is required to facilitate either veno-arterial or veno-venous bypass.

The membrane can be either the *parallel plate* type or the *hollow fibre* type. Oxygen transport occurs according to the *advancing front* theory, in which the dimensionless constant known as the *Sherwood number*, a ratio of partial pressure changes between the membrane and the bloodstream, is an important concept. Because $CO_2$ exists in three forms in the blood, its transport through a membrane is more complex (Dorrington 1989).

## *References*

**Arellano**, D. H., Tobar, E A. and Lazo, M. T. (2022) Assessment of a splitter for protective dual-patient ventilation in patients with acute respiratory distress syndrome, *Br. J. Anaesth.*, **128**(5), pp. E314–17.

**Attebo**, **L.**, **Bengtsson**, **M.** and **Johnson**, **A.** (1993) Comparison of portable emergency ventilators using lung model, *Br. J. Anaesth.*, **70**, pp. 372–7.

**Bauchmuller**, **K. and Glossop**, **A. J.** (2016) Non-invasive ventilation in the perioperative period, *BJA Educ.*, **16**(9), pp. 299–304.

**Bourgain**, **J. L.**, **Billard**, **V.** and **Desruennes**, **E.** (1994) Resonant volume amplification during high frequency jet ventilation, *Br. J. Anaesth.*, **72**(suppl. 1), p. 10.

**Campbell**, **R. M.**, **Sheikh**, **A.** and **Crosse**, **M. M.** (1996) A study of the incorrect use of ventilator disconnection alarms, *Anaesthesia*, **51**, pp. 369–70.

**Chakrabarti, M. K.** ***et al.*** (1990) A new infant oscillatory ventilator, *Br. J. Anaesth.*, **64**, pp. 374–5.

**Chang**, **H.** and **Harf**, **A.** (1984) High frequency ventilation – a review, *Respir. Physiol.*, **57**, pp. 135–52.

**Classic paper** (1995) The Manley ventilator, *Br. J. Anaesth.*, **50**, pp. 64–71.

**Crawford**, **M. R.** (1986) High frequency ventilation, *Anaesth. Int. Care*, **14**, pp. 281–92.

**Davey**, **A. J.** (2012) Automatic ventilators, Chapter 9, and Ventilation in intensive care in intensive care, Chapter 10, in Davey, A. J. and Diba, A. (eds) *Ward's Anaesthetic Equipment*, 5th edn, Elsevier, Philadelphia, PA, pp. 231–73.

**Dorrington**, **K. L.** (1989) Oxygen transfer in extracorporeal lungs; Carbon dioxide transfer in extracorporeal lungs. Chapters 5 and 6 in Gross, J. B. (ed.), *Anaesthetic and Extracorporeal Gas Transfer*, Oxford Science Publications, Clarendon Press, Oxford, pp. 203–67.

**Fludger**, **S.** and **Klein**, **A.** (2008) Portable ventilators, *Cont. Educ. Anaesth. Crit. Care Pain*, **8**, pp. 199–203.

**Gallifant, J., Zhang, J., Lopez, M.** ***et al.*** **(**2022) Artificial intelligence for mechanical ventilation: systematic review of design, reporting standards, and bias, *Br. J. Anaesth.*, **128**(2), pp. 343–51.

**Garnier**, **M.**, **Quesnel**, C., **Fulgencio**, **J.-P.** ***et al.*** *(*2015**)**, Multifaceted bench comparative evaluation of latest intensive care unit ventilators, *Br. J. Anaesth.*, **115**(1), pp. 89–98.

**Haselton**, **F. R. and Scherer P. W.** (1982) Flow visualization of steady streaming in oscillatory flow through a bifurcating tube, *J. Fluid Mech.*, **123**, pp. 315–33.

**Heinrichs**, **W.**, **Mertzluft**, **F.** and **Dick**, **W.** (1989) Accuracy of delivered versus preset minute ventilation of portable emergency ventilators, *Crit. Care Med.*, **17**, pp. 682–5.

**Kirplani**, **J.**, **Santos-Lyn**, **R.** and **Roberts**, **R.** (1988) Some infant ventilators do not limit peak inspiratory pressure reliably during active expiration, Crit. *Care Med.*, **16**, pp. 880–3.

**Kolton**, **M.** (1984) A review of high frequency oscillation, *Canad. Anaes. Soc. J.*, **31**, pp. 416–29.

**Lee**, **C. P.** and **Yip**, **Y. Y.** (2023) Understanding your bag-mask-valve resuscitator, *BJA Educ.*, **23**(6), pp. 208–11.

**Lewis**, **R. P.** ***et al.*** (1991) The use of the Penlon Nuffield 200 in a monoplace hyperbaric oxygen chamber, *Br. J. Anaesth.*, **46**, pp. 767–70.

**Martinez**, **G.** and **Vuylstecke**, **A.** (2012) Extracorporeal membrane oxygenation in adults, *CEACCP*, **12**(2), pp. 57–61

**McCluskey**, **A.** and **Gwinnutt**, **L.** (1995) Evaluation of the Pneupac Ventipac portable ventilator: comparison of performance in a mechanical lung and anaesthetised patients, *Br. J. Anaesth.*, **75**, pp. 645–50.

**Mushin**, **W. W.**, **Rendell-Baker**, **L.**, **Thompson**, **P. W.** and **Mapleson**, **W. W.** (1980) *Automatic Ventilation of the Lungs*, Blackwell Scientific Publications, Oxford, pp. 33–251.

**Petros, A. J.** ***et al.*** (1995) The Hayek oscillator. Nomograms for tidal volume and minute volume using high frequency oscillation, *Br. J. Anaesth.*, **50**, pp. 601–6.

**Plummer, A., DuBois, J. L., Flynn, J.** ***et al.*** **(**2020) A simple method to estimate flow restriction for dual ventilation of dissimilar patients: the BathRC model, *PLOS One*, **15**(11), p. e0242123.

**Pryn**, **S. J.** and **Crosse**, **M. M.** (1989) Ventilator disconnection alarm failures, *Anaesthesia*, **44**, pp. 978–81.

**Raphael, J. H.** and **Atkinson, I.** (1995) A combined high frequency oscillator and intermittent positive pressure ventilator, *Br. J. Anaesth.*, **50**, pp. 611–13.

**Roth, S.** ***et al.*** (1986) Excessive airway pressure due to malfunctioning anaesthesia ventilator, *Anesthesiology*, **65**, pp. 532–4.

**Sara, C. A.** and **Wark, H. J.** (1986) Disconnection: an appraisal, *Anesth. Int. Care*, **14**, pp. 448–52.

**Scherer, P. W.** ***et al.*** (1989) Convective mixing mechanism in high frequency intermittent jet ventilation, *Acta Anaesthesiol. Scand.*, **33**(suppl. 90), pp. 65–9.

**Schreiber, P.** (1985) *Safety Guidelines for Anaesthesia Systems*, North American Draeger, Telford, PA, pp. 31 and 51.

**Sherry, K. M.** ***et al.*** (1987) Comparison of haemodynamic effects of intermittent positive pressure ventilation with high frequency jet ventilation, *Anaesthesia*, **42**, pp. 1276–83.

**Smith, B. E.** (1990) High frequency ventilation: past, present and future? *Br. J. Anaesth.*, **65**, pp. 130–8.

**Spittal, M. J.**, **Hunter, S. J.** and **Jones, L.** (1991) The Pneupac hyperbaric variant HB: a ventilator suitable for use in a one-man hyperbaric chamber, *Br. J. Anaesth.*, **67**, pp. 488–91.

**Tipping, T. R. and Sykes, M. K.** (1991) Tracheal tube resistance and alveolar pressure during mechanical ventilation in the neonate, *Br. J. Anaesth.*, **46**, pp. 565–9.

**Wallon, G.**, **Bonnet**, A. and Guérin, C. (2013) Delivery of tidal volume from four anaesthesia ventilators during volume-controlled ventilation: a bench study, *Br. J. Anaesth.*, **110**(6), pp. 1045–51.

**Wong, L. S. S. and McGuire, N. M.** (2000) Laboratory assessment of the Bird T-Bird ventilator performance using a lung model, *Br. J. Anaesth.*, **84**, pp. 811–17.

## *Further reading*

**Davey, A. J.** and **Diba, A. (eds)** (2012) Chapter 9, Automatic ventilators (A. Davey) and Chapter 10, Ventilation in the intensive care unit (M. Street), in *Ward's Anaesthetic Equipment*, 6th edn, Elsevier, Philadelphia, PA, pp. 231–75.

# Chapter 27 **Intravenous pumps and syringe drivers**

In the past, many infusions on the general ward were given by gravity-assisted drip sets that gave a flowrate dependent on the height of the reservoir above the patient, the length of the tubing, the bore of the IV cannula, the density and viscosity of the fluid being delivered, and the patient's venous pressure. However, it is now common to use programmable volumetric intravenous pumps to deliver fluids, other intravenous drugs and epidural infusions, and to use syringe drivers to deliver intravenous anaesthesia, patient-controlled analgesia, and other drugs, which are programmable to give desired flowrates or volumes. There has been a rapid increase in the use of such devices to deliver intravenous anaesthetic drugs as a target-controlled infusion (TCI). These pumps have become so flexible that they can be programmed not only to aim for different targets (i.e. plasma or tissue target concentrations), for different patients (i.e. weight, size, gender), but also the same device can be programmed for different drugs (i.e. remifentanil or propofol).

Historically, fluid infusion devices were powered only by gravity and a manual drip rate adjuster, but the flowrate from an infusion bag is now generally controlled by a photoelectric drip rate detector in conjunction with a microprocessor-controlled drip occlusion device. The earliest volumetric pumps did not rely on a drip counter, but used a syringe driver of sorts in which fixed aliquots of fluid were drawn into a cassette for accurate delivery, to within 5–10% of the set dose, shown in Figure 27.1. Most modern devices now use a peristaltic mechanism instead, either of the linear or rotary type, shown in Figure 27.2. Syringe drivers were initially powered by clockwork motors, but most modern infusion devices use an electrically powered stepper motor, shown in Figure 27.3, which is designed so that the rotation is by a fixed amount per supplied electrical pulse, independent of the mechanical load it is carrying, transmitted to the syringe by a screw-threaded rod. The pulses are controlled by a microprocessor in the pump and the rate of infusion is dependent on the stepper motor's output. The microprocessor can accept inputs for delivery in ml/hr, mg/kg/hr or µg/kg/min, or as a target plasma or tissue concentration for a choice of drug based on a pharmacokinetic model of choice.

Syringe drivers are designed to recognise and use a range of syringe sizes and some require special delivery tubing. The flow is a continuous, pulsatile flow and accuracy is 2–5%. Modern syringe drivers are usually sufficiently accurate over the desired range of infusion. However, there may be a delay before the drug is delivered to the patient as the parts attached to the syringe take up slack. Where the bolus to be delivered is small, say 0.5 ml, as in a PCA pump (patient-controlled analgesia), it becomes increasingly difficult to be sure of the accuracy of the delivered bolus (Baeckert *et al.* 2020). The trained user must bear in mind the hazardous nature of some of the drugs being delivered, as well as the potential hazards and limitations of a syringe driver or an infusion pump. For example, if an infusion stops accidentally, it may be hazardous in causing awareness (eg propofol) or circulatory failure (e.g. noradrenaline), so it is important that alarms are appropriately set before use. Very often, when an infusion device fails to do what is expected or required, user error is found to be the cause, including poor pump maintenance (Thomas and Galvin 2008). A common error is a mistake in the drug dosage or concentration selected. Sometimes, if different drugs are being infused through a series of pumps that look the same, a parameter on the wrong pump might be altered. If a drug is being given through a different pump than the one the clinician is used to, the wrong alteration might be made. After refilling or replacing a fresh pre-filled syringe, the clinician may forget to restart the pump. Uncontrolled siphoning of the drug into the patient by virtue of gravity can occur if the position of the syringe driver is above the patient's venous cannula, although normally there is a means of firmly fixing the syringe and its plunger to the driver to prevent this. Where multiple infusion lines are connected to a single point of vascular access, and there is a distal point of obstruction, it is possible for drugs from a driver to reflux up a gravity-fed line, which might then be unintentionally given later in excess dose, after the

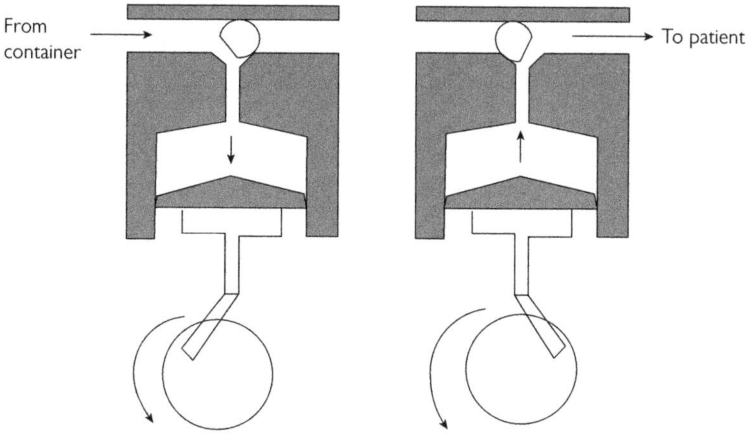


**Fig. 27.1** Syringe volumetric infusion pump.

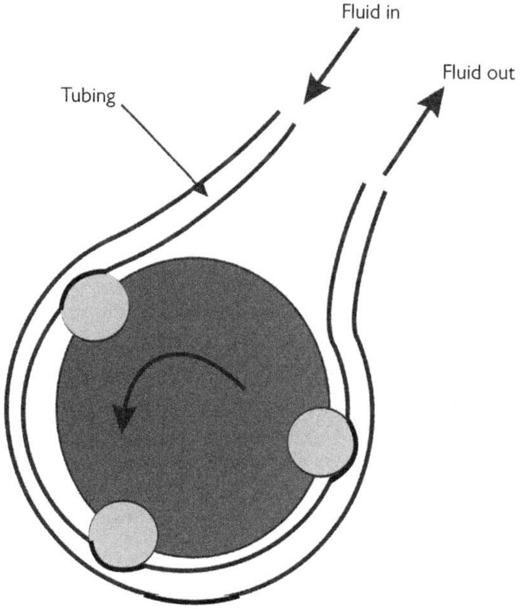


**Fig. 27.2** Peristaltic pump mechanism.

obstruction has cleared. Care must be taken to prevent air ingress into the system upstream of the pump, and modern infusion devices have either ultrasonic or optical air detection systems, usually placed downstream of the driver, connected to an alarm. Since microprocessors are subject to electromagnetic interference, it is possible for the radios of emergency services and security staff to interfere with infusion pump function, although this is much less likely with mobile telephones, and does not seem to occur with computer local area networks.

Techniques for total intravenous anaesthesia (TIVA) with drugs of short excretion half-life now exist using syringe drivers or infusion pumps. The infusion rate may be set according to a desired target

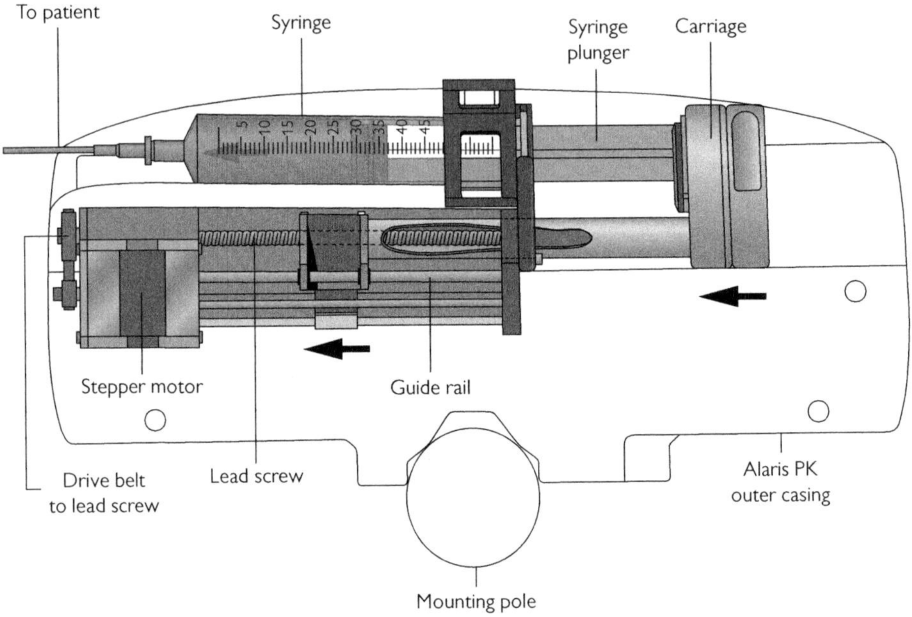


**Fig. 27.3** Syringe driver with microprocessor-controlled stepper motor connected to the syringe plunger by a carriage on a lead screw.

Reproduced with permission from Davey, A.J., and Diba, A. (2011). *Ward's Anaesthetic Equipment* (6th ed.) Elsevier.

(target-controlled infusion, TCI). With advanced software it is now possible to allow patient body parameters and desired drug plasma or tissue concentration to be entered, with the concentrations estimated from the pharmacokinetic model being used to be displayed and manual or automatic adjustment to the pump to be made according to the need to achieve the desired effect (Al-Rifai and Mulvey 2016a, 2016b). It is usually necessary to give a bolus dose initially in order to load the drug's volume of distribution in the body, and reduce the infusion rate progressively to maintain a target concentration. The devices can accommodate different-sized syringes and different drugs may be programmed for infusion; furthermore, in the case of a propofol infusion or a remifentanil infusion, the pumps may also be programmed to deliver according to different pharmacokinetic models for propofol (Schnider, Marsh), or for remifentanil (Minto). This provides a great deal of choice to the anaesthetist, but also some potential confusion in the face of such choice, with an uncertainty about what the drug concentration might be at the effector site (Absalom *et al.* 2009). One of the factors delaying a more rapid uptake of propofol TIVA has been the absence of a means of measuring plasma or tissue propofol levels; however, this matter is in the process of being addressed (Ferrier *et al.* 2022; Craft 2025). It may even be that there is a place for artificial intelligence algorithms to control the output of such pumps in the near future (Litman *et al.* 2020). Nevertheless, considerable care should be exercised using infusion devices and syringe drivers, particularly in a paralysed, ventilated patient, lest the pump should fail and render the patient aware. As well as checking all infusion equipment before use (Association of Anaesthetists of GB and Ireland 2012), it is recommended that a non-return, anti-reflux valve should be used in the line where TIVA is being given, and the IV site of administration should be continuously visible in case of inadvertent extravasation of the drug (Keay and Callander 2004).

## *References*

**Absalom, A. R.**, **Mani, V.**, **de Smet, T.** and **Struys, M.** (2009) Pharmacokinetic models for propofol – defining and illuminating the devil in the detail, *Br. J. Anaesth*, **103**, pp. 26–37.

**Al-Rifai, Z.** and **Mulvey, D.** (2016a) Total intravenous anaesthesia: basic pharmacokinetics and model descriptions, *BJA Educ.*, **16**(3), pp. 92–7.

**Al-Rifai, Z.** and **Mulvey, D.** (2016b) Total Intravenous Anaesthesia: practical aspects of using total intravenous anaesthesia. *BJA Educ.*, **16**(8), pp. 276–80.

**Association of Anaesthetists of Great Britain and Ireland** (2012) Checking anaesthetic equipment, *Anaesthesia*, **67**(6), pp. 660–8.

**Baeckert, M.**, **Batliner, M.**, **Grasse, B.**, ***et al.*** (2020) Performance of modern syringe infusion pump assemblies at low infusion rates in the perioperative setting, *Br. J. Anaesth.*, **124**(2), pp. 173–82.

**Craft, T.** (2025) Personal communication, Somnus Scientific.

**Ferrier, D.**, **Kieley, J.** and **Luxton, R.** (2022) Propofol detection for monitoring of intravenous anaesthesia: a review, *J. Clin. Monitor. & Comput.* **36**, pp. 315–23.

**Keay, S.** and **Callander, C.** (2004) The safe use of infusion devices, *CEACCP*, **4**(3), 81–5.

**Litman, R. S.**, **O'Neill, S.** and **Beard, J. W.** (2020) What can we learn from smart pump infusion data analysis? *Br. J. Anaesth.*, **125**(4), pp. 430–2.

**Thomas, A. N.** and **Galvin, I.** (2008) Patient safety incidents associated with equipment in critical care: a review of reports to the UK National Patient Safety Agency, *Anaesthesia*, **63**(11), 1193–7.

## *Further reading*

**Moyle, J. T. B.** and **Davey, A.** (2012) *Ward's Anaesthetic Equipment*, 6th edn, WB Saunders Co. Ltd, Philadelphia, PA, pp. 399–419.

# Chapter 28 Environmental safety

## Fire and explosion

For these to occur, there is a need for combustible material, oxygen and a source of ignition. The risk of these being present results from the use of high oxygen partial pressures and the use of inflammable anaesthetic agents or other inflammable materials.

If the pressure of any gas is increased, heat is liberated. If the gas is oxygen and this comes into contact with something flammable like oil or grease in a confined space, the heat liberated may cause an explosion. Hence oil or grease should be kept well away from pressurised oxygen sources. These include not only oxygen, but pressurised air and pressurised nitrous oxide, which can dissociate into nitrogen and oxygen.

Although modern anaesthetic volatile agents are not flammable, ether and cyclopropane are, and may still be used in some parts of the world. Ethyl chloride, used to test sensory perception in local anaesthetic blocks and methyl alcohol for cleaning skin, are also flammable.

Ignition sources include sparks from static electricity, or faulty electrical apparatus from the diathermy machine or from mains plugs sparking when disconnected. To prevent static electricity causing ignition, not only should efforts be made to minimise the generation of static electricity, but also to discharge any static slowly to earth. There should therefore be an upper and a lower limit to the electrical resistance between the antistatic floor and earth, of between 5 M$\Omega$ and 20 k$\Omega$ respectively. All equipment capable of generating static electricity should make electrical contact with the floor through a medium made of antistatic (conducting) rubber. Staff footwear should also have antistatic rubber soles and the tubing of breathing systems should also be made of antistatic material.

Classification of anaesthetic proof equipment is based on the ignition energy required to ignite the most flammable mixture of ether and air (IEC standard 60601-1). *'AP'* (anaesthetic proof) standard equipment can be used between 5 and 25 cm from such an inflammable anaesthetic gas mixture escaping from a breathing system; furthermore, its temperature should not exceed 200°C. *'APG'* standard is a more stringent one for equipment which already meets the AP standard; it is based on the ignition energy required to ignite the most flammable mixture of ether and oxygen, which should be less than 1 J. The equipment temperature should not be more than 90°C and the equipment can be used within 5 cm of an escaping flammable gas mixture.

## Atmospheric pollution and anaesthetic gases

There is a heightened awareness of the many ways in which human activity pollutes the atmosphere, and steps we should take to minimise, and perhaps even reverse the process (Campbell and Pierce 2015). There are two compelling reasons to be concerned. The first is the gradual increase in atmospheric temperature due to the trapping of infrared radiation within the atmosphere by so-called 'greenhouse' gases, such as carbon dioxide and methane, as well as nitrous oxide and volatile agents used in anaesthesia. The second cause for concern is the loss of the layer of ozone ($O_3$) at the top of the troposphere, which protects the Earth's surface from the damaging effects of solar ultraviolet radiation, of which the chlorofluorocarbons (CFCs) and nitrous oxide are the main culprits.

In its early evolution the original atmosphere of helium and hydrogen were lost from the Earth's gravitational field and replaced with the contents of outgassing volcanoes, such as $CO_2$ and $N_2$, and only very small amounts of $O_2$ were available to support life. Photosynthetic activity in plant life resulted in a buildup of $O_2$ as a by-product from $CO_2$ consumption. An appreciable greenhouse effect developed due to the release of methane from decaying organic plant matter, even though $CO_2$ levels themselves were falling at the time. Until the start of the industrial revolution, atmospheric $CO_2$ levels remained in the 280–300 ppmv, and have risen to 430 ppmv (Madge 2025) since then, mainly due to the burning of fossil fuels. In addition, methane levels continue to rise, as do the levels of other greenhouse gases, which include nitrous oxide with a duration in the atmosphere of 120 years and the CFCs, which last a hundred years or more, and anaesthetic volatile agents, which last several years.

Light in the visible and infrared wavebands of inbound solar radiation penetrates the atmosphere, heating the Earth's surface. A proportion of this is reflected back and escapes the atmosphere, but infrared radiation is prevented from escaping by water vapour and $CO_2$ at the top of the troposphere, whose molecules absorb infrared radiation and re-emit it at a longer wavelength. This heats up the Earth's surface by as much as 25°C, which in the early years of the evolution of life, permitted life to evolve when it might not otherwise have done so. Although methane is present in low concentrations, it is 25 times as effective in producing a greenhouse effect. This and the CFCs absorb infrared light in the 7–13 μm waveband, which is different from the wavebands of $CO_2$ and water absorption. This effectively adds extra panes of glass to the greenhouse, increasing atmospheric heating.

Oxygen absorbs ultraviolet (UV) radiation and provides protection on the Earth's surface against excessive UV radiation, but ozone does this much more effectively. Ozone has a maximum concentration of 10 ppmv at an altitude of 100 000 feet, and is formed by short-wave ultraviolet irradiation of oxygen. Below 40 000 feet the UV radiation is sufficiently weak not to catalyse this reaction, the concentration of ozone being 0.03 ppmv at sea level. Ozone itself is toxic to the human respiratory tract, causing bronchial irritation, a fall in vital capacity, FEV and diffusion capacity, and 10 ppmv can cause fatal pulmonary oedema.

Ozone levels vary throughout the year, depending on the local levels of UV radiation, but can be removed by the action of free radicals of chloride and nitric oxide. Chlorine itself is highly reactive, but does not normally penetrate the troposphere. CFCs do, and remain stable and pass freely through the troposphere to photodissociate and produce chloride radicals, each of which can destroy 10 000 molecules of ozone. Nitrous oxide will also pass through the troposphere to produce nitric oxide radicals with a similar effect on ozone. Ozone levels in the atmosphere fell from 300 units to 100 between 1960 and 1994, and continue to fall.

As anaesthetists we are therefore encouraged to use chloride-free volatiles, and to avoid nitrous oxide, even though medical use of both substances is small compared with those from older refrigerator circuits, agricultural fertilisers and other industrial sources (Brown and Sneyd 2016; McGain *et al.* 2020).

With this background, occupational exposure limits were devised under COSHH (Control of Substances Hazardous to Health) regulations in 1988. Anaesthetic gases were reviewed by the Health and Safety Executive in the 1990s, to determine if there was any link between occupational exposure to nitrous oxide and spontaneous abortions. Although no conclusive evidence was drawn, it is thought that an underlying mechanism of cell damage could be methionine synthetase inhibition, leading to impaired synthesis of vitamin $B_{12}$, folate and DNA, which could lead to subacute combined degeneration of the spinal cord. The stated 8-hour weighted average workplace exposure limit for nitrous oxide is 100 ppmv. Equivalent ppmv exposure limits under COSHH for Halothane are 10, and for enflurane and isoflurane are 50 (HSE 2020). There are no published UK workplace limits for Desflurane and Sevoflurane, but in Scandinavia, the figures are 5 and 20 ppmv (Varughese and Ahmed 2021). Manufacture of halothane, enflurane and isoflurane will stop after 2030.

## Scavenging systems

Environmental pollution from anaesthetic waste gases is a potential hazard to staff in the operating suite, as well as a longer-term issue with respect to the wider environment. Local pollution can cause staff to have chronic side effects of the volatile agents. As indicated above, CFCs, volatile agents and nitrous oxide are *greenhouse gases* and they interfere with the formation of *ozone*. 5% of the NHS's carbon footprint is due to exhaled anaesthetic agents, although all such gases from medical sources

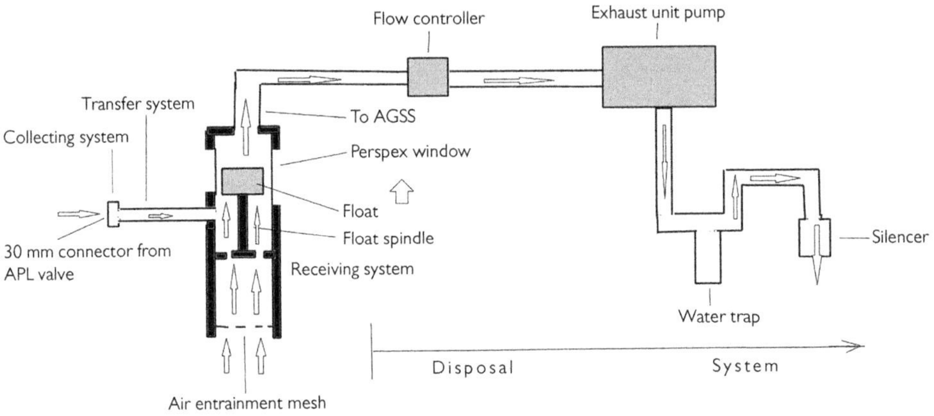


**Fig. 28.1** Components of an active scavenging system.

only account for 1% of gases from all sources. Scavenging systems can only help local pollution rather than global.

Scavenging systems are designed to transport waste anaesthetic gases from the breathing system to the atmosphere in order to avoid pollution in the enclosed environment of the operating room. They should not affect the patient's oxygenation or ventilation adversely. Systems can be either *active* or *passive*, although passive systems are seldom installed these days. Systems should contain a *collecting system, a transfer system, a receiving system* and *a disposal system*.

## Active system

This is shown in Figure 28.1. It has a collecting system, consisting of a shroud, either around the expiratory valve of the breathing system or around the APL valve of the ventilator. This is connected to the transfer tubing by a 30 mm conical connector. At the other end of the transfer tubing is the receiving system, which consists of an open-ended reservoir, shown in Figure 28.1, in which received expired gas passes upwards through a non-return valve assembly, visible through a clear tube, which is also allowed to entrain air from below. This entrainment allows uniform gas flow to the disposal system, which consists of a vacuum pump that delivers the gas to the atmosphere.

## Passive system

This consists of a collecting and transfer system similar to the active scavenging system. The receiving system consists of a reservoir bag associated with two spring-loaded valves: a positive pressure relief valve set to 1000 Pa, and a negative pressure relief valve set to -50 Pa. The disposal system is a wide-bore copper pipe leading to the atmosphere.

Some systems need to be adapted to suit circumstances that might otherwise make scavenging gases difficult, i.e. when using a Jackson–Rees modification of an Ayre's T piece (Dhara and Pua 2000).

## References


**Brown, S. M.** and **Sneyd, J. R.** (2016) Nitrous oxide in modern anaesthetic practice, *BJA Educ.*, **16**(3), pp. 87–91.

**Campbell, M.** and **Pierce, T. J. M.** (2015) Atmospheric science, anaesthesia and the environment, *Br. J. Anaesth.*, **15**(4), pp. 173–9.

**Dhara, S. S.** and **Pua, H. L.** (2000) A non-occluding bag and closed scavenging system for the Jackson–Rees modified T piece breathing system, *Anaesthesia*, **55**, pp. 450–4.

**HSE** (2020) *Workplace Exposure Limits EH40/2005*, 4th edn. HSE, London.

**Madge**, **C.** (2025) Rise in carbon dioxide off track for limiting global warming to 1.5°C *Met Office.* Available at: https://www.metoffice.gov.uk/about-us/news-and-media/media-centre/weather-and-climate-news/2025/rise-in-carbon-dioxide-off-track-for-limiting-global-warming-to-1.5c

**McGain**, **F.**, **Muret**, **J.**, **Lawson**, **C.** and **Sherman**, **J. D**. (2020) Environmental sustainability in anaesthesia and critical care, *Br. J. Anaesth.*, **125**(5), pp. 680–92.

**Varughese**, **S**. and **Ahmed**, **R. (**2021) Environmental and occupational considerations of anaesthesia: a narrative review and update. *Anesth. & Analg.*, **133**(4), pp. 826–35.

## *Further reading*

**Al-Shaikh**, **B. and Stacey**, **S.** (2002) Chapter 3 in *Essentials of Anaesthetic Equipment*, 2nd edn, Churchill Livingstone, London.

**Davey**, **A. J. and Diba**, **A.** (2012) Atmospheric pollution. Chapter 18 in *Ward's Anaesthetic Equipment*, 6th edn, Saunders, Philadelphia, PA, pp. 385–98.

**MacDonald**, **A. G.** (1994) A short history of fires and explosions caused by anaesthetic agents, *Anaesthesia*, **72**, pp. 710–22.

**MacDonald**, **A. G.** (1994) A brief historical review of non-anaesthetic causes of fires and explosions in the operating room, *Anaesthesia*, **73**, pp. 847–56.

**Mushin**, **W. W. and Jones**, **P. L**. (1987) Initiation of explosions. Chapter 22 in *MacIntosh, Mushin and Epstein: Physics for the Anaesthetist*, Blackwell Science, Oxford, UK, 4th edn, pp. 543–85.

# Chapter 29 **Imaging and radiation**

This chapter contains: radioactive decay; production of X-rays; imaging (X-rays, computed axial tomography, nuclear medicine, positron emission tomography; biological effects of radiation, radiation protection; magnetic resonance imaging, hazards; lasers.

The chapter links with: Chapter 3.

## Introduction

This chapter explains in simple terms the background physics of imaging using standard X-rays, computed axial tomography (CT), nuclear medicine (including positron emission tomography-PET), and magnetic resonance imaging (MRI). It covers the basics of ionising radiation, and also discusses lasers, which are a form of non-ionising radiation.

X-rays, CT, aspects of nuclear medicine, and lasers are covered briefly. MRI is examined in more detail. All of the modalities can require the presence or advice of an anaesthetist.

## Radioactive decay

Some isotopes are naturally occurring but many of the radioactive nuclides used in medicine are produced artificially by a nuclear reactor or *cyclotron*. Each of these will provide isotopes that are useful for different purposes. Unstable radioactive nuclides achieve stability by radioactive decay, during which they can lose energy. This occurs in a number of ways. For example, atoms can lose energy by ejection of an *alpha* particle (an extremely tightly bound basic atomic structure of 2 protons and 2 neutrons, which is equivalent to a helium nucleus). This occurs if they have too many nucleons (protons or neutrons) and results in the atomic number being reduced by two and the atomic mass by 4. Other ways that unstable radionuclides decay include: emission of an electron $(^{-})$ from the nucleus if the atoms have an excess of neutrons, or by, either emitting a positron $(^{+})$ or capturing an electron if they are neutron-deficient. Normally isotopes produced by a reactor will be neutron-rich and decay by emitting an electron and the cyclotron will tend to produce isotopes that are proton-rich and the decay will then be by emitting a positron. This is illustrated in Table 29.1.

The new nuclide formed by the decay process (the daughter nuclide) may be left in an excited nuclear state and can release this excess energy by emission of gamma ($\gamma$) radiation as shown in Figure 29.1. This example is where the electron $(^{-})$ has been emitted. The situation is more complex when a positron has been emitted. The emitted positron travels a short distance depending on the isotope (typically less than 1 mm) during which time it loses energy and interacts with an electron. This encounter annihilates both the electron and positron and the result is a pair of 511 keV gamma photons travelling in opposite directions. This pair of gamma rays are used in *positron emission tomography* (PET), discussed later in the chapter.

**Table 29.1** Mechanisms of decay

| Nuclear instability due to: | Mode of decay |
|---|---|
| excess neutrons | beta minus $(^{-})$ |
| excess protons (deficiency in neutrons) | positron $(^{+})$ or electron capture |
| excess neutrons and protons | alpha ($\alpha$) |

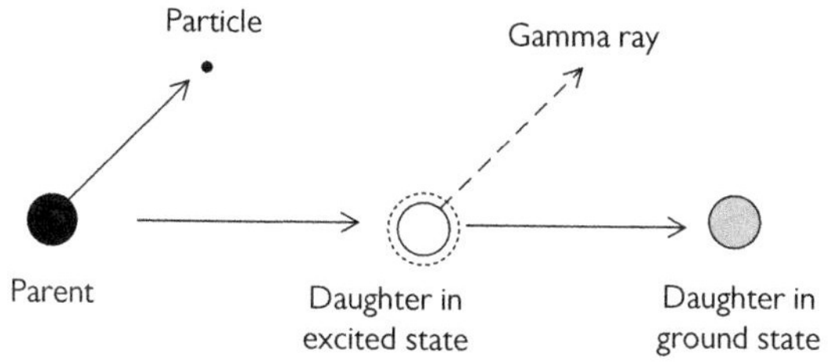


**Fig. 29.1** Radioactive decay showing gamma radiation. The parent in this example could be molybdenum-99 ($^{99}Mo$). The daughter in the excited state would be technetium-99m or $^{99m}Tc$. The ground state would be technetium-99 or $^{99}Tc$.

Gamma radiation is electromagnetic radiation like X-rays. They have similar energy and similar properties. Gamma rays come from the atomic nucleus and X-rays from changes in energy of electrons. Diagnostic radiology involves the use of X-rays produced in an X-ray tube, whilst nuclear medicine imaging detects gamma radiation emitted by a radioisotope that has been injected into the body. The amount of radioactivity is measured in terms of decay rate. A becquerel (Bq) is one disintegration per second.

## Production of X-rays

X-rays are produced when fast moving electrons are suddenly stopped by impact on a target (often metal). The kinetic energy of the electrons is converted into X-rays (1%) and heat (99%). An X-ray tube (see Figure 29.2) consists of a negative electrode (cathode) which has a tungsten filament heated to greater than 2200°C, and a positive electrode (anode) that incorporates a metal target, usually made of tungsten. Electrons leave the cathode and are accelerated towards the anode under the influence of a large potential difference of 50 000 to 140 000 volts, which is applied across the X-ray tube. These electrons bombard the target anode with a velocity of around half the speed of light.

X-rays are generated in two ways, emerging as discrete characteristic radiation and a continuous spectrum (the bremsstrahlung). Characteristic radiation is illustrated in Figure 29.3(a)–(c). When an accelerated electron from the filament collides with an electron in the K-shell (for example) of a tungsten atom in the target, an electron is ejected from this atom, leaving a *vacancy* in the K shell. The vacancy is most likely to be filled by an electron falling from the L-shell accompanied by the emission of a single X-ray photon. In this example, the energy of the characteristic photon is equivalent to the energy difference between the L and K shells in the tungsten target. A characteristic photon can only be produced if the energy of the bombarding electron is greater than the energy required to eject a K-shell

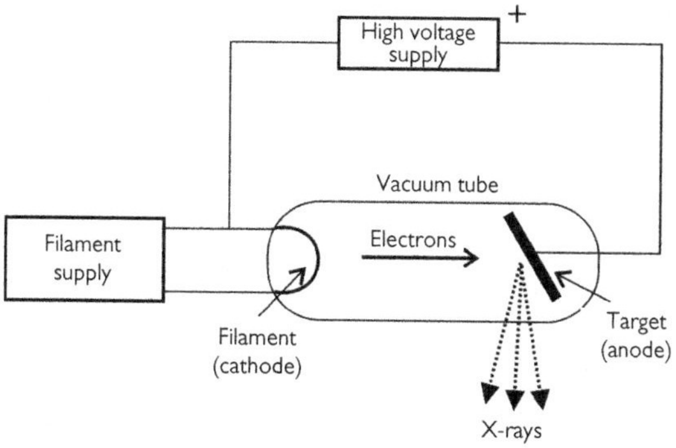


**Fig. 29.2** Diagram of an X-ray tube and the power supplies.

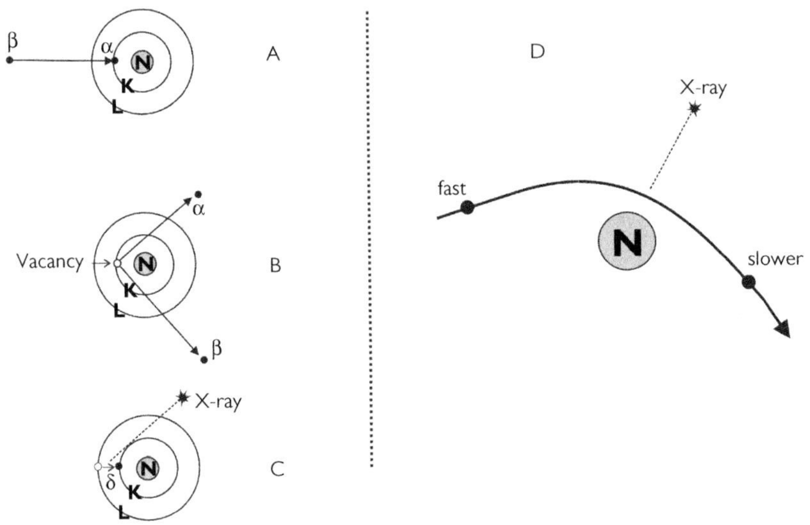


**Fig. 29.3** Production of X-rays. Characteristic radiation is shown in diagrams (a)–(c). N is the nucleus of the atom. In (a), a bombarding electron () from the filament collides with an electron in the K shell ($\alpha$). In (b), the $\alpha$ electron is ejected from the atom leaving a vacancy. In (c), the vacancy is filled by an electron falling from the L shell, which causes the emission of a single X-ray photon. In (d), N is the nucleus. The fast bombarding electron is deflected and slows down, losing some or all of its energy. This lost energy is carried away as a single photon of X-rays, as shown.

electron, and it will be characteristic of the particular target material. The mechanism for producing the continuous spectrum of X-ray energies is illustrated in Figure 29.3(d). A fast bombarding electron penetrates the K-shell and approaches close to the nucleus where it is deflected. It loses some or all of its energy in the interaction and the *lost* energy is carried away as a single X-ray photon. The process is repeated with various amounts of energy being lost in further interactions with other target nuclei. The net effect of all the electron interactions is a continuous spectrum of X-ray photon energies.

# Imaging

## *Imaging using X-rays*

When photons in an X-ray beam fall onto the patient, some pass through unchanged and some are absorbed. Overall, the X-ray beam is attenuated exponentially as it travels through the body. When the beam emerges from the patient, it carries a pattern of intensity resulting from the thickness and composition of the organs in its path. The X-rays can be captured on a large flat phosphor screen, which converts the invisible X-ray image into a visible image of light. This image is recorded and then, in computed radiography (CR) and digital radiography (DR), is viewed on a high-specification workstation. Some X-ray equipment allows the display of a 'live' image on a monitor and fluoroscopy is an example of this type of procedure. In this case, the detector is either an image intensifier or a so-called 'flat-plate' digital detector. Some computed tomography (CT) procedures (see below) also use 'real-time' image display, e.g. cardiac CT angiography.

## *Computed axial tomography imaging*

Conventional X-ray imaging produces a two-dimensional image of a three-dimensional object, which can be limiting for diagnosis. In computer axial tomography (CT, or sometimes CAT), a more detailed image of a thin slice of tissue can be obtained by rotating an X-ray tube around the patient. A narrow beam of X-ray is used and the intensity of the transmitted beam is recorded at each location around the body using a bank of highly sensitive detectors. The resultant signals are fed into a computer, which reconstructs a slice of the human body within seconds. The image is formed by a mathematical process. This is most commonly *filtered back projection* but increasingly iterative reconstruction methods are being used. As the demand for combined imaging modalities and cone-beam CT increases, there is a need for better processing algorithms, i.e. accurate and more efficient. In general the doses received by the patient undergoing CT examination are significantly higher than for conventional X-rays.

## Nuclear medicine imaging

Whereas CT and X-rays give anatomical information about the patient, nuclear medicine imaging gives dynamic information about organ function. The imaging can be two-dimensional, which is called scintigraphy, or three-dimensional, which is called single photon emission computed tomography (SPECT). A more complex form of nuclear medicine is PET, which is discussed later. In scintigraphy and SPECT, a radiopharmaceutical, normally produced by a nuclear reactor, is administered to the patient, usually by intravenous injection. This follows biological pathways and is designed to concentrate on the organ of interest. The role of the radionuclide is to signal the location of the radiopharmaceutical by the emission of gamma rays, as discussed earlier. As given in the example, Figure 29.1, $^{99m}Tc$ is the most commonly used radionuclide. It emits a gamma ray with an energy of 140 keV and has a half-life of 6 hours. Following the injection of a radionuclide, the patient acts as a source of radiation, the emerging gamma rays are detected by a *gamma camera*, and an image of the organ of interest is displayed. Depending on the isotope used, a patient can remain radioactive for a long period, ranging from hours to several days. The gamma camera consists of a number of sodium iodide crystals (or more recently, solid state devices) in a chamber. The crystals will produce light pulses when a gamma photon strikes them, and this pulse is then detected by electronic light detectors by the computer. For the 2D image, this will sit over the region of interest near the patient, and for the 3D image, the camera will normally rotate around the patient, and computer reconstruction will create the image.

## Positron emission tomography

PET is a more complex form of nuclear medicine already described. It is a 3D image process that again involves functional processes in the body, but it involves different isotopes that have much shorter half-lives, and are normally produced by a cyclotron. The PET process involves the pairs of 511 keV gamma rays already described. The radionuclides used in PET scanning are typically isotopes with short half-lives such as carbon-11 (half-life 20 minutes), nitrogen-13 (10 minutes), oxygen-15 (2 minutes) and fluorine-18 (110 minutes). These radionuclides are incorporated either into compounds normally used by the body, such as glucose, water or ammonia. The most commonly used nuclide is fluorine-18 in the form of fluorodeoxyglucose (FDG). The masses of the isotopes are small and so are their half-lives. Therefore, the cyclotron must be within a suitable travelling distance of the PET facility. The gamma camera in the case of PET is slightly different in that it normally consists of a complete ring of detectors around the patient. The PET process relies on the organ of interest in the body emitting the dual gamma rays in opposite directions, and the principle of coincidence detection will localise the object of interest. In simplistic terms, a detector will detect the gamma photon and then, at this same time, all the other detectors in the ring will be scanned to determine if they have detected a photon as well. The dual detection will be assumed to have come from the same location, but the gamma photons will have travelled in opposite directions. The place of emission will be along the line joining these two detectors. (This is shown in Figure 29.4.) PET imaging is proving very useful in neurology and oncology applications and, in particular, in the assessment of cerebral and cardiac function. It is very useful in tumour staging, in the early detection of cancer, and in the discrimination of benign and active tumours.

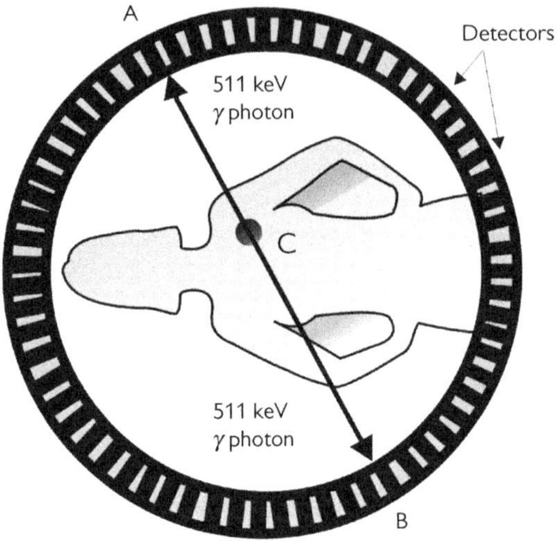


**Fig. 29.4** PET imaging. The diagram shows the emission of the gamma rays at C, travelling in opposite directions. They will be detected by the gamma detectors at A and B. The diagram shows a complete ring of multiple detectors all around the patient.

## *Biological effects of radiation and radiation protection*

Radiation can cause damage to the human body because the energy it carries causes ionisation (usually of water). Ions are produced that react with other water molecules in the body leading to free radicals and hydrogen peroxide. These produce further reactions with molecules such as DNA, which can lead to cellular and biological damage either immediately or after some time.

## *Radiation protection*

The three basic rules of radiation protection are shielding, distance and time (length of exposure). One should either move away from the source of the radiation or put an absorber between the source and the person. If, for example, a 185 kBq source from a radiotherapy machine fell on the floor about 1 m away from a person, then this person would receive a lethal dose of radiation in about 2 minutes. However, if the source were placed 4 m away, then the lethal dose would take around 32 minutes. About 30 mm of lead would be required to give the same protection as moving 4 m away. At low energies, lead screening is very effective; for example for a protective screen in a diagnostic X-ray room, 2.5 mm of lead is typically required.

## *Radiation units*

The absorbed dose is measured in terms of the energy absorbed per unit mass of tissue. Energy is measured in joules (J) and mass in kg and the unit of dose is the *gray* (Gy), where 1 Gy = 1 J $kg^{-1}$. Radiation energy is conveniently measured in electron volts and 1 J = $6.2 \times 10^{18}$ eV. A dose of 1 Gy means that $6.2 \times 10^{18}$ eV of energy has been absorbed in 1 kg of tissue.

The unit of equivalent dose, i.e. the dose that gives the same risk of damage to tissue whatever the type of radiation, has a special unit which is the sievert (Sv). An equivalent dose of 1 Sv is equal to 1 J $kg^{-1}$multiplied by a constant that depends on the type of radiation. For example, for X-rays and $\gamma$ waves this constant is 1 while for $\alpha$ particles it is 20. In most hospital situations the constant is 1. Typical doses from X-rays and $\gamma$ waves are shown in Table 29.2.

**Table 29.2** Typical figures for X-rays and $\gamma$ waves doses for different conditions

| Condition | Effective dose |
|---|---|
| Typical whole body dose due to background radiation in 1 year (UK average) | 2.2 mSv |
| Statutory dose limit to general population in 1 year | 1 mSv |
| Statutory dose limit to staff who work with radiation | 20 mSv |
| Adult chest X-ray | 0.1 mSv |
| Adult chest CT scan | 8 mSv |
| Tranatlantic flight | 0.1 mSv |
| Dose exposure that will cause nausea, sickness and diarrhoea in some people | 0.5 Sv (500 mSv) |
| Dose exposure that will kill many people in the few months following exposure | 5 Sv (5000 mSv) |

### *Measurement methods*

Various measurement devices are used for personal radiation dosimetry including the following: film badges (films exposed within screens inside a holder), thermoluminscent dosimeters, laser stimulated phosphor badges and electric dosimeters. A personal dosimetry badge is worn by the user for a set time during which the badge is affected by the amount of radiation falling on to it. It is then processed and provides a retrospective measure of the radiation dose received by that person. Electronic dosimeters give a real-time instantaneous read out and are useful when a measurement of a dose to an individual is required immediately. Although electronic dosimeters in the past were commonly based on ionisation chambers, solid state devices are now always used.

## Magnetic resonance imaging

Magnetic resonance imaging (MRI) is an imaging technique that uses the behaviour of atomic nuclei in strong magnetic fields to produce high-quality images of the human body. A patient is placed in a static magnetic field and radio-wave energy is applied. When the radio-wave transmission is turned off, the patient re-emits radio-waves, due to magnetic resonance that occurs in the atomic nuclei of body tissues. The signals from the body are detected and used to construct an image. The largest magnetic resonance signal is produced by the nuclei of hydrogen atoms (free or attached to other molecules, mainly water or fat) due to the high biological abundance of this element in the body. The nucleus of a hydrogen atom consists of a single unpaired proton and it therefore possesses the property of 'spin', essential for the magnetic resonance effect. MRI is able to measure the hydrogen content of individual volume elements, or *voxels* (e.g. a few cubic millimetres) in a slice of the patient and represent it as a shade of grey in the corresponding pixel on the image screen.

Unpaired protons *spin* continuously like a spinning top around an axis, and this causes them to behave like *bar magnets*. Normally all these individual magnets point (i.e. the direction of north–south pole axis) in a random orientation and combine to give a zero total magnetic effect. However, if a patient lies in a coil (as shown in Figure 29.5) and DC is passed through it (making it into an electromagnet and producing a strong magnetic field of 0.15–3 Tesla) the magnetic field causes the *bar magnets* to turn and point along the direction of the field in one of two stable directions: either in the direction of the applied magnetic (spin-up) or in the opposite direction (spin-down). For various reasons, there are slightly more magnets pointing spin-up than spin-down since this represents the lower energy state. MRI depends on detecting this difference although the excess number of spin-up over spin-down protons is very small.

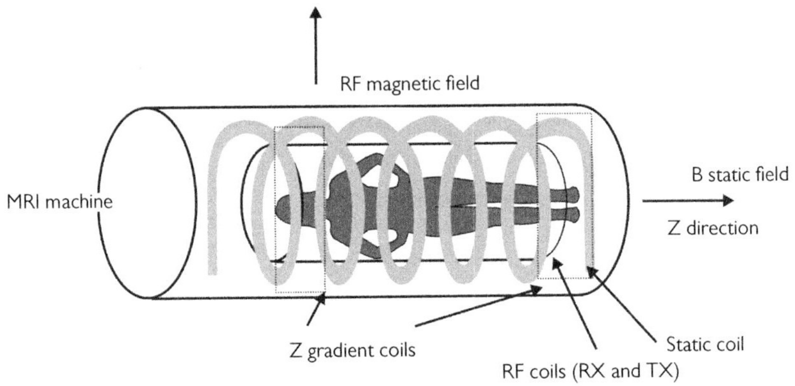


**Fig. 29.5** Diagram of the coils in an MRI machine. RF = radiofrequency, RX = receiver coils, TX = transmitter coils.

For example in a cubic millimetre of water, there are about $7 \times 10^{19}$ protons of which around $2 \times 10^{14}$ will be excess spin-up. The resulting magnetic field is not directly detectable because the direction is the same as the applied field, which would swamp this new field. As well as lining up the protons in a regular manner, the magnetic field causes the spinning protons to *precess*. This effect can be likened to a spinning top as it gradually slows down – it begins to tilt and rotate around another axis (sometimes referred to as wobble). This is illustrated in Figure 29.6. This shows the proton spinning around its own axis, and the precession axis as a separate phenomenon.

This precession frequency, the *Larmor* frequency, is proportional to both the strength of the magnetic field and a certain property of the nuclei called the *gyromagnetic* ratio. As an example, in a magnetic field of 1 Tesla, the proton (hydrogen nucleus) has a Larmor frequency of 42.6 MHz, which is in the radiofrequency range. When a magnetic field is applied, there is a net magnetisation in the direction of the magnetic field, but no magnetisation in any other direction, since all the protons are precessing independently in a random manner (out of phase). There are two potential signals but neither are yet useful: the *excess* spinning effect in the direction of the magnetic field cannot be measured as it is in the same direction and thus swamped by it, and the magnetic effect in other directions is zero because the protons precessions are out of phase. There still needs to be a method of measuring the MR signal (and obtaining an image) and this is carried out by supplying

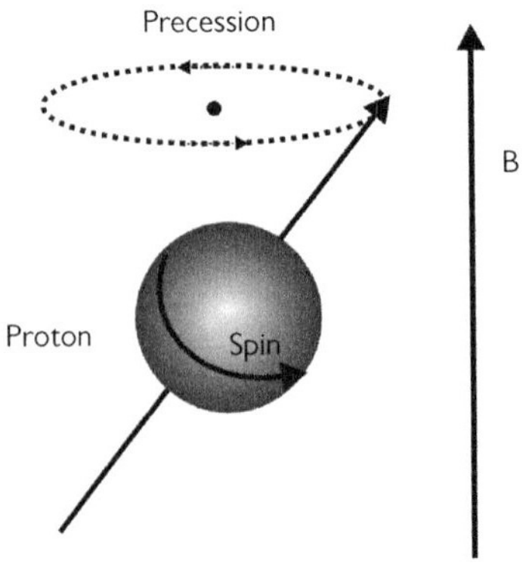


**Fig. 29.6** The precession of a spinning proton. The magnetic field direction is shown as B.

radiofrequency energy via appropriate coils, as shown in the Figure 29.5. This energy, the frequency of which is *tuned* to the Larmor frequency (resonance), is applied by a radiofrequency pulse lasting typically 1 ms and causes all the protons to precess in step (in phase). As a result, their combined spins produce a measurable magnetic pulse which is in a different direction to the applied static magnetic field. Viewed perpendicular to the applied field, this net magnetisation appears to oscillate due to the rotations of the protons. The use of a radiofrequency pulse to flip the direction of the net magnetisation, enables the magnetic resonance signal to be measured. When the radiofrequency pulse is temporarily switched off (the *off* part of the pulse), the circularly precessing magnetic field will be still present for up to 3 seconds as many of the precessions will be still in phase. This radiofrequency energy induces a voltage in the tuned receiver coils (Figure 29.5) and the effect is analogous to a radio transmitter and receiver, both tuned to a specific station. The received signal controls the pixel brightness (that makes up the image), and is dependent on the number of protons per cubic millimetre (the voxel), the gyromagnetic ratio (the magnetic properties) of the nucleus and the strength of the static field.

Only mobile protons give out signals and those immobilised in bone do not. Air in sinuses, for example, having no hydrogen, produces no signal and always appears black on an image. Tissues do not vary greatly in the proton density but fat has a higher proton density than other soft tissues and grey matter has greater proton density than white matter.

The MR signal is greatest immediately after the 1 ms radiofrequency pulse has *stopped* and it decays away due to two different processes: *spin-lattice* and *spin-spin* relaxation. Both are affected in different ways by properties of the human anatomy, and knowledge of the relaxation properties of different tissues allows images to be obtained with enhanced contrast. Water and CSF have long relaxation times (also urine, amniotic fluid, and other solutions of salts). In contrast, bone, tendons, and teeth have very short relaxations times. Different solutions in the body also have different relaxation properties (Farr and Allisy-Roberts 1998). With an understanding of the properties of different materials in the body, the contrast of each pixel can be improved to produce sharper, crisper images. Other machine related factors can also influence the image quality and contrast, such as radiofrequency pulse repetition rate, echo time and pulse sequences.

## *Spatial encoding*

An MR scan is made up of a series of parallel slices (Figure 29.7) imaged in turn. To obtain the image, it is necessary to identify the signals coming from individual pixels within each slice (and therefore voxels). Three different perturbations are applied to the magnetic field, one for each of the three orthogonal directions, and this allows spatial information to be localised within the body in three dimensions. Each direction is considered separately in the description below. The following method is used to select the signal specific to an axial slice through the body.

Since the precessing frequency is proportional to the strength of the magnetic field, applying a magnetic field gradient in the direction along the patient, allows axial position to be uniquely related to signal frequency. This is done by supplying DC through a pair of gradient coils which are in addition, but close proximity to, the main static coil (Figure 29.5). The field is made to vary from the head to the foot of the patient with a constant gradient. For example if the field is diminished at the head of the patient and augmented at the toe, accordingly protons at the head will precess more slowly than those in the middle and those at the toe will precess faster. There is therefore a corresponding gradient in the resonant frequency of the protons in the Z direction (see Figures 29.7 and 29.8). The selected slice will have a unique narrow frequency range and the radiofrequency transmitter is tuned to generate a pulse that contains this small range of frequencies. Only protons in a certain thin slice of the patient will be excited by this transmission, and will respond by producing an MR signal as described previously.

In a similar manner, the other directions (i.e. X and Y) can be selected. The Y coil, shown in Figure 29.8, identifies lines within the slice, and the X coil determines actual pixels with the line. Knowing the location of each pixel, the image can gradually be created by putting together all the pixels.

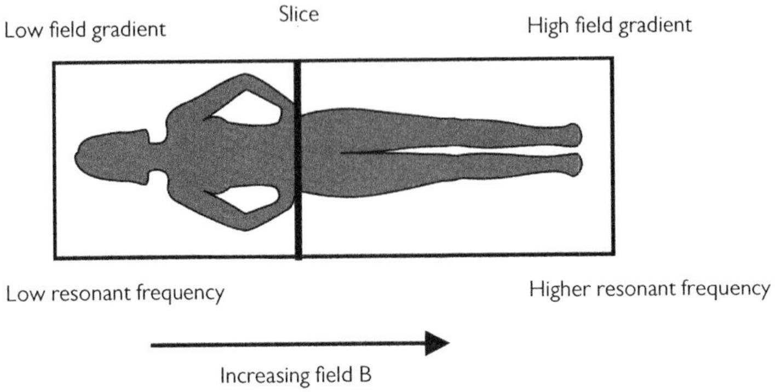


**Fig. 29.7** Diagram showing slice selection. There is increasing field strength from left to right, and this causes increasing resonant frequency from left to right of the diagram.

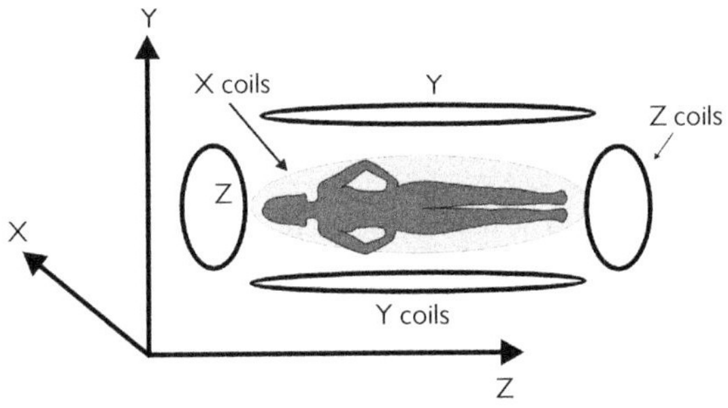


**Fig. 29.8** The various gradient coils, X, Y and Z. The Z coils cause a gradient change along the patient. The Y coils are over and under the patient, and cause a gradient change in the Y direction. The X coils (one on each side of the patient) cause a gradient change in the X direction.

## *Hazards*

MRI does not involve ionising radiation, and up to the present time there has been an absence of serious adverse health effects due to the magnetic field. In 2008 the Health Protection Agency (HPA) recommended a relaxation of the safety guidelines for patient exposure to static magnetic fields. The revised limit for patients and volunteers undergoing MRI procedures permits static magnetic field strengths of up to 4 T in routine operating mode.

Various national and international bodies have proposed exposure limits for workers in static and time-varying electric, magnetic and electromagnetic fields. For example in 2002 the National Radiological Protection Board in UK recommended a limit on magnetic flux density of 0.2 T continuous exposure throughout the working day while permitting short exposures to the head at 2 T and limbs at 5 T. The Medicines and Healthcare products Regulatory Agency (MHRA) and the Institute of Physics and Engineering in Medicine (IPEM) have produced safety notices and directives to minimise risks and improve safety. The EU Physical Agents (Electromagnetic Fields) Directive 2004/40/EC was designed to protect the health and safety of workers exposed to electromagnetic fields. The Directive was approved by the European Commission (EC) in 2004, and then revised in 2013 to the 2013/35/EU directive on electromagnetic fields. This was transposed into UK law in 2016 by the Control of Electromagnetic Fields at Work Regulations 2016 (CEMFAW regulations).

The switching of the gradient magnetic fields can create induced *eddy* currents (induced currents produced by changing magnetic fields, as in transformers), which might be induced in any biological conductor, e.g. nerve fibres, which can result in involuntary muscular contraction, breathing difficulties and possible VF. Particular care is required for patients with heart disease and MRI may not be possible on a patient with an implantable pacemaker. When very strong fields are present, staff and patients may experience flashes of light on the retina and sensations of taste. The magnetic gradient fields should not build up too quickly to avoid shock-like symptoms due to severe nerve stimulation: no faster than 20 T $s^{-1}$ and in practice, 1 to 5 T $s^{-1}$ is typical. As a precaution, MRI should not be carried out during the first trimester of pregnancy.

Microwave heating may occur with radiofrequency fields, especially at the higher frequency associated with strong static fields. It is usually compensated by vasodilatation. However both the cornea and testis have a lower blood supply and may be at risk. The specific absorption ratio is the radiofrequency energy deposited per unit mass of tissue and should not exceed 2.0 W $kg^{-1}$ for the whole body. HPA (2008) recommend a limit on the rise in core body temperature of 0.5°C and an upper temperature limit of 39°C for the trunk and the head. The radiofrequency may also affect the workings of pacemakers, computers and vacuum-related devices such as gamma cameras in the immediate vicinity. MR-compatible monitoring equipment should be used in the MRI room and patient leads must be re-directed so that induced currents are minimised.

Mechanical attraction of ferromagnetic objects varies as the square of the magnetic field and the inverse cube of the distance. The fringe field, which can extend for a few metres, may convert scissors, scalpels and ferromagnetic gas cylinders into projectiles. Therefore, non-magnetic materials should always be used. Joint and dental prostheses are firmly fixed and should present no problem. Patients should remove hair grips, ear-rings and mascara containing iron oxide. The fringe fields can also affect watches, credit cards and computers and disks. Free access of the public must be limited to areas where the field strength is less than 0.5 mT.

### *Special features of MRI*

The special features of MRI include:

- ionising radiation is not involved in producing images;
- images can be obtained simultaneously in a number of places at any angle;
- soft tissue contrast is high;
- bone and air do not produce artefacts;
- it is non-invasive.

## Lasers

As explained in Chapter 3 (see also Figure 3.7), electrons can be considered to be distributed in a number of concentric shells around the nucleus that have different energies. If electrons move from one level or shell to another, energy is consumed or liberated in steps or quanta.

If external energy, above a certain threshold, is applied to suitable gases, liquids or solids, and therefore to the atoms of these materials themselves, the atoms can leave the *ground state energy* level (resting level) and achieve an *excited* level. The level of excitation depends on the amount of applied energy being supplied by, for example, heat, light or electricity. In the excited state, the electrons move to higher energy orbits, further away from the nucleus. Once an electron moves to a higher energy orbit, it eventually wants to return to the ground state. When this happens, it releases a photon – a particle of light.

The laser is a device that controls the way that energised atoms release protons. *Laser* is an acronym: *L*ight *A*mplification by *S*timulated *E*mission of *R*adiation. In any type of laser, the lasing medium, which gives the laser its wavelength or colour, is *pumped* to get the atoms into an excited state.

Typically, intense flashes of light or electrical discharges pump the lasing medium and create a large collection of excited-state atoms (atoms with a higher than normal number of electrons in excited states). It is necessary to have a large collection of atoms in the excited state, which requires a large energy input. There is then a *population inversion*, which is where the normal ground-level electrons become dominant in the higher shells. The electrons have absorbed energy to get to the higher levels and all the atoms will have electrons at the same higher levels. These electrons subsequently are relaxed to a lower energy state and release energy in the form of photons of light of a specific wavelength or colour. For example, two identical atoms with electrons in the same higher level, pumped from the same energy source, will release photons with identical wavelengths. Laser light has the following properties:

- The light is monochromatic: it contains one specific wavelength;
- The light released is coherent: all the wavelengths are in phase;
- The light is highly directional.

To achieve these properties a process called stimulated emission has to occur. A photon emitted by an atom has a certain wavelength, energy and phase. If this photon then interacts with another atom and electron in the same excited state, stimulated emission can occur. The first photon can stimulate or induce atomic emission, such that the subsequent photon from the second atom has the same frequency and direction as the incoming photon.

The cavity containing the lasing material also contains a pair of mirrors. Photons are reflected by the mirrors and so travel back and forth through the lasing medium, constantly stimulating other electrons to make the downward energy jump. In this way a cascade effect occurs. Since one of the mirrors is not completely silvered, the laser light is able to pass through once an appropriate density of light is achieved. To give an example, Figure 29.9 illustrates how a ruby laser works. An energy source (pump), such as a high-intensity flash from a mercury vapour discharge lamp, emits radiation into the ruby rod. The light excites atoms in the ruby and some of these atoms emit photons of energy as they fall back to the lower shell. Some of these photons travel in a direction parallel to the crystal axis and are reflected by the mirrors. As they continue to travel back and forth through the crystal, they stimulate emissions in other atoms and a cascade effect occurs.

There are many types of laser and the lasing medium can be solid, liquid, gas or semiconductor. Examples are:

- solid state lasers, e.g. ruby with a 694.3 nm wavelength;
- gas lasers e.g. $CO_2$ (far infrared) 10 600 nm;
- dye lasers; complex organic dyes in liquid solution; they are tuneable between 570 and 630 nm;
- semiconductor lasers; low power, current through PN (semiconductor) junction.

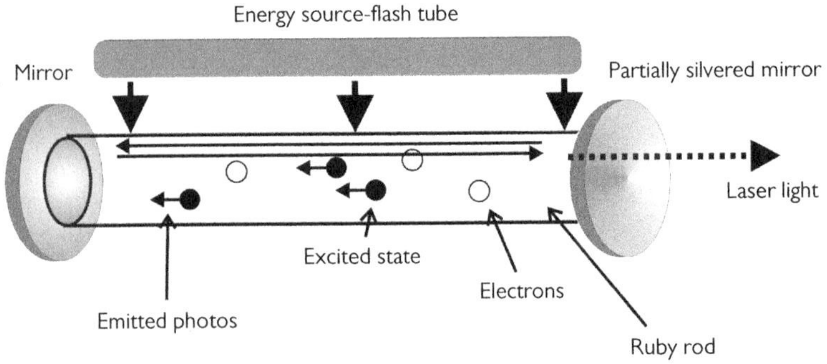


**Fig. 29.9** Simplified diagram of a ruby laser. See text for details.

The laser can be classified into four classes:

- class 1: these lasers cannot emit laser radiation at known hazard levels;
- class 2: these are low-power visible lasers, at a radiant power not above 1 mW;
- class 3: these are intermediate and moderate power lasers, and are hazardous only for intrabeam viewing;
- class 4: these are high-power lasers (> 500 mW continuous), which are hazardous to view and are a skin hazard.

### *Biomedical applications*

All biomedical applications of laser energy depend on tissue absorption. However, the particular response depends on where the absorption occurs (Cornelius 1983). There are three ranges of radiant energy (infrared, visible and ultraviolet) that produce different tissue responses. Infrared induces molecular vibration, leading to heat effects. Visible light produces photochemical effects. Ultraviolet radiation can produce molecular bond dissociation, as well as skin burns. $CO_2$ lasers are normally used for surgical applications, such as in gynaecology, and argon-ion gas lasers can be used for ophthalmology. Solid state lasers such as neodymium (Nd): yttrium-aluminium garnet (YAG) have dermatological uses.

## *References*

**Cornelius, W. A.** (1983) Applications of lasers in medicine, Australas, *Phys. Eng. Sci. Med.*, **6**, pp. 106–14.

**Farr, R. F.** and **Allisy-Roberts, P. J.** (1998) Magnetic resonance imaging, in Allisy-Roberts, P. J. (ed.), *Physics for Medical Imaging*, Harcourt Publishers, Edinburgh, pp. 215–51.

**Health Protection Agency (HPA)** (2008) *Protection of Patients and Volunteers Undergoing MRI Procedures*, HPA, London, UK.

## *Further reading*

**Farr, R. F.** and **Allisy-Roberts, P. J.** (1998) *Physics for Medical Imaging*, Harcourt Publishers, Edinburgh.

**Gibson, K. F.** and **Kernohan, W. G.** (1993) Lasers in medicine – a review, *J. Med. Eng. Tech.*, **17**(2), pp. 51–7.

**Lalabekyan, B.**, **Rennie, A.**, and **Luoma, V.** (2025) Principles of radiation safety for anaesthetists, *BJA Educ.*, **25**(5), pp. 181–90.

**Parker, R. P.**, **Smith, P. H. S.** and **Taylor, D. M.** (1978) *Basic Science of Nuclear Medicine*, Churchill Livingstone, London, UK.

**Taylor, J.**, **Chandramohan, M.**, and **Simpson, K. H.** (2013). Radiation safety for anaesthetists, *Cont. Educ. Anaesth. Crit. Care Pain*, **13**(2), pp. 59–62..

# Chapter 30 **Cleaning and sterilisation of equipment**

## Two different processes

Although an increasing proportion of anaesthetic and surgical equipment is disposable nowadays, there is still a significant amount of cleaning and sterilisation required, and with the emergence of new organisms, the methods used have come under closer scrutiny. It is worth noting, in passing, that hand cleanliness of staff coming into contact with patients has also come under close scrutiny in recent years, especially since the COVID-19 pandemic, and the wearing of clinical masks has become more common even outside the operating theatre. Cleaning of equipment involves the physical removal of as much of the infectious agent as possible, usually using water and a detergent, and is an important precursor to disinfection or sterilisation. It can be done manually where automated devices are unavailable. Ultrasonic washers are sometimes used, as are irrigation pumps for flushing out the lumina of tubes.

There is a difference in definition between disinfection and sterilisation. Disinfection is merely the killing of non-spore producing micro-organisms. It kills most bacteria except mycobacteria and spores, and it kills some fungi and some viruses. A higher level of disinfection ensures the destruction of mycobacteria, and most fungi and viruses. Sterilisation is required to kill all micro-organisms, including spores, fungi and viruses. Prions are, however, resistant to most sterilisation procedures. To disinfect or sterilise the modes of applied heat, chemicals or radiation are used.

Moist heat is much more efficacious at coagulating bacterial protein than dry heat, which requires higher temperatures for longer periods to guarantee effect. Moist heat achieves this by increasing the permeability of the organism's cellular structure to the heat. A hot water washer or low temperature steam applied to instruments for fifteen minutes kills bacteria, but not spores. Higher temperatures are achievable by pressurising the steriliser (Boyle's law). The modern autoclave uses steam at 134°C and 2 bar, when 3½ minutes is sufficient to kill all organisms, providing the steam can reach the instruments; to dry the equipment, the steam is removed and replaced with sterile air, the total cycle time being 10 minutes. Rubber and plastic materials degenerate after some time with this regime, and a combination of 121°C for fifteen minutes, or 115°C for 30 minutes can be used instead. If the equipment being sterilised is damaged by superheated steam, a low temperature of 73°C at 290 mmHg gauge pressure for two hours can be used to kill bacteria, and the addition of formaldehyde to the steam deals with spores.

Chemical sterilisation is useful for instruments such as endoscopes, which may not tolerate steam. Chemicals, which kill by protein coagulation, only act on the surface of materials, and some of them react with metals; they may impregnate rubber and plastic, which may be a source of tissue irritation on subsequent use of the equipment. Formaldehyde may be used for endoscopes and catheters, but it is hard to get rid of after the sterilisation process. Ethylene oxide is an agent that is bactericidal and toxic to humans. It is effective against all organisms and penetrates well, but requires at least 8 hours for effectiveness. It is explosive at a concentration above 3% in air, and requires 10% $CO_2$ and a humidity of between 30 and 50% for safety. Although slow, it is an efficacious method of sterilising delicate equipment, such as ventilators, other respiratory equipment and prostheses. To get rid of the ethylene oxide after the sterilisation process, six vacuum cycles are recommended.

A number of liquids are used for sterilisation, for topical use and otherwise. 1–5% phenol is used for cleaning surfaces, and should not be used on objects that contact the patient's skin; it does not kill spores. 0.5–2% iodine in alcohol irritates skin, although 10% povidone-iodine is less so. 70–80% ethyl alcohol is more effective than absolute alcohol. 0.5% chlorhexidine in ethyl alcohol, sometimes with cetrimide added, is effective for skin sterilisation. 2% glutaraldehyde solution in sodium bicarbonate is used for endoscopes and kills bacteria in 15 minutes and spores in 3 hours.

Gamma irradiation is used to sterilise equipment because it does not leave the equipment radioactive. A dose of 2.5 Mrad is bactericidal. Clearly, careful control of radiation dosing is required. It is normally used to sterilise surgical gloves, surgical instruments and orthopaedic implants.

## *Further reading*

**Davey, A. J.** and **Diba, A.** (2012) Cleaning, disinfection and sterilization. Chapter 23 in *Ward's Anaesthetic Equipment*, 6th edn, Elsevier, pp. 429–37.

**Davies, N. J. H.** and **Cashman, J. N.** (2006) Anaesthetic equipment. Chapter 2.1 in *Lee's Synopsis of Anaesthesia*, Elsevier, Philadelphia, PA, pp. 96–8.

# Chapter 31 **Medical training using simulators**

This chapter contains: simulation centres and environments; model-driven simulators, mathematical modelling; scenario-based training; surgical skills laboratories; hybrid training; virtual and augmented reality training.

The chapter links with: Chapters 1 and 11.

## Introduction

Training and education using simulation has been used extensively in many high-risk industries including aviation, nuclear power, military and rail. Repeated exposure to simulated crises and events has meant that, for example, airline crews are well prepared to face a rare disaster when it happens in real life. The use of simulation, simulators and simulation environments in medicine, to train and educate healthcare professionals is now widespread throughout the UK. The first simulation centre of its kind in the UK was the Bristol Medical Simulation Centre, which opened in 1997. After this, several more similar centres opened, but it was the Chief Medical Officer's 2008 annual report – *Safer Medical Practice: Machines, Manikins and Polo Mints* (Department of Health 2008) that caused this mode of training to gain national support and widespread adoption. There are now many similar centres in the UK and many more with manikins in simpler settings, and hundreds of centres throughout the world (Department of Health 2010). All these centres offer a similar concept to that which the high-risk industries use, where training for medical emergencies using sophisticated manikins is used in realistic medical settings, and task trainers are used to teach, for example, practical surgical skills. Additionally, medical education is also enhanced using simulation techniques and this is widespread now (Health Education England 2016). Medical simulation centres and facilities are now located in many different environments. Some are part of university healthcare facilities and medical schools, and others are located in NHS premises.

Many potential accidents in medicine are due to human error and communication problems (Kohn *et al.* 1999; Department of Health 2009). Simulators can help train teams to function optimally using *human factors* style teaching, and can help training in patient safety issues in anaesthesia (Burnett *et al.* 2024). Simulation could also be a practical solution to several current educational issues. These include the challenges faced by educational institutions in securing clinical placements, the decrease in social acceptance of trainees learning on patients, the drive to maximise patient safety, the shortage of senior clinical trainers and the shortage of traditional clinical training spaces.

## Simulation centre environments

The simulation centres consist of a number of different designated rooms, depending on which clinical or medical environment is being simulated, and the complexity of the simulation facility. For example, in the operating theatre, simulated operations and team training can be carried out in a suitably equipped theatre suite. This suite is created to be as close as possible to the modern operating rooms. It contains real equipment such as anaesthetic machines, ventilators, defibrillators, patient monitors, trolleys and drip stands. A control room is usually next to the operating room, with a one-way viewing window. This is where the manikin is controlled and where the simulation training is viewed and recorded. Tutors in the control room communicate with key personnel in the clinical rooms using radio headsets. Audio-visual facilities are located in the control room, and all of the simulation carried out in the rooms is normally recorded. The operating room can be re-configured to be other clinical rooms, such as ITU, or in some centres, the ITU is a permanent fixture.

Debriefing is essential to the simulation process, and a de-briefing conference room is essential for this. This can be connected to the simulation room by a one-way viewing window or viewed using the audio-visual facilities. Simulated episodes may be replayed and analysed multiple times by the trainee with the tutor, or independently.

There can be multi-bedded wards included in the simulation facility. These are provided with monitors, ventilators and similar equipment to that provided in the real wards.

Simulation can take place outside the simulation centres: *in-situ* simulation is where the manikins are taken to real wards, accident and emergency or other real clinical environments. The environment is real in these cases, and simulations such as resuscitation training can be very effective.

All the simulation facilities mentioned have manikin-based simulators included in them and this is what makes this type of centre or environment unique.

### *Manikins-based simulators*

These manikin-based simulators can be at many levels of complexity and levels of fidelity. The most complex high-fidelity ones are very life-like, and they can be model-driven (driven by mathematical models of the physiological systems) or non-model-driven. The model-driven ones are capable of functioning on their own with less tutor or technician involvement, whereas the non-model systems are controlled by complex software and scenario scripts. Complex non-model driven systems are more widespread, and are mainly related to the SimMan family, created by Laerdal Medical, and the more complex models are the SimMan 3G plus and the SimMan Critical Care. These are very realistic, but are not model-driven. Other complex simulators are manufactured by Gaumard.

In both these types of simulators, the human is represented by a correctly sized whole-body manikin (adult, child or baby). Furthermore, many of the ways in which the medical team interact with a patient can be simulated. The manikins can be cannulated, intubated, ventilated, and monitored (ECG or arterial waveforms, heart sounds, blood pressure, oximetry).

Less sophisticated manikins are also used in the simulation process, and these can be hugely valuable in the education process, where sometimes the level of technology is not so important (Lavoie 2020), or portability is needed, as in the in-situ simulation discussed earlier. However, anaesthetic training modalities tend to favour more high-fidelity manikins for their training.

## Model-driven patient simulators

The model-driven high-fidelity human patient simulators offer the greatest realism of the simulators (initially METI until 2011, USA, then CAE, USA until 2024, now Elevate Healthcare, USA) and are complex machines with all the physiological signals generated by the mathematical models. The human physiology and pharmacology are modelled realistically by computers that drive it. There are many advantages of using model-driven devices. They can be more dynamic and give very realistic interpretations of human physiology and the response to medication. There is less demand on the tutor or trainer, as the simulator can perform independently. Many different patient types can be created, as discussed later. An example of a model-driven paediatric simulator in an operating theatre is shown in Figure 31.1

These patient simulators have real gas exchange. Anaesthetic gases are recognised by the gas analyser in the manikin's associated electronics, and intravenous drugs are recognised by a bar-code reader, or input via the computer console. Each drug syringe has a bar code on it that relates to the strength and type of drug. The syringe contains saline. When the syringe is *injected* into the patient, the bar code reader will relay to the computer what drug and concentration is being supplied. In the same way, the gas analyser will supply the mathematical models with the data to give the correct response.

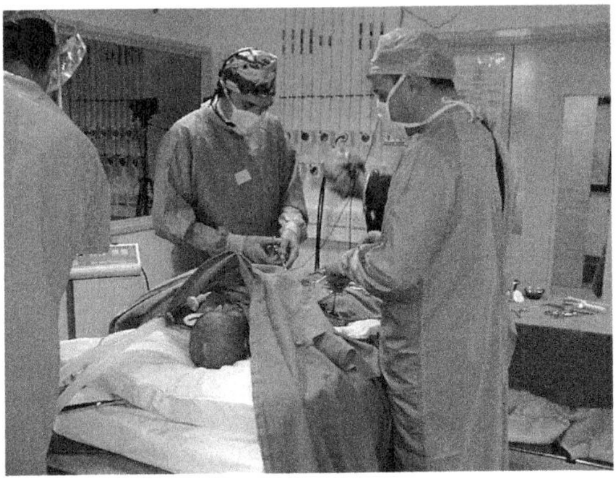

**Fig. 31.1** An example of a paediatric human patient simulator in an appropriately equipped operating theatre.

## Mathematical modelling

Mathematical models simulate the patient's physiology and pharmacology and provide responses in real time to the therapeutic interventions for the patient's clinical condition. The models rely on software to predict the manikin's responses and have great flexibility for changing the model parameters. The human patient simulator currently contains thirteen different models (van Meurs et al. 1997, 1998), but they can be grouped into three groups, the cardiovascular (the heart systems), the respiratory (the lung systems), and distribution and pharmacology (drug systems). The complete models are shown in Table 31.1.

The models receive either inputs from the outside world, e.g. gas flow measurements from the lungs, anaesthetic gas concentrations, or take outputs from another model. Many of the models, where appropriate, interact with each other.

**Table 31.1** Human patient simulator mathematical models

| Cardiovascular | Respiratory | Pharmacology and reflex control |
|---|---|---|
| Uncontrolled cardiovascular system (blood volumes, pressures, flows, wedge). | Lung and chest wall mechanics (gas volumes, pressures, flows) | Distribution of anaesthetic gases |
| Myocardial oxygen balance | Respiratory rhythm (including respiratory muscle pressure generator) | Pharmacokinetics of intravenous drugs |
| Cardiac rhythm (including contractility and ECG generators) | Pulmonary gas exchange | Pharmacodynamics and control of circulation |
| Thermodilution cardiac output ... | Distribution of respiratory gases | Pharmacodynamics and control of breathing |
| | | Pharmacodynamics of neuromuscular blockade and reversal |

Most of the models provide real outputs, e.g. breath sounds, ECG, various pulses around the body, pulse oximetry signals, blood pressure, thermo-dilution cardiac output, and temperature. These are generated independently of the operator or tutor.

## Patient types

As the simulator is model-driven, the vast number of parameters that control a typical patient can be changed at the start of a simulation session to create many different patient types. The simulator comes supplied with many people types. For example, one system has 'Standard Man' (70 kg, 25-year-old male, standard fitness, non-smoker, standard height, standard physiology), 'Standard Junior', 'Stanette' (female Stan), and 'Truck Driver' (very obese, heavy smoker, unfit, short male) and many more. The basic physiological models can be changed to create different types and many interesting people can be created.

## Scenario scripts

The simulator can be allowed to run freely on its own for tutorials on, for example, physiology and pharmacology. The models and other parameters of the simulation can be controlled in real time by the user interface. Both model-driven and non-model-driven simulators use scripts to control how they work. The computer programs (similar to high-level languages, like C++, Pascal, Python) can be used to control and modify physiological parameters and give commands to the simulator to react or respond in a certain manner. The same sequence can be used time and time again for *fair* testing of trainees.

For example, a simple critical incident scenario such as anaphylaxis (idiosyncratic, abnormal, and potentially fatal reaction to a normally innocent material, drug or foodstuff) uses a script as shown in Figure 31.2. The scripts are written by the course leader and can range from complex to very simple. Each stage or 'state' of the script contains several procedures to produce the effect, and the *begin analphylaxis* state is expanded to show this. The scenario will start at the baseline and will either progress by the operator manually advancing it or can be sequenced automatically. If a Boolean *condition* is met, such as 'IF time >60 s', or 'IF drug given', then the algorithm will automatically advance to the next state.

There are numerous crisis events that can be programmed, for example, malignant hyperthermia, asthma and major haemorrhage. These can be as complex as the imagination and skill of the course designer allows. For example, a severe crisis can be made to develop. Oxygen supply can actually run out during a Caesarean section operation, complications can occur, there is a fire alarm, a power failure, etc.

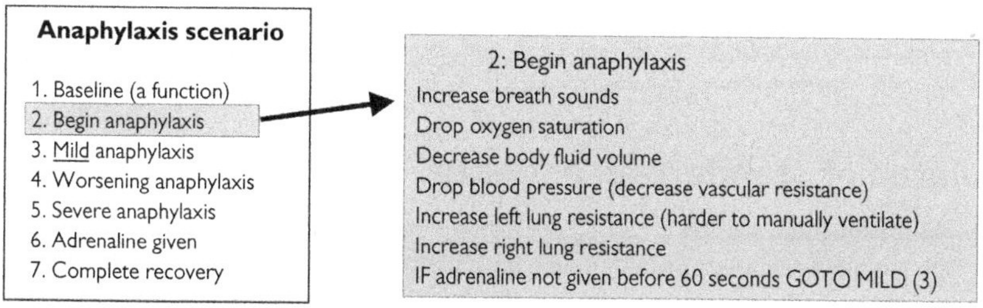


**Fig. 31.2** An example of a simplified anaphylaxis script.

## Scenarios

The scenario computer script must be accompanied by a *play* or scenario to give some background so that the medical *team* and controllers know what is happening. For example, to go with the anaphylaxis script, there can be the following scenario in a GP course:

The delegates are told that an 18-year-old man has been rushed into the emergency room having accidentally eaten a sweet containing peanuts. The man has a known allergy to peanuts and carries an *EpiPen* (a source of readily available injectable adrenaline). The delegates now attend the manikin, which has oral itching and swelling, which rapidly progresses to severe stridor (upper airway obstruction). The patient cannot be intubated and requires a surgical airway. The delegates have to deal with this situation!

### *Educational opportunities*

The educational opportunities are many with human patient simulators. Trainees can be taught at the bedside by the tutor who can run the simulator from a handset. Equally, the simulator can be run from a hidden control room so that the trainees are unaware of how the tutor is programming the simulator. This allows a range of educational packages to be developed. These range from simple human physiology and pharmacology tutorials to the practice of emergency protocols that involve the whole operating team, e.g. the response to a fire in the theatre complex. In all situations, the advantage of simulation is to allow trainees to investigate human physiology and responses or practice the management of medical crises without danger to patients.

Simulators can also be used in examinations, such as the Royal College of Anaesthetists' Objective Structured Clinical Examinations assessment station within the primary fellowship examination. This was introduced initially as a fully assessed pilot scheme (McIndoe 2012) and fully implemented in the examination process (RCoA 2018).

Simulators can also be used in teaching medical students in novel ways. A team has been using a physiological model-based virtual simulator to teach large classes of medical students physiology (Helyer *et al.* 2024).

## Surgical skills laboratory

Another area where simulation can be useful is in surgery and surgical training. The surgical skills laboratory can contain many different devices to teach and provide objective evaluations of the trainee surgeons' technical abilities, and teach new techniques to qualified surgeons. These simulation devices range from the simple plastic device that teaches medical students how to stitch wounds, to complex, sophisticated devices that combine mechanical models with computer stations. Both can be used to teach basic skills and surgical tasks through repetitive proctored challenges, and will enable detection and analysis of surgical errors and near-miss incidents without risk to patients. These simulators are wide-ranging and include laparoscopic, cardiac simulators and robotic simulators. Most of the simulation systems include sophisticated measurement systems, which measure, for example, time to completion, number of errors, accuracy, economy of motion, and tracking of hand and limb movement.

## Simulated or standarised patients

This is when a simulation session is carried out without using a manikin. Instead, a skilled actor is employed, who has been carefully coached to simulate a patient so accurately that a skilled clinician cannot detect the simulation. This type of simulation can be very useful in certain teaching situations such as team training, but less useful for training in the anaesthetic process. However, actors are used to simulate preoperative patients in the FRCA examination.

## Hybrid training

Hybrid training has a couple of definitions: it can be when surgical trainers and wearable technology are combined in either manikins or strapped to actors, but in a realistic environment, so that team training using human factors and crisis events can be practised during 'real surgery' (Kneebone *et al.* 2005; Brown *et al.* 2020). It is also taken to refer to the combination of different modalities, such as using manikins, simulated patients and virtual or augmented reality.

## Virtual and augmented reality training

Simulation task and team training can be provided in a complete virtual world (such as the still-used Second Life, Kamel Boulos *et al.* 2007) that contains virtual patients and virtual medical devices within a very realistic three-dimensional clinical environment. Advanced computer models mean that the virtual patients behave very realistically, although there is no actual physical, hands-on experience. The trainees normally wear advanced headsets and can have sensors in their gloves. Augmented reality is where the digital information is overlaid onto the real clinical environment, enhancing the trainee's situational awareness.

### *Simulation miscellany*

Artificial Intelligence (AI) is likely to play a significant role in simulation training and is being utilised in research environments. It could help with personalised learning experiences and produce adaptive programs that adjust the difficulty of scenarios based on the trainees' or teams' performance.

Simulation centres can also provide test-beds for introducing new technologies and medical devices into a clinical environment, by monitoring how the team accesses and uses the novel equipment, under realistic, stressful conditions. The full team can be monitored using wearables to determine their stress and reaction levels to the novel equipment.

### *References*

**Brown, W. J.** and **Tortorella, R. A. W.** (2020). Hybrid medical simulation – a systematic literature review, *Smart Learn. Environ.*, **7**, p. 16.

**Burnett, G. W.** and **Goldhaber-Fiebert, S. N.** (2024) The role of simulation training in patient's safety in anaesthesia and perioperative medicine, *BJA Educ.*, **24**(1), pp. 7–12.

**Department of Health** (2008) *Safer Medical Practice: Machines, Manikins and Polo Mints. Annual report of the Chief Medical Officer*. Department of Health, London

**Department of Health** (2009) *150 Years of the Annual Report of the Chief Medical Officer*, Department of Health, London.

**Department of Health** (2010) *NHS Simulation Provision and Use Study Summary Report*, Department of Health, London.

**Health Education England** (2016). *Enhancing UK Core Medical Training through simulation-based education.*

**Helyer, R. J. *et al.*** (2024). Virtual patients to teach large classes: the University of Bristol experience. Available at: https://simzine.news/experience-en/did-you-know-en/virtual-patients-to-teach-large-classes-the-university-of-bristol-experience/

**Kneebone, R. L., Kidd, J., Nestel, D., *et al.*** (2005) Blurring the boundaries: scenario-based simulation in a clinical setting, *Med. Educ.*, **39**(6), pp. 580–7.

**Kohn, L. T., Corrigan, J. and Donaldson, M. S.** (1999) *To Err is Human: Building a Safer Health System, Institute of Medicine (U.S.), Committee on Quality of Health in America*, National Academies Press, Washington, DC.

**Kamel Boulos, M. N., Hetherington, L.** and **Wheeler, S.** (2007) Second Life: an overview of the potential of 3-D virtual worlds in medical and health education, *Health Info. Libr. J.*, *24*(4), pp. 233–45.

**Lavoie, P. et al** (2020). Beyond technology: a scoping review of features that promote fidelity and authenticity in simulation based health professional education. *Clin. Sim. Nurs.*, **42**, pp. 22–41.

**McIndoe, A.** (2012). *High stakes simulation in anaesthesia. Cont. Educ. Anaesth. Crit. Care Pain*, **12**(5), pp. 268–73.

**Royal College of Anaesthetists** (2018), *Simulation Strategy 2018–2023*. Royal College of Anaesthetists, London, UK.

**van Meurs, W. L., Good, M. L.** and **Lampotang, S.** (1997) Functional anatomy of full-scale patient simulators, *J. Clin. Monit.*, **13**, pp. 317–24.

**van Meurs, W. L., Nikkelen, E.** and **Good, M. L.** (1998) Pharmackinetic-pharmacodynamic model for educational simulations, *IEEE Trans. Biomed. Eng.*, **45**(5), pp. 582–90.

## *Further reading*

**Elendu, C., *et al.*** (2024) The impact of simulation-based training in medical education. *Medicine*, **103**(27), p. e38813.

**Henson, L. C.** and **Lee, A. C. (eds)** (1998) *Simulators in Anesthesilogy Education*, Plenum Press, New York and London.

**Riley, R. H.** (2008) *Manual of Simulation in Healthcare*, Oxford University Press, Oxford.

## *Useful simulation societies*

SESAM: Society for simulation in Europe. Contact sesam@sesamsociety.org

ASPiH: Association for simulated practice in healthcare. Contact admin@aspih.org.uk

# Index

*For the benefit of digital users, indexed terms that span two pages (e.g., 52–53) may, on occasion, appear on only one of those pages.*


## A

absolute blood flow 117
absolute humidity 95
absolute pressure 83
absolute temperature 89
absolute zero 90, 93
acid-base balance 177
actor-based simulation 296
adiabatic compression 91
advancing front theory 267
air compressor 217
Airtraq 236
airway management devices 225–34
  artificial airway 225
  checks 224
  endotracheal tube 229–34
  facemask 226–27
  I-gel 228–29
  laryngeal mask airway 226–28
  monitoring the airway 122
  nasopharyngeal airway 225
  oropharyngeal airway 225, 229
alarm systems 120, 220, 222, 258
α-error 26
alpha particle 278
alternating current/voltage 53–54
amplifiers 60–64
anaesthetic gases
  checks 222–23
  Entonox 217
  environmental pollution 274–75
  flow control 219–20
  gas cylinders 218–19
  medical compressed air 217
  nitrous oxide 216
  occupational exposure limits 275
  oxygen 121–22, 215–16
  piped medical vacuum 217–18
  pressure regulators 219–20
  scavenging systems 223, 275–76
anaesthetic machine
  checklist 222
  safety features 219–20
anaesthetic monitoring 119–24
  AAGBI recommendations 121
  airway and ventilation 122
  alarm systems 120
  blood pressure 123
  carbon dioxide 122
  cardiac rate and rhythm 122–23
  checks 223
  circulation 122–23
  depth of anaesthesia, *see* depth of anaesthesia monitors
  neuromuscular function 124
  oxygenation 121–22
  postanaesthesia care 124
  temperature 123–24
  tissue perfusion 123
analogue-to-digital converter 64, 65
analysis of frequency tables 33–34
analysis of variance 31
anatomical dead space 155–57
aneroid barometer 149–50
arterial blood pressure 123, 131–32
artificial airway 225
artificial intelligence 199–200, 264, 272, 297
Association of Anaesthetists of Great Britain and Ireland (AAGBI)
  checklist for equipment 220–22
  recommendations for monitoring 121
atmospheric pollution 274–75
atmospheric pressure 83–85
atomic structure 43–44
auditory evoked response 187–90, 198
augmented reality training 297
auscultation 127–28
autoclaves 290
averages 19
averaging 188–89
Ayre's T piece 246–47

## B

bag-in-bottle ventilator 259–60
Bain system 245
band-pass filters 58
Baralyme 249
base excess 179
Beer–Lambert law 160, 168
Bernoulli equation 82
β-error 26
biological signal processing 64

biphasic defibrillators 206–8
bipolar diathermy electrodes 212
bipolar pacemaker leads 202–3
bispectral index monitor 196
black-box concept 40
blinding 36
blood flow 114–17
blood gas analysis 177–80
blood-gas partition coefficient 99
blood pressure measurement 127–41
  auscultation 127–28
  central venous pressure 140–41
  cuff size and site 130
  diastolic blood pressure 127–29, 130
  direct methods 131–39
  Doppler ultrasound 130
  during anaesthesia 123
  non-invasive (indirect) methods 127–31
  oscillometry 128–30
  palpation 127
  plethysmography 130–31
  systolic blood pressure 127–29, 130
Bodok seal 219
body plethysmograph 155
Bohr's equation 156
boiling 103
bougies 240
Bourdon gauge 149
Boyle's law 89, 150
bradycardia, pacemakers 202–4
breathing systems 241–50
  Ayre's T piece 246–47
  Bain 245
  checks 223
  circle system 247–50
  enclosed afferent reservoir 243–44
  Humphrey ADE 247
  Jackson Rees modification 246–47
  Lack 242
  Magill 241–42
  Mapleson classification 241–47
  Miller modification 243–44
  parallel Lack 242
  T pieces 244–47
  Venturi 247
bridge circuits 51–53
buffer base 178–79
Bunsen solubility coefficient 99

## C

calculus 6–11
capacitive transducers 68
capacitors 54–55
capnography 122
carbon dioxide absorber 223, 241, 249–50
carbon dioxide monitoring 122
carboxyhaemoglobin 162–63
cardiac defibrillators 204–8
cardiac output measurement 143–45
  echocardiography 145–46
  pulmonary artery catheter 143–45
  pulse contour analysis 146–47
  thermodilution catheter 9, 144
  transthoracic electrical impedance 147
cardiac rate and rhythm monitoring 122–23
cardiac vector 181–82
categorical data 17, 33–34
catheters 240
CAT scan 276
centiles 20–21
central range 20
central venous pressure 140–41
cerebral function (analysing) monitor 194
Charles' law 90
checklists 220–24
chemical sterilisation 290
chemical transducers 68
chemoluminescent sensors 175
circle system 247–50
circuit breakers 74–76
circulation monitoring 122–23
Clarke electrode 174, 177, 179
class 1 equipment 69–70
class 2 equipment 70–71
class 3 equipment 71
cleaning equipment 290–91
clinical trials 36
C-MAC 236, 238–39
Coanda effect 82–83
colour flow Doppler 115
Combitube 229
common mode rejection (ratio) 62
compliance 253
compressed air supply 217
compressed spectral array monitor 194–96
computed axial tomography (CAT) 280–81
conduction 94
confidence interval 25
confusion matrix 29
contingency table 33–34
controlled ventilation 242–44, 245, 246, 247, 249
convection 94
Cook catheter 240
correlation 31
COVID-19 264
cricothyrotomy tube 233
critical flow rate (velocity) 78–79
critical pressure 92

critical temperature 92, 100
CT (computed tomography) scan 280–81
cuffed oropharyngeal airway 229
current density 76–77, 210
cyanosis 119, 160
cycling 253–54, 257

## D

Dalton's law of partial pressures 85–86
damping 134–39
dead space 155–57
decompression sickness 98–99
defibrillators 204–8
degrees of freedom 25
density spectral array monitor 195–96
deoxyhaemoglobin 160–61
depth of anaesthesia monitors 194–200
  artificial intelligence 199–200
  auditory evoked response 198
  bispectral index 196
  cerebral function 194
  compressed spectral array 194–96
  electrocardiogram (ECG)-based 199
  electroencephalography (EEG)-based 194–98, 199
  entropy 197–98
  fuzzy logic 199
  Narcotrend 198
  non-physiological systems 199
  patient state index 198
  Quantium consciousness index 199
  recommendations 124
  respiratory sinus arrhythmia 199
diagnostic tests 29–31
diathermy, *see* surgical diathermy
differential amplifier 62–64
differential equations 9–11
differentiation 6–7
diffusion 86–87
digital signal processing 64–65
dimensions 38–40
direct current/voltage 53–54
disinfection 290–91
Doppler ultrasound 113–17
  blood flow 114–17
  blood pressure measurement 130
  colour flow 115
  echocardiography 145–46
  frequency shift (power) spectrum 115–17
  gas flow 154
  pulsed 114–15
double-lumen tubes 233–34
draw-over vaporiser 107–8
drift 40
dynamic viscosity 78

## E

earth faults 72–73
earth-free supplies 76
earth lead 69
earth leakage current 71
echocardiography 145–46
eddy currents 200
electrical circuits 50–53
electrical safety 69–77
electric charge 48
electric current 48
electricity supply 69
electrocardiogram (ECG) 181–84
  cardiac monitoring 122–23
  depth of anaesthesia 199
electrodes 65–67
electroencephalogram (EEG) 184–87
  depth of anaesthesia 194–98, 199
electrolysis 77
electromotive force 48–49
electromyogram (EMG) 190–92
enclosed afferent reservoir system 243–44
endotracheal tube 229–34
energy 45–47
Entonox supply 217
entropy 197–98
environmental safety 274–76
ethylene oxide 290
evidence-based medicine 36
evoked responses 187–90, 198
exercise testing, preoperative 175–76
explosion risks 274
exponential function 10
extracorporeal membrane oxygenation 267
extrapolation 2–4

## F

facemask 226–27
false positive/negative 26
fibre optic systems 236–38, 239–40
Fick's law of diffusion 86–87
Fick's principle 144
filters 58–60
Finapres 130
fire risks 274
Fleisch pneumotachograph 151–54
flow generator 253–54, 255–56
fluid flow 78–88
  diffusion 86–87
  laminar/turbulent 78–80
  measurement devices 80–83
  osmosis 87–88
  pressure 83–86

force 44–45
Fourier analysis 6, 42
Fowler's method 155–56
frequency domain analysis 186–87
frequency response 41–42
fuel cells 174
functional residual capacity 155–57
fundamental frequency 41–42
fuzzy logic 199

## G

gamma camera 281
gamma radiation 278–79
gas; *see also* anaesthetic gases; respiratory gas analysis
  cylinders 218–19
  flow control 219–20
  laws 89–92
  pressure measurement 149–50
  pressure regulators 219–20
  solubility in gas 99
  solubility in liquid 98–99
  volume and flow measurement 150–59
gauge pressure 83
Gay-Lussac's law 90
Glidescope 236, 238–39
goodness of fit 33
Graham's law of diffusion 87
graphs 1–4, 18
greenhouse gasses 274–75
Guedel airway 225

## H

Hagen–Poiseuille equation 40, 79
half-cell potential 66
harmonics 41–42
heart rate variability 199
heat and moisture exchangers 96
heat sterilisation 290
heat transfer 94
helium dilution 156–57
Henderson–Hasselbalch equation 178
Henry's law 98
high frequency ventilation 265–67
high-pass filters 60
histogram 18
hot wire anemometry 154
human factors 119–20
humidification 95–96
humidity 95–96
Humphrey ADE system 247
hybrid training 297
hyperbaric atmosphere 84–85
hypobaric atmosphere 84–85
hypothesis testing 26
hysteresis 40

## I

I-gel 228–29
imaging methods 280–87
  computed axial tomography/computed tomography (CAT/CT) 280–81
  magnetic resonance imaging (MRI) 283–87
  nuclear medicine 281
  positron emission tomography (PET) 281
  single photon emission computed tomography (SPECT) 281
  X-rays 280
impedance 55
implantable cardiac defibrillators 205
inductive transducers 68
inductors 54–55
infrared spectroscopy 168–69
infusion pumps 270–73
integration 7–9
intensive care ventilators 262–64
intermittent blowers 260–61
interpolation 2–4
inter-quartile range 20–21
intravascular blood gas analysers 179
intubation aids 236–40
isotopes 44

## J

Jackson Rees modification 246–47
Joule effect 94

## K

Kelvin 89, 90, 91, 93
kinematic viscosity 78
kinetic energy 45

## L

Lack breathing system 242
laminar flow 78–80
lamination 217
Larmor frequency 284–85
laryngeal mask airway 226–28
laryngoscope 236–40
lasers 287–89
latent heat of crystallisation 93
latent heat of vaporisation 93, 100
leakage currents 71
LiDCO 147
linearity 40
linear regression 33
linear scale 18
liquid oxygen 215
lithotripsy 117
live lead 69

logarithms 11–16
low-pass filters 58–60

## M

Macintosh laryngoscope 236
Magill breathing system 241–42
magnetic resonance imaging (MRI) 283–87
magnetism 49–50
mains electricity supply 69
manikin-based simulators 293
Mann–Whitney U test 29
manual resuscitators 265
Mapleson breathing systems 241–47
mass 44–45
mass spectrometry 169–71
mathematical models 294–95
McCoy laryngoscope 236
McGrath laryngoscope 236
mean 19
mechanics 44–47
median 19
median power frequency 186–87
medical compressed air 217
meta-analysis 34–35
methaemoglobin 162–63
microshock 74
Miller modification 243–44
minute volume divider 259
mode 19
model-driven simulators 293
moist heat sterilisation 290
monophasic defibrillators 206–8
monopolar diathermy electrodes 212
MRI (magnetic resonance imaging) 283–87

## N

Narcotrend 198
nasal oxygen 226–27
nasopharyngeal airway 225
natural logarithms 13
nebulisers 96
needle positioning 113
negative end expiratory pressure 257
nerve stimulator 190
neuromuscular blockade monitoring 190–92
neuromuscular function 124
neutral lead 69
Newtonian fluid 78
Newton's laws 45
nitric oxide measurement 175
nitrous oxide 216, 275
nominal data 17
non-linear scale 18
non-parametric methods 28–29
normal distribution 23–24
nuclear medicine 281
null hypothesis 26
numerical data 17–18
Nyquist rate 65

## O

Ohm's law 50
oil–gas partition coefficient 99
one-sample t-test 27
operational amplifiers 60–61
ordinal data 17
oropharyngeal airway 225, 229
oscillometry 128–30
osmolality 87–88
osmolarity 87
osmosis 87–88
Ostwald solubility coefficient 99
Overton–Meyer hypothesis 99
oxygenation monitoring 121–22
oxygen concentrator 215–16
oxygen failure warning 220, 222
oxygen saturation 160–61, 163
oxygen supply 121–22, 215–16
oxyhaemoglobin 160
ozone layer 274, 275

## P

pacemakers 202–4
  codes 203–4
paired t-test 27–28
parabola 2
parallel circuits 50–51
parallel Lack breathing system 242
paramagnetic oxygen analyser 172–74
parametric methods 27–28
partial pressure 85–86
partition coefficient 99
patient isolated differential amplifiers 62–64
patient monitoring, *see* anaesthetic monitoring
patient state index 198
$pCO_2$ electrode 178
peak expiratory flowmeter 157
PEEP 257
Peltier effect 94
Penlon Nuffield ventilator 260
peripheral nerve stimulator 124
PET(positron emission tomography) scan 281
pH 12
pH electrode 177
photoconductive cells 68
photoelectric transducers 68
phototransistors 68
photovoltaic cell 68
physiological dead space 155–57
PiCCO 146

pie chart 18
piezoelectric effect 110–11
piezoelectric gas analysis 171–72
piezoelectric transducers 68
pin index system 219
piped medical vacuum 217–18
pitot tube 152
plethysmography 130–31, 155, 160–61
Pneupac 260–61
$pO_2$ electrode 177
Poiseuille's equation 38–40
polarographic electrode 174
Polio laryngoscope 236
pollution, atmospheric 274–75
polynomial 2, 33
population mean 24–25
positive end expiratory pressure 257
positron emission tomography (PET) 281
postanaesthesia monitoring 124
post-tetanic facilitation 190
potential energy 45
power (electrical circuits) 49
power (statistical) 26–27
power (ventilation) 256–57
power (work) 47
powers 11–16
Poynting effect 217
preoperative exercise testing 175–76
pressure 45, 83–86
pressure generator 253–54, 255
pressure–volume curves 89–92
probability 21–25
Proseal 227
pseudocritical temperature 217
pulmonary artery catheter 143–45
pulsatility index 116
pulse contour analysis 146–47
pulsed Doppler 114–15
pulse oximetry 119, 120, 160–63
*P* value 26, 27

## Q

quadrupole mass spectrometer 170–71
Quantium consciousness index 199

## R

$R^2$ 33
radiation protection 282–83
radiative heat loss 94
radioactive decay 278–79
Raman spectroscopy 171
range 20–21
Raoult's law 88
Rayleigh refractometer 166–67
reactance 54–55
receiver operating characteristics curves 30–31
rectangular hyperbola 4
refractometry 166–67
regression 33
residual current device 74–76
residue 33
resistance 50–51
resistive index 116
resistive transducers 67
resonance 134–39
respiratory gas analysis 165–76
  fuel cells 174
  infrared spectroscopy 168–69
  mass spectrometry 169–71
  nitric oxide measurement 175
  paramagnetic oxygen analyser 172–74
  piezoelectric methods 171–72
  polarography 174
  preoperative exercise testing 175–76
  Raman spectroscopy 171
  refractometry 166–67
respiratory sinus arrhythmia 199
Reynolds' number 78–79
root mean square 53
Rotameter 80–81, 157–58, 220

## S

safety
  anaesthetic machine 219–20
  electrical 69–77
  environmental 274–76
  magnetic resonance imaging (MRI) 286–87
  radiation protection 282–83
  surgical diathermy 213–14
  ventilators 257–58
sample mean 24–25
sample size 26–27
saturated vapour pressure 100, 103
scatter diagram 18
scavenging systems 223, 275–76
SCOTI device 233
Seebeck effect 94
sensitivity 29
series circuits 50
shear stress 78
Sherwood number 267
signal processing 64–65
simple harmonic motion 6, 10
simulators 292–97
  actor-based 296
  artificial intelligence 297
  augmented reality 297
  educational opportunities 296
  hybrid training 297
  mannikin-based 293

mathematical modelling 294–95
model-driven 293
patient types 295
scenarios 296
scenario scripts 295
simulation centres 292–93
surgical skills laboratory 296
virtual reality 297
sine wave 6
single-ended amplifiers 61–62
single photon emission computed tomography (SPECT) 281
sinusoidal waveform 6
SI units 38–40
skewed distribution 21
soda lime 249
solubility 98–99
specific heat capacity 76, 92–93
specificity 29
SPECT (single photon emission computed tomography) 281
spectral edge frequency 186–87
spectroscopy
infrared 168–69
pulse oximetry 160
Raman 171
spirometer 150–51
splitting ratio 104
standard bicarbonate 179
standard deviation 21
standard error of the mean 25
star point 69
static electricity 48, 77, 274
statistics 17–37
clinical trials 36
correlation 31
data types 17–18
diagnostic tests 29–31
evidence-based medicine 36
frequency analysis 33–34
hypothesis testing 26
incorrect use 36–37
meta-analysis 34–35
non-parametric 28–29
parametric 27–28
power calculation 265
probability 21–25
regression 33
study design 35–36
variability 18–21
steam sterilisers 290
sterilisation of equipment 290–91
gamma irradiation 291
straight line graph 1
stray capacitance 71, 213–14
Student's t-distribution 25
Student's t-test 27–28
study design 35–36
sublimation 92
surgical diathermy 210–14
bipolar electrodes 212
blended modes 212
coagulation 212
current density 76–77, 210
cutting 210–11
desiccation 212
fulguration 212
interference with other equipment 214
monopolar electrodes 212
safety 213–14
stray capacitance 213–14
surgical skills laboratory 296
syringe drivers 270–73
systolic blood pressure 127–29, 130

## T

tachyarrhythmia, pacemakers 212
target-controlled infusion 271–72
temperature 93
blood gas analysis 179
critical 92, 100
monitoring during anaesthesia 123–24
tension 99
Tensymeter 131
test statistic 33–34
thermistor 94
thermocouple 94
thermodilution catheter 9, 144
thermodynamics 89–96
gas laws 89–92
heat transfer 94
humidification 95–96
latent heat of crystallisation 93
latent heat of vaporisation 93, 100
specific heat capacity 76, 92–93
temperature 93–94
thermometry 94
Thompson effect 94
time domain analysis 185
tissue perfusion monitoring 123
total intravenous anaesthesia 199, 271–72
touch current 71
T pieces 244–47
tracheostomy tubes 233
training simulators, *see* simulators
train-of-four stimulation 190
transcutaneous blood gas analysers 179
transducers 42–43, 67–68, 132–34
transformers 55–56
transthoracic electrical impedance 147

trigonometry 4–6
triple point 92, 93
turbulent flow 78–80
two bag test 223
two-sample t-test 27–28
two-sided t-test 27
Type I/II error 26
type B/BF/CF equipment 71

## U

ultrasonic flow transducer 154
ultrasound 110–13, 117; *see also* Doppler ultrasound
unidirectional valve 241, 247–48
unipolar pacemaker leads 202–3
units 38–40

## V

vacuum insulated evaporator 215
vaporisation 94, 100–2
vaporiser 102–9
  checks 223
variability 18–21
variance 21
ventilators 253–68
  alarm systems 258
  bag-in-bottle 259–60
  checks 223
  classification 253–58
  cycling 253–54, 257
  extracorporeal membrane oxygenation 267
  flow generator 253–54, 255–56
  high frequency 265–67
  inspiratory/expiratory phase 253–54
  intensive care 262–64
  intermittent blowers 260–61
  manual resuscitators 265
  minute volume divider 259
  monitoring ventilation 122
  paediatrics 258–59
  PEEP/NEEP 257
  Penlon Nuffield 260
  Pneupac 260–61
  portable 265
  power 256–57
  pressure generator 253–54, 255
  respiratory mechanics 253
  safety features 257–58
  sharing 264
  testing 258–59
Venturi device 247
Venturi flowmeter 81–83
Venturi mask 226–27
videolaryngoscopy 238–40
virtual reality training 297
Vitalograph 151
voltage (volts) 48–49
voltage dividers 51

## W

warming patients 95–96
washout method 155–56
Wee device 233
weight 44–45
wet and dry bulb hygrometer 95
Wilcoxon signed rank sum test 28
work 45–47
Wright's respirometer 151

## X

X-rays 279–80

## Z

zeolite 215–16